D1233794

Defy Aging

Defy Aging

A Beginner's Guide to the New Science of Longer Life and Better Health

Beth Bennett

ROWMAN & LITTLEFIELD
Lanham • Boulder • New York • London

Published by Rowman & Littlefield
An imprint of The Rowman & Littlefield Publishing Group, Inc.
4501 Forbes Boulevard, Suite 200, Lanham, Maryland 20706
www.rowman.com

86-90 Paul Street, London EC2A 4NE

British Library Cataloguing in Publication Information Available

Library of Congress Cataloging-in-Publication Data Available

978-1-5381-5514-1 (cloth)
978-1-5381-5515-8 (electronic)

I am grateful to the many wonderful scientists who have spent their careers pursuing truth, sometimes in the face of disdain and even ridicule. And to my friend Julie Brugger, who asked so many of the questions I've tried to answer in this book.

Contents

1

What Is Aging, and Why Do We Get Old?

The beautiful chariots of kings wear out, this body too undergoes decay.
—Samyutta Nikaya, Pali Canon

Old age is like a plane flying through a storm. Once you are aboard there is nothing you can do. —Golda Meir

WHAT IS IN THIS BOOK AND HOW TO USE IT

Popular books on aging abound, especially on how *not* to age, but this is not one of them. My goal in writing this book is to provide a guidebook to the aging of the body.

We are all familiar with guides to roads, trails, mountain peaks, hot springs, and the like. You use a guide book to get information about possible destinations: how to get there and what to find when you get there. We are all taking another kind of journey along the aging trajectory with little information as to how to go and what to expect along the way. Some stops along the way can range from mildly amusing to absolutely debilitating. Astonishingly, age-related declines begin to show up in our cells in our late twenties and early thirties but accelerate to observable changes in our forties and fifties.

One major difference exists between a travel guide and this one: I provide annotated sign posts telling you why you are experiencing novel events as you age and information about how to arrive at a different destination. My goal

1

is twofold. First, I give you background detail about the biology of your body to explain the aging process. Then, I describe new research that exploits the biology to slow or reverse the changes that aging can cause.

An important point to keep in mind while reading this book is that aging is not a disease, although some scientists are beginning to argue that maybe we should think of it as one. Aging is a normal process that we all—inevitably— experience. However, age is a risk factor for many chronic diseases that plague industrialized societies. In fact, age is *the* major risk factor for many diseases such as cancers and heart diseases—the main causes of death in the United States and other developed nations. Because of this correlation between advancing age and chronic disease, the community of geroscientists (researchers who study aging) is increasingly discussing whether aging should be considered a disease. I'll return to this idea in the final chapter. Although it's not possible to turn back the clock, it is possible to slow—even reverse—many of the deleterious changes that occur with age and predispose us to those chronic diseases.

By the time you read this, those aged sixty and over will outnumber children under five years. By 2050, nearly a quarter of the world's population will be over age sixty.[1] With this unprecedented change in age groups, we are faced with a critical question: Will longer life mean a longer healthy life, or will we see increases in chronic disease?

Our quality of life as we age depends not on our chronological age (i.e., the number of years we have been alive) but on the interaction of numerous cellular, molecular, and genetic events that give us our biological age (i.e., how old we seem to be). You may be sixty but look and feel forty whereas someone who is forty may look and feel much older for this reason. And, naturally occurring events, such as injuries, diet, and other lifestyle factors, can interact with diseases to worsen age-related declines.

Yes, I did just say declines. Many positive changes accompany the ticking clock of chronological aging, but the unfortunate physical reality is that the body deteriorates. These positive effects include a broadened perspective from a lifetime of experience (some might call this wisdom)[2] and an improved ability to accept the hard knocks that come hand in hand with life's wonders. But in the context of the body, the changes that occur with age represent declines from our physical peak.

I discuss how and why these declines occur in the next chapters. For now, let me just say that I don't intend a value judgment here. Our society is very much biased toward youth, with enormous emphasis placed on looking young and attractive. I disagree with this bias, but that is not the point of this book.

I want you, the reader, to understand what is happening in your body. Once you have a basic understanding of the processes at work over the decades, the new scientific findings that illustrate the potential for slowing or reversing those changes will make sense to you. Then, you can make informed choices whether to pursue some of those findings. To reiterate, although I use the terms age-related declines and deterioration throughout the book, please don't interpret these as value-laden, just with reference to a physical peak that inevitably occurs in our twenties to thirties. Conversely, I label many of the strategies to counter these declines as antiaging. This term is not popular with some geroscientists, possibly because it implies turning back the clock. I simply use it as shorthand to describe a potentially beneficial action or drug.

But don't just take my word for this usage. Recently, the World Health Organization (WHO), the agency of the United Nations focused on global public health, added the term "aging-related" disease to its massive twenty-eight-chapter volume that classifies all known diseases.[3] This modification means that scientists and physicians are increasingly realizing that age may be something that can be treated, leading to therapies and interventions. We probably won't modify our language to say that we've been infected with age or come down with a bad case of it, but this is exactly the approach I explore in this book. If it's possible to determine the changes that occur in our cells and the molecules that build them as we age, it can be possible to "fix" those changes. I will show you that new research is identifying those processes. And, once identified, it becomes possible to modify them. Exciting new research is focused on exactly that: reversing or slowing some age-related changes.

Personally, I have experienced some unpleasant surprise visits from the aging fairy. These range from the cosmetic, wrinkles, and gray hair, to the more serious, osteoporosis and skin cancers. Being a scientist, I delved into the scientific literature to try to make sense of what is happening. After reading and digesting hundreds of technical papers, and talking to friends and colleagues about this research, it became clear to me that people are curious about what will happen in the second half of life. And most of us don't have the time and expertise to digest the scientific literature. Sure, you can do Google searches. But more likely than not you will end up with popular websites disseminating a little fact mixed in with a lot of hand waving at best and total fiction at worst.

In the past decade, research into the underlying physiology and genetics of aging has exploded. Numerous journals focus on gerontology research, defined as the multidisciplinary study of normal aging and older adults. Of the dozen that publish primarily in the biological (as opposed to psychological) arena, seven have been established since 2000. The recent journals focus on the field of geroscience, an interdisciplinary field combining the study of normal aging with related events in other areas such as the biochemistry and molecular biology of age-related disease. These journals publish technical papers describing new findings, but often this information stays in academia. The time lag between "bench" (i.e., laboratory research) and "bedside" (i.e., clinical care) means that much of this information has not yet been passed along to health-care professionals. Some recent research findings have identified new biochemical mechanisms underlying aging. Each embodies the possibility of potential mitigations or even fixes. I endeavor in this book is to provide an easy-to-read understanding of why age-related changes are happening and what the new science tells us can be done about them.

As you read this book, you will tour the systems of the body (skin, muscle, skeletal, cardiovascular, etc.) and preview how aging affects each one. I will also digest the relevant scientific literature to tell you how and why aging alters these systems. When therapies or drugs to minimize or reverse the aging effects exist, I will describe them, how they work, and possible side effects. Similarly, when genes are known that affect aging of the body system being described, I will discuss them and their roles. I will try to keep technical jargon to a minimum, but for the interested reader, I will provide additional sources in notes following each chapter. I give the technical references, gleaned from academic journals. I also include popular science books, articles, and websites that more clearly explain the science for a nonscientist. To alleviate the annoyance of flipping back through pages to find the definition of an acronym, I include a table of those used in each chapter at its end.

What you won't find is any presentation or discussion of currently used medical technologies, devices, treatment modalities, or pharmaceuticals. These areas have many valid and important methods for treating age-related declines, but I leave these for you to discuss with your health-care provider. I will focus on new and novel therapies and methods to slow or even reverse age-related declines, but—and this is a big but—only those that have what I consider to be solid experimental evidence. This support often is preliminary, often coming from animal experiments, which have big caveats (discussed below).

In the time between this writing and your reading, things may have changed—in either direction. Thus, if you find a preliminary intervention you wish to pursue, you should do a little research to find possible further information. One way to do this is to take the reference(s) I give in the note and enter it into the search field in Google Scholar (https://scholar.google.com), which will search forward from its publication date. This search will give you later references to the study I cited. In the final chapter I give a brief primer about how to take this information and self-experiment if you are so inclined.

In the next chapter, I start with a brief history of the theories as to why we age. These are relevant because they attempt to explain the aging process. If we understand that, maybe we will be better equipped to fight it. If it's not interesting to you, skip it. Much of the book is structured so that you can pick and choose what to read: find what is important and interesting to you.

Then in chapter 3, I define some commonly accepted mechanisms underlying the aging process. These are the *how* of aging. Again, these are relevant because they represent the main targets for novel approaches to reduce the damage of aging. If they are overly complicated, again, skip them and return as needed. I will reintroduce relevant mechanisms in each chapter on the various body systems. This revisiting may be redundant to some of you but essential to others. If it's annoying, my apologies. In my experience as a university instructor, I found repetition helpful to students. In each chapter when I introduce and define jargon terms, they will be shown in bold type.

Chapters 4–8 cover individual body systems, starting with the external covering, the skin, and progressing through muscle, bone, cardiovascular, and nervous systems. You can pick and choose areas of interest. In each chapter, I start with some basic anatomy (structure) and physiology (function) so that you will know the names and uses of the most important components. The meat of the chapter follows, which is what happens to these structures and functions as they age. Interspersed, I summarize some of the latest research on possible interventions for the system addressed in that chapter. Much new research was sparked by a consideration of mechanisms, so you can return to chapter 3 if you need a refresher on those. For the interested reader, I include a section on the few genes known to affect the system and the potential benefit of testing for those genes.

The final two chapters introduce you to the concept of what I call interventions. These are actions or drugs (and drug-like compounds) that may slow or even reverse some age-related events. Although some are more speculative than others, all of these ideas have experimental support. Most have been tested in human trials, but I do include promising suggestions with data only from animal studies.

References, to research or resources that may be helpful or interesting, are relegated to the end of the book. Most of these come from peer-reviewed papers published in reputable scientific journals. Peer review is the process, considered essential in modern science, for ensuring that only high quality, verifiable scientific studies are published. Peer review means that when a paper is submitted to a journal for publication, several independent and presumably unbiased scientists with credibility in that area will review it. Only when the reviewers approve, or the author(s) can stave off the criticisms, is the paper accepted for publication. Of course, the process has glitches, but by and large, it ensures the publication of solid science.

Occasionally I will reference a website, press release, or Wikipedia link, as these can provide clear, elementary prose. If the website is that of a ".com," be aware that the information is not unbiased. That said, I have found some exceptionally clear and accurate science writing and beautiful graphics on many of these sites. Keep in mind, too, that some authors of scientific papers have connections to commercialization of their work, which, though they are required to disclose such "conflicts of interest," may bias them. I attempt to point out some of these connections in the final chapter, where I focus on current and soon-to-be-available interventions.

My linking to these sites, including some popular websites such as WebMD and LiveStrong, does not mean that I endorse all of their content or their commercial backing, simply that it is well-written and easy to understand. Nor am I suggesting that you purchase any products that have been commercialized. I include mention of a product because, in my mind, solid scientific data supports its proposed use. That said, it might not be right for you. Each of us is genetically and experientially unique. Our response to any given drug or therapy may vary. As with any health or lifestyle decision, you should weigh the costs and benefits. And, as I describe in the final chapter, experiment on yourself.

HOW TO INTERPRET SCIENTIFIC STUDIES
AND NOT-SO-SCIENTIFIC RESULTS

Everywhere you look—books, newspapers, magazines, social media, websites—you see "scientifically based" claims for all kinds of outcomes. Weight loss, hair growth, virility, antiaging—you can find "proof" for it all. How can anyone evaluate these claims?

Keep in mind that science is a way of answering questions about the world. We have many ways of doing that. You may remember the "scientific method" from middle school as a recipe for doing science: you make an observation, then come up with an explanation for the thing you observed (hypothesis), which is then supported (or not) by experiment. This approach is known as hypothesis-driven science, and it can be done in a lot of ways. When you realize that many alternative hypotheses can explain a given observation, the method becomes more complicated.

What I'm saying is this: we have many ways to get to an answer about how the body works—or doesn't. You can experiment to test a hypothesis. This is the "scientific method" I mentioned above. But we have other ways to do science. One is to look at a lot of people and search for correlations between the issue you are interested in and possible causes. This observational approach is less discussed in the popular press but frequently used. It got its start in epidemiological studies in the nineteenth century, when physicians were trying to pin down the causes of diseases such as cholera. Because they didn't know the causal agent, they had to look for patterns and correlations. I'll give you examples of both approaches, as applied to studies of human health.

HOW HUMAN STUDIES WORK

Take the story about coronary heart disease (CHD; more on this in chapter 7). In the 1940s, CHD had become the leading cause of death in adults (i.e., observation). Many explanations (i.e., hypotheses) were proposed: age, high blood pressure, high cholesterol, smoking, weight, and others. But how do you test hypotheses in humans? In some cases, it is ethical to enroll subjects in a study, bring them into the lab, and expose them to a specific treatment. This approach has many problems. It's expensive, time-consuming, and difficult to standardize the subjects, especially their behavior outside the lab. And if your method involves an unpleasant treatment, observational studies are more likely to get more recruits than experimental studies. Would you rather sign up to have a big needle stuck into a muscle to provide a tissue sample, or to have the muscle measured and that measurement correlated with your activity level? When you think of heart disease, which takes decades to develop, the problems of the experimental approach are enormous.

So, scientists turned to the observational approach to design the Framingham Heart Study. This method is similar to what epidemiologists use to identify the cause of an epidemic because you can't just inject people with suspected infectious agents. The Framingham study is a longitudinal study that recruited more than five thousand adults and has followed them (and their children and grandchildren) since 1950. Every two years, each subject is evaluated on a battery of physiological tests, such as blood pressure, cholesterol levels, and heart pathologies, as well as lifestyle assessments such as diet and exercise.

As individuals age and develop CHD, the data from their prior tests is analyzed to test the hypotheses. But note: lacking experimentation, this approach doesn't fit the classical scientific method. Also note, connecting lifestyle or physiological data with heart disease in this way gives an association, not necessarily a cause, which I will return to shortly. And a final note: many potential confounding factors, such as microbiome activity, genetics, and a host of other unknown and potentially unknowable variables, are not taken into account in these studies. Nonetheless, a lot of valuable information has been collected, and the significant associations could then be tested experimentally for a causal role in CHD.[4]

Before I go on to describe how these associations can be followed, let's digress into what exactly an association is and why it can be weak and even misleading. When scientists try to figure out what may cause a specific event such as a disease in humans using the observational approach, they come up with a list of possible causes. Because this is not an experimental approach, the causes may not make any real contribution to the disease.

Here's an example from a study looking at what might affect the sex of a child at conception. The authors tabulated the sex of children of 740 mothers along with the results of a food questionnaire, containing 133 different food items. Only one of these, breakfast cereal, showed an association with sex. Specifically, moms who ate cereals for breakfast had more boys. Scientists call this kind of association a correlation. Figuring the degree of correlation requires some calculations and can be expressed as a percent or proportion. Two things that are perfectly (or 100 percent) correlated always go together. If everyone ate bacon and eggs together for breakfast, these two foods would show a 100 percent correlation for that meal.

It's important to keep in mind the truism that correlation does not equal causation. In other words, just because you see a connection between two things does not mean one causes the other. One of these famously spurious correlations is the link between the number of churches in a city and the amount of crime there. Obviously, another variable causes the connection, possibly the population size of the city.

Going back to the breakfast cereal story, a major problem with this correlation is that a child's sex is determined by which of two possible sex chromosomes, the X or the Y, is present in the father's sperm. The mother's diet has nothing to do with it! Including a variable like what the mother ate in this study is an example of a hypothetical explanation that is not plausible. In other words, scientists have to be careful to screen their hypotheses for biological validity before looking for an association. This and other features of observational studies have been known for more than fifty years when they were first formalized by a British epidemiologist.[5]

Clearly, to investigate causality, you have to do experimental science. How do you design experiments to test hypotheses in humans? You can't take people and put them in cages and experiment on them. Faced with this kind of ethical issue, scientists turn to animal models.[6] Although humans are similar in many ways to rodents, they have some major differences. Nonetheless, a lot can be learned from laboratory studies on rodents (and other species). Then, promising results can be extended into humans in a complicated and expensive series of *clinical trials*. These trials can have a lot of permutations, depending on the nature of the intervention (drug, procedure, device) and the population for which the intervention is intended (healthy, terminally ill, surgical patient).

In general, the series of trials follows a three-stage process to determine safety, dose, and efficacy (how well does the intervention work compared to placebo, which is a similar but inactive treatment). Sometimes a fourth type of trial is done to test the previously determined dose in other patient populations. These trials are really expensive because they take years and involve a lot of people—both study subjects and testing personnel. Thus, clinical trials are mainly limited to drugs or devices developed by big companies or venture capital start-ups.

In order to run a clinical trial, the applicant, whether a corporation or university researcher, must apply to the Food and Drug Administration (FDA) for approval. FDA regulators review the application for a new drug or device. Approval at this stage is based primarily on safety considerations determined by description of the manufacturing process and the characterization of the new drug, and studies performed in animals. Then, the three-stage process described above is designed. Each stage is developed using information from the preceding trials. Each stage must meet requirements to protect the rights, safety, and privacy of human subjects. The regulatory agency assesses the scientific design of the trial to confirm both the safety of the subjects and the generation of data that will justify approval.

An additional level of regulation is the requirement for approval from an independent ethics committee, which is called an Institutional Review Board (IRB) in the United States. This approval is required to run a trial anywhere in the world. The IRB looks at ethical aspects of the research to assure that the rights of the human subjects are protected.

Subjects for trials are enrolled in a variety of ways, including newspaper ads, signs in clinics or hospitals, or the internet (more on this below). These research trials almost never include a fee, and trial subjects often are reimbursed for their time and efforts. Studies designed and paid for by corporations testing drugs or devices follow the same rigorous study design, but read on for a discussion of the effect of conflict of interest. Trials performed by research scientists at universities or in government labs to test new treatments for diseases or medical conditions face an additional level of scrutiny. Government-funded studies are subject to review by the National Institutes of Health (NIH), which funds most biomedical research in the United States. All clinical trials are listed on and enrolled through a government-curated website (clinicaltrials.gov).

Another variation on the clinical trial is conducted by clinics using new and relatively untried methods such as stem cell injections or blood transfusions.

This type of clinical trial typically charges participants. If these trials are listed on the government website, their design and test substance were reviewed by the FDA. However, the consumer should be aware that some substances, such as blood products, may not be subject to the same consideration as drugs. Essentially, the reason is that if your blood is removed, then reinjected, it's assumed to be safe. For reasons I won't get into here, this assumption is not always valid.

A final factor to consider in evaluating clinical trials is who pays for the study. Because these are big, expensive studies, they are increasingly funded by the companies likely to benefit from the drug or device being studied. Conflict of interest? You bet. So, it's not surprising that one analysis of this conflict found a strong effect of funding on outcome. In other words, you get what you pay for. In addition, the analysis found that pharmaceutical companies are not very likely to pay for studies evaluating the effects of traditional medicines or alternative therapies that could not be patented.[7] This finding would suggest increasing government funding for these sorts of trials (which I suggest in later sections when I present novel interventions), but in the current environment in Washington, funding for science is being cut.

WHAT STATISTICAL SIGNIFICANCE MEANS

Another example of a large human observational study is the Women's Health Initiative (WHI), begun in 1991, designed to examine major health issues in postmenopausal women. Their health outcomes (such as cancer, heart disease, etc.) were correlated with hormone replacement therapy (HRT) and other interventions (calcium, vitamin D, low-fat diet). In the past sixteen years, the study enrolled more than 160,000 "healthy" postmenopausal women. One of the striking conclusions of the WHI was that HRT *significantly* increased the risk of heart attacks, strokes, and breast cancer.[8]

Now, what *significant* means to you and what it means to me may be rather different. Statistical analysis is designed to identify differences between a control group (not taking the drug or other therapy) and a treatment group (taking the drug or therapy) that are not due to chance. The traditional cutoff for significance when deciding that a treatment has a real effect compared to the control is 5 percent or less. In other words, if you repeated the experiment many times, you would find that the treated group had the same outcome as the untreated control less than 5 percent of the time. Scientists don't always use 5 percent; and in fact, the idea of relying on a somewhat arbitrary cutoff is hotly debated at this time. That said, the 5 percent level is pretty standard.

Think about an experiment as like flipping a coin. You expect 50 percent heads and 50 percent tails on a series of coin tosses. But you might find a string of 50 heads before a tail flips up. You know this is a rare outcome and intuitively realize that it's a fluke. You don't have the same intuitive expectation regarding what experimental result is equivalent to a rare outcome.

Enter the statistical analysis tool kit. In the world of statistical analysis, the more individuals in your sample, the more powerful your test can be in terms of determining a fluke outcome. The flip side of this is that even a small difference between the control and the treatment group can emerge as a statistically significant outcome when you have a lot of people in your study. Or, if you flip a lot of coins, you could decide that 49 percent heads and 51 percent tails is a fluke.

In the WHI, this meant that for every ten thousand women taking the hormone therapy, compared to an equivalent control group not taking the hormones, there were seven additional heart attacks, eight additional strokes, eight additional cases of breast cancer, six fewer colorectal cancers, and five fewer hip fractures. And these numbers were statistically significant because of the large number of women in the study, though I have some doubts about the interpretation of these results. In other words, how important is seven additional heart attacks out of ten thousand, especially if this may be balanced by reduced hip fractures while taking hormones. Hormone therapy may have other benefits as well, some of which I will address in later chapters, but the WHI was designed and interpreted mainly to look at risks.

One final point, from large observational studies such as the WHI or Framingham, is the large number of variables evaluated. In WHI, for example, the scientists looked at numerous health outcomes. The Framingham study scored hundreds of potential causes of heart disease. This makes sense intuitively: how do you know up front which variables are important? But from a statistical perspective, every time you ask another question of your data, you lose some power of the data to answer. A very rough analogy is trying to figure out how many suits of cards are in a deck. By dealing a lot of hands of only two cards, eventually you can get an answer. But if you mix different decks that have different numbers of suits you won't be able to get a reliable answer using only two cards.

OTHER CONSIDERATIONS OF SCIENTIFIC STUDIES

My point in discussing human studies is that you have to know a little bit about the study that made the claim you are interested in. For example, maybe you've been hearing that curcumin, an anti-inflammatory agent in the spice turmeric, may reduce heart disease. You go to a website that sounds reliable and read that "Researchers in France fed 20 mice a diet supplemented with curcumin or a comparison diet not supplemented with curcumin. After 16 weeks, mice fed on the curcumin-based diet had a 26 percent reduction in fatty deposits in their arteries compared to mice on the comparison diet."[9] What to think? Well, first, think ten mice in each group is a pretty small number. Next, mice and humans are often very different when it comes to metabolizing food and drugs. Better to see similar results in people, but I still wouldn't trust a sample of ten.

Now, because it's expensive to experiment on people, a lot of studies have small samples. And you now know that small samples are not very powerful in confirming a hypothesis. But we don't have to throw out all these studies. It's possible to combine them using statistics. The main problem with combining study results is that different researchers often use different methods to collect their data. Statistical methods attempt to correct for that weakness, but keep that issue in mind when reading about these so-called meta-analyses. Nonetheless, we can get useful information from meta-analyses, and I will present some of them.

Bottom line: you have to look somewhat closely at the study design to evaluate the results. Personally, I believe that no right or wrong way exists to do science. What is important is to design studies carefully. By this I mean two things. First, the researcher should ask a clear and answerable question. (In the context of the scientific method, this means being able to reject a hypothesis that is incorrect.) Second, the study should minimize variability. In other words, every test or experiment should be conducted using exactly the same conditions. These criteria are not always possible to evaluate, especially by nonscientists; this evaluation is one big plus of the peer-review process, as the reviewers should dig into the study design before giving a thumbs-up to publication.

Finally, in most interventions being proposed now for mitigating the deleterious effects of aging, we have no large controlled trials in humans, only a growing number of small studies with a limited number of subjects. We have a lot of intriguing animal results, many of which are currently in *translational* clinical studies in humans. Neither of these will give a definitive answer to the question "How well does this intervention work?" I present both types of findings in this book, but if we have no human studies supporting animal results, regard them as very preliminary.

That said, if many independent studies corroborate each other, this is suggestive. The preliminary interventions I describe in the final chapters (as well as throughout the book) have come out of good research by dedicated scientists who have published their work in peer-reviewed journals. Be aware, as I am, that although these interventions have some support, either in animal studies or limited human trials, they may not stand up to further investigation. Further, some may work in small populations but not in most people, due to poorly understood effects of genetic variation. It's a very exciting time in aging research, but we have few good fixes yet.

I want to finish this mini-course on how science works with one important point. It may seem from what you have read in the past few pages that science doesn't work very well. It's tempting to paraphrase Winston Churchill's famous quote that "democracy is the worst form of government except for all the others"; but that's not the case for science. Science is a great way of trying to figure out what is going on in the universe. As you have seen, we have many ways to do this.

But we don't stop with one experiment and its analysis. Each experiment or observational study should be replicated to verify the results. Then, we learn from each study and can refine our questions and methods in the next one. In other words, science is an iterative process. Because of this aspect, it may seem that the scientific method is weak, but the opposite is true. We build on previous studies to refine our understanding of the world. This is an exciting time in science, with new techniques being developed almost daily, allowing us to refine our methods. That means that we are early in the process of applying these methods to issues of aging. It may seem, then, that we don't have firm answers, but the process is still young.

BEFORE YOU READ MORE

I want you to treat the book like a smorgasbord of aging information, picking and choosing topics that interest you. In each of the subsequent chapters on the various body systems (chapters 4–8), I will give you an overview that gets progressively more detailed. On my deepest dives into the weeds, I will warn you by using the header *A Deep Dive*. That section may be too detailed for you. If so, skip it. You can always return to it, or if not, I give you the take-home message in the first section and the overview. You can also visit my website (www.senesc-sense.com), which I continue to update, for additional information.

Finally, I hope you take away an appreciation for the amazing complexity of the body and its ability to regenerate. Although this ability declines as we age, it persists, and we can take actions that will encourage and prolong it.

2

The Why of Aging, or Evolutionary Explanations for Why We Grow Old

If you don't know why, you can't know how. — Anonymous

OVERVIEW

Aging is a natural biological process that occurs in almost all species of animals—usually after they can't reproduce anymore.[1] In Western medicine, aging is not considered a disease per se, but it does increase our vulnerability to many diseases. As we age, we see a progressive physiological decline accompanied by that increased risk of age-related diseases. In fact, aging is *the* major risk factor for the chronic diseases (e.g., dementias, atherosclerosis, diabetes, blindness, kidney dysfunction, and osteoarthritis) that contribute to most of the pain, suffering, and death of old age. This inevitable deterioration is what **gerontologists** (scientists who study aging in humans; a newly introduced term for those studying aging in a variety of animal models is **geroscientists**) call **primary aging**. In other words, it is inescapable. Additional deleterious effects can pile on from disease, poor lifestyle choices, or environmental factors. This "secondary aging" is much more amenable to mitigation or even reversal.

More than 75 percent of older Americans suffer from at least one of those chronic diseases, and more than half have more than one. As aging is the shared risk factor for all these diseases, increasing our knowledge and awareness of the role it plays can reduce the associated suffering and costs. Modest increases in health span could significantly reduce the social (i.e., human and economic) costs associated with aging.[2]

In our aging lexicon, a new concept is **health span**: the number of years lived relatively free from disease, during which daily activities and independence continue.[3] Many scientists are working on antiaging strategies. The goal of most of these interventions is not to prolong life span per se, although this may be a desirable side effect, but rather to extend health span.

A jargon term often used synonymously with aging is **senescence**. Senescence, or aging, is associated with the deterioration we experience later in adult life. An important point is that each of us ages at a different rate because of our genes. In other words, some of us have genes that protect us from senescence whereas others have genes predisposing us to deteriorate more rapidly. Huh? Yes, you may well wonder; read on.

LIFE SPAN

The controversy is widespread over why we age and deteriorate as we do. Some animal species, such as lobsters, don't appear to deteriorate as they get older. Lobsters continue to grow as they get older, and they eventually hit a wall where it is just too metabolically expensive to build a bigger, new shell. Lobster babies, known as larvae, are vulnerable to all kinds of predation, so they die at a high rate while young. Humans, on the other hand, at least developed countries, don't have high death rates while young. For species such as ours, the death rate speeds up in the final third of life, where the curve drops steeply—meaning that the percentage of people surviving is falling. Birds are intermediate because death is just as likely at any age.

There is a lot of variation in what biologists call **life history**: the pattern and timing of life events stretching from birth through reproductive maturity to death. Given that similar species can have very different life histories and life spans (e.g., mice, which are short lived; and bats, which are much longer lived), the inevitable conclusion is that our genes determine our life spans.

At advanced ages, your risk of death actually declines. In other words, if you make it past, say, eighty, you are more likely to reach ninety, one hundred, and beyond. This slowdown in mortality at older ages is seen in the three species in which really large, careful studies have been conducted (fruit flies, nematode worms, and humans).

The reason for this counterintuitive slowing is a mystery. One unsatisfying explanation is that less healthy individuals die off at younger ages, leaving the remaining population to age more slowly. But in humans, hints are that some "good" genes may predispose their bearers to longer lives by reducing the physiological effects of senescence. The effects of these genes seem to be more important at later ages, especially in humans. Gerontologists studying **centenarians** (people living to one hundred) and **supercentenarians** (those living past 110 years) reached this conclusion because they, like many people, noted that long lives seem to run in families. The scientists went on to study these people and found that parents and siblings of centenarians also tend to live longer. In addition, they tend to be healthier. We will return to the specific genes and how they might influence life and health span in the next chapter.[4]

Here I should introduce one potentially confounding factor to this "good genes" idea: the finding that in some areas people routinely exceed the average life span, living long—and importantly—healthy lives. These areas, called blue zones, are extensively studied by gerontologists.[5] This finding suggests an important role of the environment, perhaps mediated by diet or pollution. However, genes are not ruled out, as the individuals living in these blue zones share ancestry as well as environment.

Average human **life expectancy** at birth in the United States has increased dramatically in the past one hundred years, from 49 at the turn of the twentieth century to 77 for men and 81 for women (and it's slightly higher in Canada and Japan).[6] But this remarkable increase has not been accompanied by an equivalent increase in health span. Most of us would rather extend our health span than our life span. This rational desire has motivated a significant amount of recent research into the biology of aging. In this book, I will focus on many of the exciting recent results in this field, which suggest some easy (and some not-so-easy) ways to live healthier while living longer.

WHY DO WE DETERIORATE WITH AGE?

So why do we, unlike lobsters, senesce as we get older? It's tempting to say that we are like our cars: they get old. And even though we take them in for periodic tune-ups, they eventually fall apart, or senesce. We are like cars in a certain sense; that is, we and cars are complex systems that deteriorate with age (though we are infinitely more complicated). Unlike cars, we have built-in repair and maintenance systems. We are constantly replacing cellular components and checking and rebuilding the molecules that make up our cells. That would be like your car growing new tires or belts as the factory-installed parts aged. Unfortunately, these repair systems, too, deteriorate with age. The next chapter details the main processes that are damaged or lost with age.

Biologists have puzzled over this issue of aging for a long time. A few, not mutually exclusive, theories from evolutionary biologists try to explain why we, unlike lobsters and some other creatures, senesce. I'll briefly summarize them and refer the interested reader to additional sources.[7] If I were more philosophical, I would puzzle over whether aging should be considered a disease. Should the president declare a war on aging as Nixon declared a war on cancer? Being more of a pragmatist, I prefer to try to understand the reasons underlying why we age. To explore this issue, we have to delve into evolutionary biology.

EVOLUTION OF AGING

From an evolutionary perspective, you are really important when you are young and not at all after you pass your reproductive years. This idea follows from the premise central to Darwin's evolutionary theory. **Natural selection** gets rid of genes that reduce reproduction or survival throughout one's reproductive span. In other words, individuals (in any species) who don't pass on their genes by not reproducing can't contribute to subsequent generations. It's the genes from the successfully reproducing ones that persist. The individuals who survived to reproduce likely had genes that helped them do so. And these genes will influence all later generations. Natural selection ignores genes with bad effects that show up after the reproductive years. This concept has been expanded into two theories of aging: the **mutation-accumulation theory** and **antagonistic pleiotropy**.

Here's what those theories mean.

First, the mutation accumulation idea. Most mutations (changes in your DNA) are not good for you. Some of them even manage to evade the excellent DNA repair mechanisms of the cell. Imagine that some of these affect genes that are bad for you when you are older but are either beneficial or neutral regarding your ability to reproduce. Then mutations deleterious to survival at older ages will persist, because natural selection, which acts during the portion of your life when you can reproduce, is not clearing them away. Genes predisposing to cancers are often used as examples of this mutation accumulation theory. Advancing age is the greatest risk factor for cancer.[8] If cancers had been common at young ages in the past, there would have been selection to protect us against this disease. In fact, this is exactly what we find when examining the mechanisms of aging in the next chapter: most of us are protected against the uncontrolled cell growth that is cancer when young. Sadly, we lose the protections with age.

Second, the antagonistic pleiotropy notion is an extension of the observation (called **pleiotropy**) that single genes can have multiple effects. One example is the gene for the enzyme that, in a mutated version, causes albinism. This so-called albino gene has effects on many body parts, including hair, skin, and eye color. If we have genes that have positive effects on reproduction and negative effects on post-reproductive survival, these effects would be antagonistic, or opposite at different ages. Because these genes support reproduction, individuals with these genes will pass them on to their offspring as natural selection will favor these genes. This "antagonistic pleiotropy" results in a trade-off between health and survival in young (pre- and reproductive individuals, as these ages matter to natural selection), and older (post-reproductive individuals, who don't matter to natural selection). In other words, a gene that helps you survive to reproduce successfully may cause later disease and death. Thus, the antagonism between its early effects and late effects.

Let's put this in the context of human evolution. Most people reading this book were born in the developed world. Consequently, we take for granted medical care, adequate (of course, this is a relative term) nutrition, and shelter. Keep in mind that this type of lifestyle has become more commonplace over just the past few generations of humans in industrialized societies. For the vast majority of our history, during which time natural selection was picking and choosing the genes to pass down through the generations, humans lived as hunter-gatherers. Several diverse lines of evidence indicate that during these hundreds of thousands of years, physical trauma, and consequent infections, were the most likely cause of death. Most of our ancestors probably didn't make it much past thirty years of age.[9]

For these people, genes that helped them survive through puberty to reproduce and raise offspring were chosen by natural selection to proliferate. If some of those genes caused cancer at later ages, no problem, as most humans did not survive to those later ages. If others of those genes caused the immune system to falter after the age of fifty, again, natural selection was unconcerned, as reproduction and offspring rearing were complete well before then. And, of course, if we had mutated genes that only showed their effects after reproduction, such as causing heart disease, again, these genes were not seen by natural selection for most of our evolutionary history.

One question these aging theories raise is why we live past reproductive age. A lot of evidence from species other than humans shows that post-reproductive individuals can contribute to the survival and success of their relatives. Consider that in most mammal species females don't experience **menopause**, when they stop producing the hormones that orchestrate ovulation. In humans and a few other species, menopause occurs in midlife. Why would this evolve by natural selection? Doesn't this limit a female's reproduction? But the older female may be more important, from a natural selection perspective, when she helps her offspring and other relatives survive. The positive effect of the older female has been demonstrated in pilot whales. Female pilot whales can live to one hundred years in the wild, in groups consisting mainly of their daughters and other relatives. Even before menopause, the pilot matriarchs reproduce less and help their offspring more.

Then, we have the **disposable soma** theory, which essentially says that we have a limited energy budget to cover reproduction, growth, and maintenance. Due to the preference of natural selection for increasing reproductive output at the expense of longevity, animals should invest more resources in avenues that increase reproductive potential. This idea gets support from the observations that animals, when stressed (e.g., by starvation), redistribute their resources into maintenance. The reallocation strategy delays reproduction until food resources are available to support it. This outcome is seen in the many species that have been experimentally subjected to caloric restriction. I have a lot more to say about caloric restriction below, as it is one of the best-studied experimental approaches for life- and health-span extension.

A Deep Dive into Our Reproductive Cells

Before leaving the disposable soma idea, I want to make one more point. In multicellular organisms such as ourselves—it's estimated that the human body contains some thirty-seven trillion individual cells, not to mention the fivefold or so more microbial cells living in or on us—we see a lot of specialization. We have nerve cells, muscle cells, bone cells, skin cells, just to name a few. But, with a few exceptions, these cells are always dying and being replaced. None of us is made up of the same cells we had at age six or sixteen.

But so-called **germ cells** are different. These cells are used for reproduction: the eggs and sperm. In order to produce a new human, egg and sperm must be combined at fertilization. In order for this combination to maintain the correct number and sets of chromosomes, each germ cell has half of a complete set of the forty-six chromosomes of our species. The process that produces the germ cells essentially sets back the age clock of those cells to zero. Unlike the cells of the body that have gone through numerous cycles of cell divisions to maintain our adult selves, our germ cells are birthed just once, in relatively protected sites, from progenitors that remain ever young. How do they do this? The special cells that produce the germ cells are essentially a type of stem cell, ever able to give rise to increasingly specialized subsequent generations of cells but maintaining their youthful lack of specialization.

I know that was a lot of detail about germ cells, but here's the thing: this one cell type, of all of our trillions of cells, is essentially immortal. In concept, germ cells don't age and die. They carry on the species. Of course, the occasional mutation occurs and causes problems or, more rarely, provides advantage. And environmental insults can affect the germ cells. By and large, they are protected and cosseted because of their passage through time. Evolution discards the individual organism that will wear out and die but its essence—the genes—moves through the generations.

This protection is not free. The egg and sperm cells are some of the only cells in the body (stem cells are the others) that continuously manufacture an enzyme called **telomerase**. You'll hear more about this in the next chapter. For now, it's enough to say that this enzyme constantly monitors and maintains the ends of the chromosomes so that they don't break. Any damage to the chromosomes would mean potential damage to the genetic integrity of that cell. Given what you've read in the past few paragraphs, you know that this damage is unacceptable in the eggs and sperm. The rest of the body cells just have to risk it. One unfortunate result is cancer.

Along this line of thought, every living organism today can be placed in an unbroken line of descent from the very earliest cells. Keep this in mind in the next chapter, when I introduce some ways in which our cells age. Both protective and damaging mechanisms have been around for the entire history of life. This thought also has implications supporting the use of simple organisms, such as the single-celled yeast, or the microscopic nematode worm (a type of roundworm) with fewer than one thousand cells, for studying aging and other physiological functions in humans.

Finally, a personal favorite evolutionary explanation for senescence is the idea that the old die to make room for the young. This somewhat altruistic explanation for senescence, and death, is based on an evolutionary explanation called **group selection**. Remember, natural selection favors the individuals carrying the genes for successful reproduction. Group selection picks the groups that survive better, unlike natural selection that acts on individuals. This makes it more complicated to test and ultimately to support, because you have to be able to identify a lot of groups in different environments. So, although this theory may have some appeal, it is pretty speculative.

Why bother with the evolutionary explanations? Personally, I find them fascinating. But a practical reason affects understanding why we have to age. And remember, many people, especially the centenarians, don't suffer from the diseases associated with aging that typically cause death. But still they die.

It may be that in order to understand why most living things die, we have to go back to the most ancient life forms: bacteria. In a way, bacteria are truly immortal. One cell splits into two, each divides again, and so on. Barring accident or predation, all of these cells, which are genetically identical (except for mutations), keep on keeping on in this fashion. Every so often, however, a big change in their environment means that most of the bacteria will not prosper or will be killed off. In this situation, it makes sense for the ones fated to die anyway to take themselves out of the picture, leaving the stage to their mutated cousins more adept at dealing with the new environment. In fact, bacterial cells carry the cellular equivalent of a cyanide pill, allowing them to commit suicide should conditions warrant. Amazingly, we also carry these little time bombs in our cells, and they are increasingly, perhaps erroneously, activated as we age.[10]

Recall that successful reproduction is the basis for natural selection. The critters that leave the most offspring win the genetic lottery by being over-represented in following generations. Then, it follows that trade-offs between physiological investments favoring reproduction and those favoring longevity will be biased toward the former.

ANIMAL STUDIES TELL US ABOUT AGING— BUT NOT EVERYTHING

One more thing to take into account is that much of the research on aging has been done in animals, for reasons I introduced in the first chapter. Our evolutionary relationships support the validity of animal research, but clearly natural selection has acted differently on mice and humans. Small vulnerable animals such as mice have a dangerous lifestyle with numerous predators and scarce resources. In these species, natural selection has favored a "fast" life history. In other words, to pass on their genes, mice should breed early and often. Mouse genes won't care about longevity. In larger animals such as humans, elephants, and whales, or for animals such as lobsters, bats, and birds that have evolved strategies to reduce the risk of predation, natural selection has favored a "slow" life history. These animals show adaptations leading to longer potential life spans.

Let me give you an example of that by explaining some emerging evidence from **geroscience** (the study of aging). Many of these new results, most from the past decade, have grown out of findings first reported almost one hundred years ago that **caloric restriction (CR)** increased both life span and health span in rodents. Since then, this finding has been extended to every species in which CR has been applied. In mice, for example, life span is extended 30–40 percent, and aged animals fed the CR diet had the physiological characteristics of much younger animals. A three-year-old lab mouse is ancient, kind of a rodent Methuselah, lacking hair and hardly able to move. But a three-year-old CR mouse looks and acts like a middle-aged, active animal: with healthy skin, hair, and vascular systems, and even able to reproduce.

CR in the lab is a pretty severe restriction. The animals are fed about 60 percent of what they would normally eat on a daily basis, supplemented with adequate levels of vitamins and other micronutrients. Most people would not voluntarily sign up for CR even though the health benefits are quite amazing in other mammals. These include improved insulin sensitivity (i.e., the opposite of type 2 diabetes), reduced body fat and cancer risk.

Not surprisingly, many scientists began investigating the cellular mechanisms underlying CR. The reasoning goes like this: if we know how CR works, then we can re-create it and get its benefits without all the agony of starving ourselves. Lots of studies in rodents, primates, and other critters showing the myriad benefits of CR vis-à-vis aging, but the jury is still out on humans. A number of "natural" experiments have been done with CR in humans (e.g., Biosphere 2 and wartime famines); these support the health and longevity effects but lack experimental rigor. Recently, a multiyear study on humans and the effect of CR was started, but, as yet, few definitive results from old folks have emerged.[11] It does seem that human CR doesn't have the same impact on life span as in shorter-lived animals. However, it does provide numerous benefits, such as a greatly lowered risk for most degenerative conditions of aging and improved measures of health. I revisit this topic in more detail in chapter 9.

A Deep Dive into Caloric Restriction

A lot of complicated and interconnected mechanisms seem to account for what goes on during CR. In a nutshell, CR is a form of stress telling the body that times are lean and our systems should hunker down and turn on their defensive mechanisms. The underlying goal, from an evolutionary perspective (yes, getting back to this idea), is to ensure that reproduction can occur eventually. Our ancestors had plenty of lean times, when they had to go hungry. In order to ensure future reproduction, ancestral organisms of all species would have delayed it during lean times and shifted their metabolic resources toward maintenance and survival.

Specifically, two **hormones**, **insulin** and **insulin-like growth factor 1** (a mouthful, so let's lump them together and call them **IGF-1**) are released by the body when food is plentiful. Hormones are chemical messengers that carry information through the body, so these two tell your cells that food is available, and a bunch of programs are then started up to build more cells and tissues. Clearly, it's an important message. But as we all know, too much of a good thing can go awry. Too much cellular activity, and growth can increase the production of damaging compounds. Think of the runaway growth that many of us see in our hometowns: lots of pollution, traffic, and other associated ills of unregulated growth. CR has the opposite effect of these pro-growth hormones: it activates pathways that slow growth, allowing time for repair systems to kick in and clean up damage.

The IGF-1 system (which includes the aforementioned insulin, IGF-1, and **growth hormone [GH]**, of which I have a lot more to say in later chapters) was the first to be shown to affect life span in lab animals.[12] An interesting example of this is the Chihuahua, the little dog with a surprisingly long life span. This breed, and some other small dogs, have a mutated form of the gene for IGF-1, so they don't make much of it and are kind of in CR all the time.[13]

Also, CR increases a process called **autophagy**. Autophagy is the way in which cells remove damaged components in order to recycle the materials into new replacement parts. When these damaged items (like proteins) accumulate, much like trash in your basement, they can contribute to age-related decline and damage to the rest of your body's machinery. Increasing autophagy may help reduce this contribution to the aging process and extend life. Much more on this process in later chapters also.

This is all well and good: natural selection chooses the favored genes, which are packaged together in the germ cells and move through time. But why does the individual organism itself age and die? Death seems to be an inevitable consequence of multicellular life. Single-celled organisms such as bacteria can split, and each half perpetuates the life of the progenitor. But big, complicated creatures like us can't do that.[14] Some scientists suggest that with corrective therapies, we may be able to extend human life span indefinitely. This idea, to maximize longevity, is popular with Silicon Valley billionaires who are funding this type of research. Personally, I think we are a long way from achieving this, if ever. However, some of their findings are accessible to the rest of us and may allow us to extend our health spans. I will cover some of these new findings in the final two chapters. Read on in the next chapter about the ways in which we deteriorate, and hints as to how to mitigate them.

ACRONYMS

CR: Caloric restriction
GH: Growth hormone
IGF-1: Insulin and insulin-like growth factor

3

The How of Aging

OVERVIEW

The prevailing view of aging is that it is caused by the accumulation of damage to cells. A few initial types of damage act like dominoes, knocking down additional systems and causing further damage. Which of these damages are more important than others, and just how they tie into age-related diseases, is prompting a lot of debate, but the basic set is pretty well agreed on.[1]

In this chapter I give you the full list of what goes wrong at the level of our cells and molecules. Each system can interact with others in complicated ways that I won't delve into too deeply. Each is amazingly complex and intricate, but we don't need that level of detail to understand, first, what the system is supposed to do and, second, what can go wrong as it ages. I will refer back to these in subsequent chapters, as they will be the usual suspects in all kinds of age-related diseases. In this listing, I'll give you a broad description of each system, hint at possible fixes that are addressed in detail in the final chapters, and in the last paragraph of each system I'll give you a brief summary.

If the information is too overwhelming, just skip this chapter. I will define these mechanisms briefly when I introduce them in later chapters, and you can return here for more detail.

In figure 3.1 is an example of a series of reactions. This type of interconnected reactions is called a **path**. The diagram here shows several interlinked pathways involved in an important process called methylation. I refer to this process in several chapters and won't spend much time on it now, but basically it involves sticking a little modifier called methyl onto one of many compounds. Figure 3.1 gives you an example of one of many thousands of biochemical paths our cells are constantly using. These paths interact in the key systems involved in maintaining the complex bodies we have. Failures at any level can have profound consequences with respect to health and longevity.

Don't look at the figure and try to follow the links. The takeaway is that there are numerous interacting components. Each small text item is a compound that acts in a chemical reaction, indicated by the direction of the arrow, to produce the next compound. Building the two end products, methionine and homocysteine (bottom right), takes place in a series of small steps, kind of like building a complex structure from simpler Lego pieces. Just like in your car, you don't have to understand how all the individual mechanical devices, such as belts, pumps, and chips, function in order to have a higher-level grasp of how the internal combustion engine works. For the interested, both methionine and cysteine are amino acids, used in building our proteins.

Homocysteine is another amino acid, one not used in proteins. The B vitamins, which include folate, play important roles in this pathway to facilitate the reactions. If you are deficient in one or more of the B vitamins (note how many of them are involved in these reactions), your homocysteine levels can

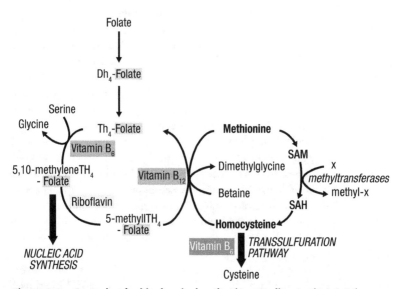

Figure 3.1. Example of a biochemical path. Linus Pauling Institute's Micronutrient Information Center.

rise. As elevated homocysteine can have some negative consequences as we age, especially in the brain, many physicians monitor it in their patients.

One way to think of these systems, how they interact, and how they can deteriorate, is to think of traffic flow in your neighborhood. Numerous systems influence traffic flow, from the engine in your own vehicle, to the integrity of the road surface, the electrical grid controlling traffic signals, and the signal mechanisms themselves. All of these systems will deteriorate with time if not maintained. If one goes out, or behaves erratically (e.g., a signal), then traffic flow is affected, and downstream injuries may occur.

GENETIC DAMAGE

Every living creature experiences damage to its **genes**, and its **DNA**, throughout its life. DNA refers to the genetic material; each gene is a small piece of the total. The integrity and stability of your DNA are constantly being threatened by external forces such as environmental chemicals, viruses, and UV radiation as well as by internal factors such as mistakes in DNA copying during cell division and oxidation damage (more on this later). DNA can be damaged in numerous ways; I'll just refer to all of them collectively as mutations, though some different types can have different consequences. A mutation changes the **DNA sequence** (the identity of the individual units of DNA, like the letters in a word). Thus, the mutant form of the gene is one variation in DNA sequence, called an **allele**, whereas the normal sequence is another allele of the same gene.

One example of a premature aging disease is Werner syndrome. This disease is characterized by extremely rapid aging. Werner syndrome is caused by a mutation in a gene that is involved in repairing DNA damage. Insidious? Yes, and certainly tragic for those suffering from it. But one bright spot is that experimental treatments that enhance DNA repair can extend life in laboratory animals.

One final note on genes involves terminology. Let me use Werner syndrome (WS) as an example. The gene that, when mutated, causes WS, is found on chromosome 8. In other words, every gene has its unique "genetic address" on a chromosome.

Each of us has twenty-three pairs of chromosomes. The members of each pair are like the two shoes or gloves of a pair: they clearly belong together but are not the same. One chromosome can carry one allele while the other chromosome can carry the same, or a different allele.

Alleles that have a large enough effect to be noticeable, such as the WS form, typically cause terrible diseases. Other, more familiar examples are cystic fibrosis and sickle cell anemia. The alleles in most of these diseases code for a protein that doesn't work. This type of genetic disease is called recessive because the mutant form can be masked by one normal form. To have the disease, a person has to have the dysfunctional allele on both chromosomes. Fortunately, these diseases are rare.

More common diseases, such as cancer and diabetes, as well as our body systems, are determined by a combination of many genes, as well as lifestyle factors such as diet or environmental chemicals. This makes the underlying genes more difficult to identify. In addition, because many genes influence these so-called **complex traits**, most of us get combinations of "good" and "bad" genes. Think about playing poker: no one card is especially good or bad; the cards in your hand combine for a good or bad hand. But the genetic hand can consist of hundreds of genes as opposed to the five or seven you get in a poker hand. Identifying the many genes that can influence a complex trait requires some DNA sequence information and a population of people (or plants or animals) who have different forms of the trait.[2]

New technologies have made this problem more solvable. In humans and a variety of other species, the DNA sequence and chromosomal address of most genes are known. Now, researchers can look for alleles of each gene, and there can be a lot of them. These can be identified by sequencing all of the DNA of a person, called their **genome**. This process would be like spelling out all the text in the New York City phone book. Once you have that, then you can go to any given gene and see the letters, called bases, that spell it out. Alternatively, alleles can be identified by examining small sections of specific genes. This latter process, used by companies such as 23andMe and Ancestry, would be analogous to having a few letters in a person's name and using that as a search string in a program such as Excel.

Most of us are probably more interested in what genes might put us at risk for developing some of the common diseases, such as cancer or diabetes. Or, you might be interested in genes that protect you, or cause a body system to work better. Although many known alleles cause recessive diseases, far fewer are known to influence normal function and aging-related declines. This is because most of these so-called **risk alleles** have only a small influence on each trait or disease, much like an individual card in a player's hand.

I expect this situation to change in the near future. Recall that you need a population to identify these genes. The bigger the population, the better. Several really big publicly funded research efforts are proposed in the United States and ongoing in the European Union and China to sequence the genomes of a million people each. And privately funded efforts by companies such as 23andMe look for relationships between alleles and function. Because the small-effect alleles produce, well, small effects, you have to look at a really big population to find them.[3]

The flip side of risk alleles is the protection that some genes confer. Studies of centenarians who have had their DNA sequenced have revealed some intriguing possibilities of longevity alleles. The role of genes in longevity is strengthened by the observation that many centenarians don't live particularly healthy lifestyles. But keep in mind the conclusions from studies on identical twins, who have the same DNA: they can have widely differing life spans. In other words, the environment, or the lifestyle choices you make, are important.

In each chapter, I will tell you about some of the genes known to affect the function of the system in that chapter. These genes may put you at risk or protect you from diseases of the system of that chapter. I'm not advocating that you have your genome sequenced—it's still not cheap—or even have your DNA analyzed by one of the companies that do this. But, if you have a family history of a condition you are concerned about, DNA analysis is one way to get more information on your risk. And as the knowledge base of our genome is increasing literally by the day, more and more factors, both protective and causal, are being identified.

At the risk of sounding repetitive, I will continue to remind you that these are very preliminary lists. Researchers can readily determine that many genes may contribute to a certain aspect of the body. But it's much more difficult to identify the actual genes, and even more difficult to figure out how they act.

TELOMERE LOSS

Telomeres are the tips of chromosomes. Their job is to protect the integrity of the functional middle section of the chromosome. They do this by losing some of their length each time the cell divides. This happens because of the way the chromosome is copied prior to cell division. The enzyme that duplicates the DNA has to have a piece of the template chromosome to attach to; this attachment region thus can't be duplicated and is lost. The telomere is basically a sacrifice zone. After a certain number of cell divisions, the telomere region is depleted, and the cell stops dividing. Thus, telomere loss is a precursor to genetic damage as well as other age-related damages such as cellular senescence, which I discuss further below. Telomere loss does correlate with these cellular events associated with aging, but is not highly correlated with chronological age. Experiments with mice have shown that lengthening telomeres can delay aging, although the equivalent experiment has not been done in humans. I should note that different types of cells lose telomeres at different rates, so it's difficult to generalize across all cell types to draw a unitary conclusion about the significance of this occurrence. Elizabeth Blackburn, who won a Nobel prize in 2009 for her work on telomeres, has written an excellent, accessible book on the subject.[4]

An important point to remember is that telomere length can and does change with environmental factors such as diet and stress. This flexibility means that we can actively work to improve telomeres. But it also means that testing your telomere length to try to predict your biological age is probably not a winning proposition.

EPIGENETIC CHANGES

Let's start here by talking about genes. You know that you get one copy of each of your two chromosomes from your mom and the other from your dad. And the genes on these chromosomes are made of a molecule called DNA. Your DNA doesn't change much over the course of your lifetime. You may get the occasional mutation here and there, but by and large your genome, as it's called, is pretty stable.

A gene is a stretch of DNA on a chromosome. Its exact layout from start to finish is called its sequence. When genes are active, they are copied into something called **RNA**, and this RNA is then "read" to produce proteins. Genes can be turned on or off, in which case they respectively do, or do not, produce their proteins.

As life goes on, our DNA gets tagged with other compounds that turn them off, on, up, or down. These are called **epigenetic markers**, because they are attached to (epi-) the DNA. Think of these things as volume controls for your genes. We are born with a set of these markers containing instructions for the specialization of different cell types. This is necessary because every cell of your body has all your DNA, known as your genome, but each type of cell, such as muscle, bone, heart, turns on different genes. In addition to these specialization markers, we acquire a whole other set as we go through life. These acquired epigenetic markers allow our external environment to activate certain genes that may enable us to react to conditions in a favorable way.

A remarkable set of experiments with baby rats illustrates the role of these epigenetic changes. Researchers used two inbred strains of rats for these studies. Within a strain, the rats are all genetically identical, in essence, like a whole bunch of identical twins. One strain was characterized by normal mothering, in which mothers lick and cuddle with their infants. Mothers in the other strain were much less caring.

The scientists wanted to look at the effect of early life stress. To do this, they focused on mother rats with infants. In each of the two strains, half the mothers and their babies were raised normally. These were the controls. In the other half, for the first week of life, the babies, called pups, were removed from their mothers for about fifteen minutes. The pups were isolated and kept warm to ensure that the stress was due to the separation, rather than physical discomfort. In the nurturing strain, when pups were returned, mothers were immediately attentive and licked and nursed the pups extensively. In the less caring strain, the mothers were not attentive and essentially ignored the pups.

When the pups were grown, they were tested on a variety of behavioral measures. Animals from the inattentive strain, who had been separated as infants, were more anxious, aggressive, and likely to be attracted to drugs of abuse such as alcohol and cocaine. Careful mothering seemed to protect pups from these adult problems.

Turns out the effect of good mothering is transferred to the genes that control stress responses via epigenetic markers. When stress response genes are activated by separation, nurturing by mothers will cause an epigenetic marker to be attached to these genes, turning them off. Those pups then grow up without the adverse consequences initiated by stressful early life events.

A lot of different epigenetic markers can affect our genes throughout life. Aging appears to be associated with specific changes in one of these epigenetic signals, called a methyl group. When a methyl group is attached to a gene, it turns the gene down or even off completely. (This is one reason the methylation path, shown in figure 3.1, is an important pathway.) Different environmental events can attach completely different epigenetic markers to the same gene. Things such as diet or parenting can cause really different epigenetic marker patterns. Some of these epigenetic signals can initiate premature aging syndromes such as Werner's in mice.

A researcher at UCLA had the clever idea to look for specific genes that were turned off or on with age. Amazingly, he found a group of about 350 genes that were consistently turned down with increasing age. By analyzing all of these simultaneously, he devised an **epigenetic clock** that predicts biological age remarkably well. You have probably noticed some people who look much older, or younger, than their chronological age. These people may have variations in the clock genes that make their biological age more, or less, than their birthdays would suggest. Although it's not known exactly what these 350 genes are doing, they do predict mortality at later ages quite well. One company will even take a saliva sample and tell you your epigenetic age.[5]

Here is just one spinoff from the clock study. Liver cells from overweight individuals tend to be older than other body cells but younger than the rest of the body in people who are underweight. This relationship wasn't found in other tissues. For example, fat cells don't show older epigenetic ages in the overweight. Unfortunately, weight loss did not undo the accelerated epigenetic age in the liver cells. A number of labs are currently researching ways to reverse the epigenetic changes, in hopes of reversing aging.[6]

A group of enzymes called sirtuins (if you have read about the longevity effect of red wine, sirtuins are believed to be involved in that) are involved in turning genes on and off via the epigenetic path. When sirtuins are active in mice, they live longer; conversely, when sirtuins are inactivated in mice, they die younger. There is a lot of current research into the role(s) and effects of sirtuins in humans; more on this when we discuss antiaging interventions in chapter 10.

Keep in mind that epigenetic marks are added to our genes throughout our lives. Although it may be tempting to conclude that stressful life events cause deleterious epigenetic changes, we don't know enough about the nature and action of these markers to say that definitively.

LOSS OF PROTEOSTASIS

Wow, that's a mouthful. What exactly does this mean? You may have heard the term **homeostasis**. That refers to the body's ability to maintain a set point for a given factor. Think about the thermostat in your house, which maintains a specified temperature. Most homeostatic systems in the body use negative feedback processes similar to the way your thermostat works to hold the various parameters (temperature, blood pH, blood levels of many nutrients such as glucose and calcium) within a narrow range.

Back to the thermostat. Say it's set at seventy. A thermometer inside is constantly monitoring the temperature. If it dips below seventy, the connection to the furnace kicks on, and the temperature in your house goes up. Once it goes above seventy, the furnace connection is shut down, and eventually the temperature will drop. Then the cycle starts over again. Negative feedback in the body works in a similar way, but typically more monitors are controlling the process to achieve a finer control.

Let's go back to **proteostasis**, a shorthand way of saying protein homeostasis. This just refers to the way that cells maintain the stability and quality of the proteins that they rely on. Proteins are a group of biological molecules with a wide array of functions, but in general they are the workhorses of our cells. They are used to build the skeletons of cells, to run the chemical processes in the cells, and to attack and remove foreign invaders. So, staying on top of protein quality is a big deal. It should come as no surprise, then, that aging and some aging-related diseases, such as Alzheimer's disease, Parkinson's disease, and cataracts, are linked to problems with proteostasis. Further, some exciting new experimental results in mice show that genetic modifications that improve proteostasis delay aging.

What do our cells do to maintain proteostasis? There are a lot of interrelated processes, much like the many systems in your car that operate jointly to keep the car moving down the road. Briefly, these processes identify, tag, and break down proteins that have something wrong with them. The general term for these processes is **autophagy** (literally, "self-eating," introduced in the last chapter), but this subsumes numerous actions, some of which also have other functions. Keep in mind that once the proteins are broken down into their components, these building blocks can be, and are, recycled into new protein.

MITOCHONDRIA AND MITOCHONDRIAL DYSFUNCTION

The **mitochondria** are the cellular power plants, taking the fuel in food and breaking it into smaller chemicals, like burning coal in a power plant, which produces CO_2. In the process, energy is released and stored in other chemical compounds, especially one called **ATP**, like the electricity released from the power plant where the coal is burned. ATP is a common energy currency, like dollars, that your cells use whenever energy is required. Then the mitochondria are like banks, exchanging all kinds of input currencies for the dollars used in each cell. But there's a price, a bit like the exchange fee that the bank charges. You can see the structure of the mitochondrion in figure 3.2.

To illustrate the importance of ATP and its production by the mitochondria, consider the toxicity of cyanide. Just a spoonful of potassium cyanide will cause death in a few hours. Cyanide blocks the formation of ATP. Without ATP, life won't go on, as ATP is used in virtually every chemical reaction in the body.

Another illustration of the significance of ATP, if you need more, is the sheer quantity used in the body. At any given instant, you have about a gram of the stuff scattered throughout your cells. But over the course of a day, because it's constantly being used up and then regenerated, mostly by the mitochondria, you will go through more than one hundred pounds of it.

The mitochondria use the oxygen that we breathe in to do their magic. Inevitably, some of this oxygen is converted to bad forms, known as free radicals,

MITOCHONDRIA

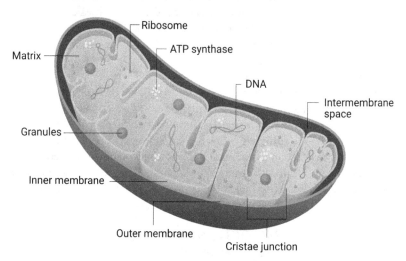

Figure 3.2.   **Mitochondrial structure. Cristae are the folds; the inner membrane separates the internal matrixfrom the rest of the structure.** © iStock / Vitalii Dumma.

or **reactive oxygen species (ROS)**. ROS can damage cellular components, including DNA, by a process called oxidation. Stay with me! The ROS can also cause the immune system to produce another type of damaging substance, so-called inflammatory compounds. I'll come back to them, too.

The Dr. Jekyll side of the ROS damages cellular DNA, lipids, and proteins, but they also have a Mr. Hyde good side. ROS act as signals, telling other parts of the cell what is happening in the mitochondria. Don't underestimate the significance of the mitochondria. Each cell has thousands of them, especially cells that use lots of energy such as muscle and liver cells. Amazingly, they take up about 20 percent of these cells' volume, or about 10 percent of your body's weight. Our cells, not surprisingly, have built in security systems to tell them about the level of ROS. This is a bit like having a motion detector outside your home to tell you when someone or something is moving around outside. So, we don't want to get rid of the ROS produced in the mitochondria entirely.

As we age, our mitochondria, which are constantly reproducing by dividing (as well as some other weird things they do), accumulate mutations, which are disruptions in their DNA. Yes, mitochondria do have some of their own DNA, although most of their genes migrated into the cell's chromosomes long ago (in evolutionary time). The mitochondrial genome is not large (only thirteen genes that code for proteins), but enough that if it's damaged, the mitochondrion doesn't function as well. In fact, impaired mitochondria are a ubiquitous sign of an aging cell.

Another type of damage that can occur in mitochondria is oxidation of their membranes. The mitochondrion has a lot of membranes. And, of course, because of its role in energy processing, a lot of oxygen is being used in the neighborhood. There's plenty of opportunity for oxidation. Different species have different types of membranes, and some of these membranes are more vulnerable to oxidation than others. Interestingly, it turns out that longer-lived species, such as naked mole rats, have membranes that are more resistant to that type of damage.[7]

Damaged mitochondria release even more ROS, resulting in even more age-related damage. Dysfunctional mitochondria can then result in a dysfunctional (senescent) cell and damage that can spread out into surrounding tissues. Mitochondrial dysfunction is found in many age-related diseases such as diabetes, cancer, and neurodegenerative disorders such as Parkinson's. In fact, one of the most typical events of aging is a progressive decline in mitochondrial functioning, which affects the entire cell and thus one's health and well-being. Even in healthy individuals, old mitochondria don't work as well, producing less energy from the same amount of food. We are gradually starting to understand how damaged mitochondria can cause these events.[8]

Young, healthy cells have mitochondrial repair mechanisms. As we age, so do these repair systems, but they don't work well. Because our cells are clever, mitochondria have a suicide mechanism programmed into them, so they self-destruct when they start to damage their environment. Damaged mitochondria become "leaky," and bits and pieces of their membrane break off into the cell where they should trigger the suicide pill. Ironically, in older cells this suicide path doesn't work as well, increasing cellular damage in a vicious cycle. And to add insult to injury, those loose bits of mitochondrial flotsam also trigger inflammation.

One proposed solution to the downward spiral instigated by increased ROS is to modify genes in the mitochondria to increase levels of their innate antioxidants. An experiment has been done in mice, modifying the gene for one specific antioxidant. The oldest mice responded best, living about 20 percent longer than their siblings without the treatment.[9] This strategy is a little like inserting a stent (a tube to open up a blood vessel) that releases anti-clotting drugs into clogged arteries feeding the heart. In other words, the fix is put at the source of the problem. Of course, altering the DNA makes for a more permanent effect than a stent, which can degrade over time.

Weirdly, as mitochondrial activity rises, life span increases. And interventions that increase mitochondrial activity, including some drugs such as metformin (more on this in chapter 10) and physical exercise, also increase life span. But this makes sense when you realize that active mitochondria (which produce the potentially damaging ROS) also stimulate the production of the naturally occurring protective chemicals known as antioxidants. Remember the beneficial role of stress in the form of CR. Well, ROS can be seen as intracellular stresses that will also elicit compensatory survival mechanisms. But, much like with the insulin story, too much compensation can cause other problems and aggravate age-related damage.

Keep in mind that your mitochondria are essential structures that are always affecting you. As their function declines with age, age-related problems can increase. Some researchers are looking into the possibility of augmenting old mitochondria, which seems to extend life in mice.

DEREGULATED NUTRIENT SENSING

I introduced the idea of caloric restriction (CR) in the previous chapter, but let's revisit it. To summarize briefly, eating fewer calories increases life and health span. (Recent studies have found that changing eating patterns to incorporate some fasting, and even limiting certain types of foods, can have the same life- and health-span extension; I discuss these in chapter 9.)

Let's look at it from the perspective of the mitochondria. Think of the fuel-conversion process in the mitochondria as a pipeline: food goes in the front end, and ATP comes out the back end. If you have plenty of fuel, aka calories, from food but don't use the energy, the pipe can get backed up. Your mitochondria are taking in more energy than they can release at the end of the process and, consequently, they release more ROS. But if you are exerting yourself, ATP is constantly being sucked out of the end of the pipeline, and fewer ROS are released. Of course, overflow valves at the front of the pipe are diverting extra calories to fat storage, but inevitably the mitochondria are overloaded, too. Adjusting either end of the pipe, fewer calories in (CR), or more energy (exercise) out, will reduce ROS. Thus, the beneficial effects of both CR and exercise. This idea is also a basis for so-called cold therapy or ice baths, cold plunges, and so forth. When your body temperature drops, the mitochondria can generate heat by diverting the flow through the pipe to a different spigot than the ATP end, one that increases the heat in the cell.

Another, seemingly counterintuitive effect of caloric restriction, in experimental animals is increased activity of mitochondria. CR does this by increasing the signal in the cell (called **NAD$^+$**, essentially a shuttle for electrons, carrying them around the cell) that turns on mitochondrial genes. When these genes are turned on, the machinery in the mitochondria that release ROS gets a tune-up, resulting in fewer ROS. NAD$^+$ also activates genes in the cell nucleus that control a number of stress responses including antioxidants that, of course, decrease ROS. NAD+ is another one of those things that, sadly, declines with age.[10] A lot of researchers are looking at ways to prevent or reverse this decline; I'll talk more about this in chapter 10.

After a meal containing carbohydrates, cells in the pancreas release the hormone **insulin**. (In general, hormones are substances that are released from the gland that makes them, travel through the body, and can affect many downstream targets.) The insulin rushes through the blood stimulating fat cells to stockpile fat and other cells to build protein and string sugar molecules together in glycogen, the storage form of carbohydrates.

Insulin also regulates the action of a similar hormone, **IGF-1**, that we met in the previous chapter. To explain the intertwined roles of insulin and IGF-1 on nutrient sensing, I have to introduce you to **growth hormone (GH)**. Yes, another hormone, which you may suspect tells your body to, well, grow. Actually, the story is not that straightforward. GH does stimulate the body to grow, especially when we are young, and when we are recovering from injuries. But another way that GH stimulates growth is by causing the release of IGF-1. I'll tell you more about GH shortly, but let's stick with insulin and IGF-1 now.

IGF-1 can have the same effect as insulin, that is, to open the cellular doors to the fuel molecules (glucose and fats) from food. In addition, this pair of chemical messengers tells your cells that nutrients are plentiful, and they should grow and divide. For brevity, let's call these two **IIS (Insulin and IGF-1 Signaling)**. The series of events, called a path (which is illustrated in figure 3.1), initiated by IIS, is found in most living cells, including single-celled organisms such as yeast. But IGF-1 is the workhorse of the pair, relaying the message to many different cells to use the newly available nutrients to build proteins and divide to make new cells.

The IIS messengers (insulin and IGF-1) act on many cellular systems involved in aging in humans as well as other organisms. Because of this commonality, scientists can study this path in simpler organisms, such as yeast, and their findings can translate into humans.

This is an ancient evolutionary path allowing animals to feast on the seasonal abundance of plants. Plant calories are high in carbohydrates, which are readily broken down into the type of sugar, glucose, that our cells use. When the glucose in your blood goes up after a carbohydrate meal, cells in the pancreas release insulin. Insulin tells different tissues to do different things. For example, adipose (i.e., fat) tissue begins to store excess calories as fat for what could be lean times ahead. For our ancestors, plant calories declined after the growing season and so did insulin. The drop in insulin in animals during winter tells the mitochondria to increase their energy-generating activity. This may seem counterintuitive but, in fact, would facilitate the ability of animals to search for more limited food sources. Interestingly, when animals are really food stressed (i.e., starving), they need less sleep so they can spend more time searching for food.[11]

Of course, in modern industrialized societies, we rarely experience lean times and the seasonal drop in insulin. If caloric intake, especially in the form of carbohydrates, stays high, the growth signals stay on.

Reducing IIS is an adaptive response aimed at minimizing cell growth and metabolism during times of stress, such as times when food is scarce. Animals with a decreased IIS survive longer because they have lower rates of cell growth and metabolism. These lower metabolic activities produce lower rates of cellular damage (more on this below). Thus, lowering IIS should extend life span. However, taken to an extreme, this defensive response may cause other, unintended problems (think of the systemic damage starvation causes) that actually speed and exacerbate aging.[12]

IGF-1 naturally decreases as we age. Its production is controlled by the master chemical of development, growth hormone (which is produced by a gland called the pituitary that sits at the base of the brain). Because we don't grow our entire lives, GH drops with age, and the concomitant decline in IGF-1 makes sense. But GH also maintains muscle size and strength, and unfortunately these decline with age, too—lots more on this in later chapters.

In mice, dogs, humans, and other animals, when the effects of GH are inhibited by mutations in genes affecting its function, life span is extended. An example of this role of growth on life span is seen in mice engineered to lack either growth hormone or the **receptors** for GH. The receptors, of course, are the gateways into the cells, without which GH can't act. These mice hold the record for longevity in that species, living 70 percent or so longer than their unmodified siblings. Not only do they live longer, but they are also healthier due to many interacting mechanisms such as increased stress resistance and stem cell activity, reduced inflammation, and better DNA repair.

In mice, these mutations make for smaller body size. This makes sense: if your growth pathways are suppressed, you won't get as big. This phenomenon is seen in people with a type of dwarfism called Laron syndrome. These individuals are small because, like the mice, they don't respond to GH. Not only do they live longer, but they also don't suffer from many of the chronic diseases associated with aging such as cancer and diabetes. However, current debate centers on the overall health of people with Laron syndrome, as they appear to be more at risk of non-age-related diseases such as alcoholism.

A second major nutrient sensor is called m**TOR**, for **target of rapamycin**. TOR is a master switch that regulates protein synthesis and overall cell growth. Inhibition of mTOR, by rapamycin, has been found to extend life span and reduce age-related disease in experimental animals. Currently, using this drug in people is attracting a lot of interest. You can appreciate the many processes controlled by TOR in figure 3.3. Rapamycin was first used clinically to suppress the immune system in transplant patients. Many of these patients showed lower than expected rates of cancer and osteoporosis, which are normally common in immunosuppressed people. Rapamycin itself has some unpleasant side effects, so a number of related compounds are being tested. More on this in chapter 10.

A similar phenomenon is seen in centenarians, those folks living to one hundred and beyond. Most of these individuals, even at one hundred years of age, are still sensitive to the effect of insulin, meaning that they rapidly and efficiently pull glucose out of the blood. Although it may seem counterintuitive, reduced IIS activity extends life span; conversely, insulin resistance leads to type 2 diabetes. (In type 2 diabetes, your pancreas releases insulin, unlike the situation in type 1 diabetes, but your cells don't respond; i.e., they are resistant.)

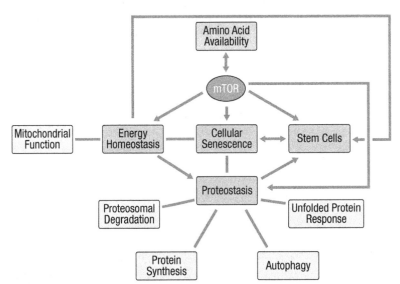

Figure 3.3. **TOR is involved in many of the processes affected by aging. Papadopoli, David et al. mTOR as a Central Regulator of Lifespan and Aging.**

More effective insulin responses reduce all those bad effects of glucose when it hangs around in your blood, as well as keeping the centenarians from putting on a lot of fat. If we dig deeper into the effects of insulin and IGF-1 (IIS), they stimulate TOR. So, it makes sense that less insulin means less TOR activity, which means less of the growth pathways that TOR controls.

Keep this in mind: in general, growth activities in cells accelerate aging whereas decreased nutrient signaling extends life and health span. Actions such as CR mimic the latter. A great deal of research is going into finding drugs that will do the same.

OXIDATION DAMAGE

Also known as oxidative stress, it results when an electron is pulled off a molecule. Sorry, but I have to introduce a little chemistry here. Electrons are the negatively charged pieces of an atom that build chemical bonds, the molecular glue holding together our chemical pieces. So, if electrons are lost from molecules, those molecules won't behave normally in our cells. Oxygen is usually the electron thief—think about how cut apples and potatoes turn brown when sitting on the cutting board—although other substances (nitrogen, lipids) can do the same thing. Oxygen is critical to our metabolism, allowing us to "burn" fuel in our cells, like we burn fuel in our auto engines. During this process, oxygen normally picks up electrons that are moving through the mitochondria, the energy processing structures of the cell.

But oxygen, and other compounds, can also grab extra electrons, producing an imbalance. These unbalanced compounds are generically called free radicals, but the ones that the mitochondria produce involve oxygen, so they are specifically known as **reactive oxygen species (ROS)**, meaning that they can react with and damage other molecules in our cells. ROS can initiate a chain reaction of electron transfers, ultimately resulting in oxidation damage when an electron is pulled from a key cellular component. This damage can be especially harmful when DNA or mitochondria are damaged. Because oxygen is a constant danger, our cells have many naturally occurring antioxidant defenses. Because these defense systems decline with age, oxidation damage increases with aging.

Key points to remember: ROS are normally produced within cells, but we have defenses against them. Unfortunately, these antioxidant defenses decline with age. ROS-lowering interventions were widely proposed as an antiaging strategy. Antioxidants, synthetic or naturally occurring compounds, that can remove ROS have been studied in this role. Unexpectedly, most studies found no health promotion in humans. Some studies even showed that taking antioxidants worsen the outcome in cancer and other age-related diseases.[13] I talk more about this surprising result in chapter 5.

INFLAMMATION

This is a response by the immune system to pathogens or damaged cells. Its role is to get rid of the pathogen or damaged cells and stimulate repair. **Acute inflammation** occurs when immune cells are recruited to an area of infection or tissue damage. Proteins (called **cytokines**) released by these first responder cells cause the local blood vessels to become porous, allowing plasma and additional immune cells to reach the injury site. This migration produces the familiar feelings of swelling and heat we associate with injury and inflammation. As the role of acute inflammation is to destroy foreign or damaged cells, it would damage normal tissue if allowed to continue for long, so feedback mechanisms turn it off. I discuss some of these in chapter 10.

Chronic inflammation is believed to underlie many age-related diseases and syndromes. This phenomenon is so pervasive that the term **inflammaging** is now used to emphasize that many of these disorders, including cancers, susceptibility to infections, and dementia, can get a jump start when inflammation is present. Unlike acute inflammation, the chronic version is not associated with infection or injury. Thus, it is sometimes called sterile inflammation.

Although the cause of chronic inflammation is not known for sure, one likely cause is overstimulation of the immune system by the cumulative effect of long-term oxidation damage. Remember, one job of the immune system is to start the healing process when it detects damage. When the immune system is overactivated, it damages the tissues it is trying to heal. Then, the immune system itself becomes dysfunctional due to a chronic activation, causing its failure to deal effectively with real pathogens and damaged tissues. Ironically, an increasingly disabled immune system produces more inflammation.[14]

Another cause of inflammaging is the signals that senescent cells release. These chemical messengers call the immune system to try to get rid of the aging cells. Of course, because we get more and more senescent cells as we get older, the immune system gets overactivated trying to clear them out.

Further overstimulation of the immune system may be caused by leakage of gut bacteria into the bloodstream. I know, it sounds disgusting, but remember that all of our systems experience some deterioration as we age, and the gut is not spared. The intestinal wall loses its remarkable self-healing ability as it ages and gets leaky, allowing some bacteria to escape. Of course, the immune system detects these foreign creatures and mounts a defense.

A related cause of inflammation is our mitochondria. I haven't forgotten that I introduced their ROS as a likely villain in the aging process, but they play another role. Specifically, mitochondria, which are akin to bacteria, carry some chemical tags that label them as such. If they leak out of the protective environment of our cells, as can happen when they or their home cell are damaged, they also can stimulate an immune response.

What happens when inflammation gets out of hand? It is known to be involved in the development of obesity and type 2 diabetes, two conditions that contribute to and correlate with aging. And it goes both ways. Many, though not all, obese people show higher than normal levels of inflammation and the chemicals that cause it. That inflammation then affects their metabolism to cause insulin resistance, which results in type 2 diabetes. In mice, high-fat diets alter the bacterial species of the microbiome living in the gut, resulting in additional inflammation. Conversely, high fiber in the diet affects the microbiome, resulting in effects on the immune system that decrease inflammation.

Likewise, defective inflammatory responses can contribute to atherosclerosis and cancer. Inflammation and stress can also shut down activity in the hypothalamus, a brain region that controls numerous hormones affecting your physiology, including growth hormone. This effect in the brain can contribute to age-related changes such as bone fragility, muscle weakness, skin atrophy, and reduced nerve cell regeneration. An exciting result of these new findings is that treatment with a hypothalamic hormone prevents the damage to nerve cells and slows aging in mice. Other findings of note indicate that blood-borne factors can slow, even reverse aging in laboratory animals following blood and plasma exchanges between young and old mice.[15]

A key point regarding inflammation is that it is an umbrella term. As I suggest above, different types of inflammation (many more that I can describe here) have different roles. Any instance of inflammation can have either good or bad outcomes depending on circumstances. And the factors that influence inflammation can themselves be influenced by other factors, such as oxidation damage. Finally, remember that rapamycin suppresses the immune system. As such, some of its beneficial effects can be explained, though, of course, too much suppression of your immune system is not good.

CELLULAR SENESCENCE

Most cells have a natural limit to the number of times they can divide. Cell division is the way we replace damaged cells and build tissues and organs. When your cells stop dividing because they've hit that limit, and start releasing some new compounds, they have become senescent. The end of the ability to divide is mainly due to telomere loss, but other factors can also induce senescence, such as radiation damage or inflammation. An intriguing new hypothesis suggests that as cells age and incur DNA damage, they pause the cell division program but growth programs continue unabated. The result is that these cells get bigger. Once a cell passes a certain size, the instructions (produced by its genes) that control internal functions get diluted. The result? This bigger cell starts to deteriorate and voila, it has entered senescence.

Cells are programmed to die once they have stopped reproducing, but sometimes they manage to escape that fate. These **senescent cells** that linger release a cocktail of chemicals that affect surrounding cells. As with inflammation, the changes in senescent cells can be either beneficial or harmful, depending on the situation. For example, by entering a nondividing state, senescence inhibits the development of cancer, which is characterized by unrestricted cell division and proliferation.

As you may have guessed from their name, these cells accumulate as we age and often become enlarged, probably because of their increased secretory activities. Ironically, senescent cells eventually can contribute to cancer risk because of some of the compounds they release. In other cases, senescent cells can contribute to healing tissue that has been inflamed. But if the immune system fails to remove them, they can aggravate the inflammation. And, of course, our immune systems get worse at cleaning them up as we age.[16]

Many compounds released by senescent cells cause inflammation (more about this in the next section). These chemicals are believed to be a major cause of the damage to surrounding cells. Thus, anti-inflammatory drugs are one approach for reducing the effects of cellular senescence. Remember the "aspirin a day" saying? Seems that our grandmas knew something. (For the pros and cons of this treatment, hold on or skip ahead to chapter 10.) Another approach is found in a new class of drugs called senolytics, which target and remove or kill senescent cells.[17] This new, promising approach for delaying, preventing, or reversing many of the conditions associated with cellular senescence may be in clinical trials by the time you read this.

Some key points to remember about senescent cells: these cells secrete molecules called growth factors (recall IGF-1) that tell cells around them to grow. As you now know, active cells produce more ROS. Senescent cells also release compounds that stimulate the inflammatory response, which damages cells directly and also decreases the anticancer activities of the immune system. If that isn't enough, they also release compounds that break down the goo that holds cells together (if you're curious, this is called the **extracellular matrix**, or **ECM**). This damage to the ECM can facilitate the spread, or metastasis, of cancers. And finally, they can stimulate the production of new blood vessels, a process called angiogenesis. Wait you say, isn't angiogenesis a good thing? Well, as always, it depends. When we are children getting bigger, or as adults, enlarging muscles, yes, it's a good thing. But if we are just making new blood vessels randomly, these bring more oxygen and release more ROS and provide nutrients for any cancers in the area.

An interesting thought regarding senescent cells is that they may be due to the continuation of developmental processes that were beneficial when we were young and growing to maturity. But, like a furnace whose thermostat doesn't shut it off, when unchecked, these processes can result in some unintended and undesired consequences. This suggestion explains the observation that senescent cells continue to grow despite the lack of the external signals, such as growth hormone, that normally tell cells to grow and divide. As I said earlier, these cells don't divide (because they have reached their limit on division), but as they continue the internal growth processes (illustrated by the activities of mTOR), they get bigger and produce substances that may be harmful to cells around them.

Like many of the processes in this section, cellular senescence is a good thing (i.e., the termination of cell division) gone bad. So, it's probably not a process that should be completely eliminated. A promising research avenue is the removal of senescent cells by drugs as mentioned above, or by filtering the blood because these cells are larger than normal cells. A number of clinical trials, and a few start-up biotech companies (e.g., Oisin, https://www.oisinbio.com; Unity, https://unitybiotechnology.com) are focused on this approach to treat specific age-associated diseases, which I address in more detail in chapter 10.

STEM CELL EXHAUSTION

Stem cells are cells in which no specific genetic program has been turned on. In other words, they are not yet specialized into any of the many cell types we have. You can think of them as precursor cells in the body that can continue dividing forever and subsequently can develop into other types of cells. Because stem cells can become bone, muscle, cartilage, and other specialized types of cells, they have the potential to treat many diseases, including Parkinson's, Alzheimer's, diabetes, and cancer.

Let's address two types of stem cells. First, in the developing embryo are **embryonic stem cells (ES)**. This makes sense, because each of us started life as a single cell, a fertilized egg cell, that started dividing. All of these early cells were ES—that is, they divided to produce more ES and cells that became more specialized, to produce the tissues and organs of the developing embryo. ES are called **pluripotent**, meaning that the cells resulting from their divisions can ultimately produce any kind of cell ranging from nerve to muscle to skin. The second kind of stem cell is the adult stem cell. We all have these in our tissues and organs where they produce new cells to repair and replace cells in *that* specific organ or tissue.

Pluripotent ES cells clearly could be useful to treat all kinds of diseases. They can keep dividing almost indefinitely and give rise to any other cell type. To get this type of cell from an embryo, you must destroy the embryo, thus the controversy around the use of ES. Another problem with the use of ES to treat disease is that the stem cell comes from a different individual than the one getting the treatment. This difference could cause rejection by the treated person's immune system.

But we have another way to get pluripotent cells: **induced pluripotent stem cells (iPSCs)** can be generated from adult cells. Researchers in Japan developed this amazing trick about ten years ago. They showed that by putting just four genes that are active in early embryos into adult cells, those adult cells would be converted in pluripotent cells. IPSCs can be produced from adult cells, meaning they bypass the need for embryos. And they can be made from your own cells. These **autologous** (literally, from yourself) cells could be used for transplants without risk of rejection.

Another way to use adult stem cells is to harvest them from our own bodies, then grow them in the lab to increase their numbers before reinjecting. This method, which is not allowed in the United States, is used in Europe and other countries with good results in many conditions. Because of the myriad ways these and other stem cells (e.g., from placentas) are used in the United States, it's difficult to compare the results from the numerous stem cell clinics springing up.

Using stem cells to treat degenerative processes is called regenerative medicine. This approach has been demonstrated in the laboratory to heal broken bones, bad burns, macular degeneration, deafness, heart damage, worn joints, nerve damage, the lost brain cells of Parkinson's disease, and other conditions. Less complex organs such as the bladder and the trachea have been constructed from a patient's cells and successfully transplanted.

Stem cells in the adult body gradually lose their ability to repair and maintain as we age. In other words, they wear out or run out. Eventually tissues and organs fail because they are not rebuilt. Recent research has shown that this occurs because increasing numbers of stem cells become dormant as age-related cellular damage of the type described in this section accelerates. Dormancy probably reduces the chances of cancer due to a damaged stem cell running amok but at the cost of failing tissues. Researchers have found that by infusing old tissue with young blood, aged stem cell populations can be restored to action, and some of the impact of aging on our tissues is reversed. This treatment is called **parabiosis**. Current research focuses on identifying the signals in blood that talk to the stem cells to revive them. Drug therapies are also being explored to improve stem cell function. In particular, rapamycin (see chapter 10), which can delay aging by improving proteostasis and by altering nutrient sensing, may also improve stem cell function.

Keep in mind that stem cell exhaustion is probably a result of the action of several to many of the processes described above. But because the loss of our regenerative cells defines the look of aging in many tissues (skin and muscle are obvious examples), this system is an obvious target for minimizing the deleterious effects of aging.

AUTOPHAGY

I debated including this topic as it is potentially confusing. But increasingly it seems that many mechanisms described here either include this or lead to it, so I decided it's really important to discuss. And more and more proposed interventions involve ways to get this process going. So just what is **autophagy**?[18] Well, remember that auto- refers to self and -phagy to eating. Eating myself? I know it sounds crazy, but consider this: each and every cell has limited resources with which to carry out a lot of different functions. So, if one process isn't being used, any materials invested there essentially are not available for other functions. These materials can be recycled by autophagy and put to better use elsewhere. Also, molecules, especially proteins, that have been damaged or corrupted during assembly can be recycled. And structures such as mitochondria, which could harm the cell if damaged, can also be recycled. Autophagy is enhanced by CR (caloric restriction) and exercise, and inhibited by high levels of dietary protein.

Keep in mind that this is not one of the major proposed routes by which aging occurs. Rather, autophagy is an important process of cell well-being that can be enhanced by lifestyle choices. Increasing this vital activity seems to play a key role in minimizing many of the deleterious age-related changes discussed above.

HORMESIS

Similarly, this is not a process that causes aging, but it is a normal and important cellular stress response involved in aging and defenses against aging, so I should introduce it. This seems like a good place, because **hormesis** ties into the other processes I discussed in this section.

It makes sense that cells and organs would have evolved mechanisms to identify and minimize the effects of stresses such as starvation. All cells and organisms, from single-celled yeast (a favorite study organism of biologists) to humans, show graded responses toward stress, such that low levels of stress induce defense and repair whereas high levels of the same stress can be toxic or lethal. A benefit, such as longevity, resulting from a low level of stress, is called hormesis. External stresses that elicit a hormetic response include radiation, oxidation stress, and prolonged exposure to high temperatures and noxious chemicals. In fact, muscle growth is a kind of positive response to stress from low-level damage to muscle cells incurred while working out.

Many of these stresses share a cellular pathway controlled by something called **PGC-1α**, which is kind of a gateway to the programs that repair and maintain as opposed to those that build and develop. Going back to CR, for example, insulin and IGF-1, which are present at high levels during times when food is plentiful, turn down PGC-1α. Various environmental stresses, such as those in the preceding paragraph, and including oxidation damage, turn up PGC-1α, eventually culminating in increased production of mitochondria. Unfortunately, PGC-1α levels drop off with age for reasons that are not understood.

Keep in mind that all organisms, including us, engage in trade-offs. When nutrients are plentiful, cells go on a building spree. But overly ambitious building can produce toxins or damage the cellular environment, much like rapid growth in urban centers. From an evolutionary perspective (aha; if you skipped that chapter, you may want to go back now) the organism can justify rapid growth early in life because reproduction is coming up. The trade-off is that later in life, some of the repair processes may be compromised.

CONCLUSION

It's complicated. But living things are complicated. We consist of lots of interlocking systems that typically all work together. Mitochondria produce energy that is used to build proteins from which we are made, and the energy also fuels autophagy and proteostasis to keep everything in good working order. Age means that these systems start to break down, but not necessarily simultaneously, and differently in different individuals. Diseases and injuries accelerate some of the breakdown. All of these insults and damages can increase the amount of TOR the cells produce in an effort to make things right. Remember, this is the master switch for the growth trajectory of the cells, but too much growth, like always driving your engine at high RPMs, can burn us out.

Tempted to throw up your hands and say it's too complicated, so pass the chocolate cake? Read on, because new developments in biochemistry and cellular biology are teasing apart the complicated threads that produce the aging tapestry and providing tantalizing hints at how to maintain health span. I will redefine these concepts in the chapters that follow as I show you how these mechanisms affect your body as you age. In each chapter I will offer a few of the new ideas on how to counter these mechanisms to keep you healthier. In the final chapters, I'll pull together many of the new interventions. Finally, I include a few general sources in the notes that cover these basic concepts in more detail for the interested reader.

ACRONYMS

ATP: Adenosine triphosphate
CR: Caloric restriction
DNA: Deoxyribonucleic acid (if you really want to know)
ECM: Extracellular matrix
ES: Embryonic stem cells
GH: Growth hormone
IGF-1: Insulin-like growth factor
IIS: Insulin and IGF-1 signaling
iPSC: Induced pluripotent stem cells
mTOR: Mammalian target of rapamycin
PGC-1α: You don't want to know
ROS: Reactive oxygen species
WS: Werner syndrome

4

Skin

OVERVIEW

The skin is a wondrous structure: loaded with a variety of sensory detectors, it covers you head to toe in a protective but permeable barrier comprising about 16 percent of the weight of the average adult—roughly twenty pounds, making it the largest organ of your body. (Unless your body fat outdoes it—more in later chapters on how our fat can have surprising effects on us as we age.) Removed—yes, I know, that's a grisly thought—and stretched out, it would cover more than twenty square feet. The skin also holds the nail beds, which produce finger and toenails, and the hair follicle cells that birth our hair.

The skin is the boundary between you and your environment, so it gets hammered from both sides: the aging processes from within, and external stresses from outside. As we all know, wrinkles, age spots, thinning, sagging, color changes, and skin cancers proliferate with advancing years. The outward face of the skin makes these signs of aging easy to see. The internal factors (genetic mutations, increased inflammatory signals, decreased **lipid** production—these are fats—and decreased hormone levels) combined with external factors (ultraviolet [UV] radiation, lifestyle [e.g., diet and smoking], and pollution) all contribute to age-related skin damage.

This damage is not limited to the loss of your smooth youthful skin. Physiological functions are affected as well. These include: **permeability** (i.e., how various things you put on your skin move through it), **vascular** (i.e., blood vessels) maintenance, sweat (and related lipid) production, **immune** function (your body's ability to defend and repair itself) and **vitamin D** (involved in maintenance of many body systems) synthesis. What you get: impaired wound healing, sagging, bruising, skin diseases, and cancers.

Even without external stresses such as UV radiation, you can see age-related changes in your skin in protected places such as the armpit. Here you find fine wrinkles, loss of elasticity, and thinning of the skin. Places that have been exposed to the sun will experience compounded damage (jargon term: **solar elastosis**), where the skin becomes yellow and thickened as a result of sun damage.

We all know people with skin that looks much younger than their age would suggest. News flash: researchers recently found that genes associated with being younger are turned on in those people. Not surprising, but dig a little deeper, and we see the significance of lifestyle and the environment we live in. Be sedentary, age more rapidly. Take up smoking, and age more rapidly. In the context of skin, sit around in the sun too much and age more rapidly. All of these lifestyle choices will affect the genes we are born with. This idea is the basis of the new science of epigenetics that I introduced in the previous chapter. In other words, we can alter the way our genes affect our skin.

WHAT IS SKIN?

Anatomy. Before I can discuss what aging does to the skin, I have to introduce you to the structural terms for its three layers (look at figure 4.1). The outer layer, the **epidermis**, creates a waterproof barrier. It is continually regenerated by cells at its base, while the upper layer is constantly sloughed off. This outer portion of the epidermis consists of 15–20 layers of flattened, dead cells. These cells contain a **protein** (a kind of microscopic scaffold) that absorbs water and prevents water loss from the body. This part of the skin is encased in a fatty layer contributing to its elasticity, and also contains more **cholesterol**—a fatty, and thus waterproofing, substance—than any other part of the body.[1] In addition, the **pigment** cells that produce the color of the skin are located here.

The next layer down, the **dermis**, holds a layer of connective tissue made up of two major proteins. Most of the protein in the dermis, more than 75 percent, is **collagen**, an important structural protein that looks kind of like a braided rope. Collagen is found in many body structures and provides structural support—like the framing of a house. Collagen is a really important protein in the skin. It acts like a thickly woven rug, with lots of fibers that are connected to make a 3-D matrix holding the other skin components in place. It's a strong yet flexible weave giving the skin its fantastic ability to protect you from injury but also be elastic. **Elastin** is a second protein in the dermis,

STRUCTURE OF THE SKIN

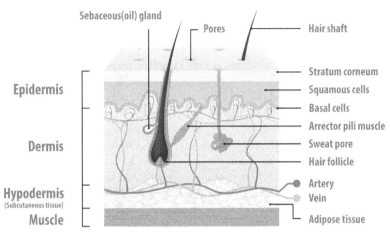

Figure 4.1. The three layers of skin. © iStock / Paladjai.

which, as the name implies, gives the skin its elasticity, allowing it to return to its original shape when stretched or squeezed. Sadly, elastin is only produced during our early years and gradually deteriorates as we age.

The dermis also contains nerve cells, hair follicles (the roots of hairs), sweat glands, nail beds, and lymph and blood vessels. The lowest layer, the **hypodermis**, contains half the fat in the body, cushioning (sometimes more than we need) the tissue beneath.

Age-related skin changes begin at about the age of thirty. What you see is increased susceptibility to injury, slower healing, reduced barrier protection, and delayed absorption of drugs and chemicals placed on the skin. You can also blister more easily.

Regeneration in the outer layer—the epidermis—slows for two reasons. The parent cells grow more slowly, and they migrate to the surface more slowly. Turnover drops by about half between the third and seventh decades of life, meaning that the cells are replaced much more slowly. We get thinner skin that is torn, bruised, or cut more easily. The production of protein and fats, which absorb and hold water here, are also reduced, and the skin becomes drier and rougher. The connection between the epidermis and dermis weakens with age, resulting in separation of these layers and increasing fragility of the skin.

As the outer epidermis loses its connections to lower supporting layers, some of our sensor cells, which are nerve cells, can be damaged and stop working as they should. A particularly bizarre manifestation of this is called **notalgia paresthetica**. Although the official term is a mouthful, many of us experience some form of this itching in a particularly hard-to-reach place on the back, typically below the left shoulder blade. Because it is caused by loss of the nerve connection, there is no cure. An anti-inflammatory gel helps some people, as may some CBD products.

The number of pigment cells in the epidermis falls off with age by about 20 percent per decade after the age of thirty. Let me put that another way: between thirty and sixty-five years of age, you lose almost 80 percent of the pigment-producing cells of the skin. Consequently, the skin gets much paler. Despite this almost unbelievable loss of cells—or maybe because of it—some of the remaining pigment cells get a lot bigger. These larger cells produce more pigment, and voila: age spots! The enlarged cells are typically found in areas most commonly exposed to sunlight, including the back of the hands, the face, arms, and legs. Because the role of the pigment in the skin is to protect from UV damage, falling pigment levels mean reduced protection from harmful solar radiation. The overall loss of pigment and the reduced immune capacity of the skin combine to increase the risk of skin cancer with age.

A little further down, the dermis is also losing cells and blood vessels. The number of **fibroblasts** (cells making collagen) decreases. The total amount of collagen decreases by about 1 percent per year after thirty. Individual collagen fibers get thicker, making it harder for the repair processes of the body to remove them from the skin. This thickened collagen is less flexible and predisposes the dermis to tearing injuries. Elastic fibers within the dermis lose their elasticity. What do we get? Sagging and wrinkling. Creases and lines appear in areas of expression and high use: frown lines on the forehead and crow's feet at the corners of the eyes. Those elastic fibers get a lot of wear and tear and stretch out earlier than in other parts of the body.

Another region that gets cut back with age is the fatty layer of the hypodermis. This also makes for wrinkles. Your face gets more than its share of wrinkles because the skin here gets a lot of sun exposure. UV radiation from sunlight damages DNA in the skin cells responsible for maintaining and repairing the skin, and then they don't do their work. The loss of subdermal fat in the extremities makes aging arms and legs look thinner and adds to the risk of hypothermia, skin tearing, and other traumatic injuries.

A Deep Dive into the Protein Structure of the Skin

Collagen is one of the strongest proteins the human body makes. In the skin, it is a supportive framework for cells and tissues. (Tissues are structures in organs made up of several different types of cells that work together.) Over time, collagen, like other proteins, can become stuck to other proteins through a process called **glycation**. These connections between adjacent collagen molecules make it stiffer and less flexible. So what, you ask? Well, then your skin becomes easier to tear or bruise and less able to rebound from stretching, making, well, wrinkles. Think of a deep, plush rug, with long and springy fibers. Now imagine the rug matted with dirt and mud, no longer springing back as you walk over it. That's a glycated collagen matrix. Glycated collagen makes its first appearance at the tender age of twenty, increasing its spread by about 4 percent each year. Doesn't sound like much? Well, by the time you're eighty, more than half of your skin collagen will be stuck and matted together.

There's more: We used to think that excessive sun exposure damaged skin primarily because of inflammation, oxidation damage, and increased rate of mutation (DNA damage; all of which I talked about at length in chapter 3). But sun exposure on young skin can cause glycation of proteins. Further, smoking, another thing that aggravates skin aging, accelerates glycation of collagen and other proteins.

As if that's not enough to think about, collagen and other support proteins in the skin are very long-lived. That means that they hang around for years or even decades before your body worries about replacing them. Once the repair system gets activated, it's usually too late if glycation has already occurred. Some good news is on the horizon, though. Researchers are working on finding tags that will distinguish between undamaged and glycated collagen so that the damaged variety can be targeted and removed. And as I discuss in the final chapter, exercise and dietary restrictions can reduce glycation.

Another important environmental factor contributing to aging skin is what you eat. Glycation takes place during cooking, in a process remarkably similar to the chemical reaction in the body that cross-links the proteins. Frying and barbecuing food, especially meat, produces more glycation than boiling or steaming. For the interested reader, this process is called the **Maillard reaction** and specifically involves a chemical reaction between sugar, present in muscle for fuel, and protein. (When this happens to meat as it is barbequed or fried, the surface caramelizes, which is one reason we like these foods.) Approximately 10–30 percent of glycated proteins in the food you eat are absorbed in the blood and can wreak additional havoc in the skin, probably by causing an inflammatory response. So, changing the way you prepare food could reduce wrinkles.[2]

And here's another "wrinkle" in the aging skin story. Measures of skin damage discussed above, such as wrinkles, uneven pigment, and sagging, can also indicate that a similar type of damage is occurring in the heart.

Just as in the skin, where these symptoms are due to unrepaired damage to its protein structure, when the structure of the heart is damaged and not repaired, problems result.

Another Deep Dive: The Vascular System in the Skin (Blood Supply)

The blood carries nutrients, oxygen, and immune system cells, which repair injuries. As we get older, blood flow to the skin decreases, as do the number of small blood vessels. The remaining blood vessels have weaker walls. These can break more easily, causing bruising. With loss of blood vessels, and decreased blood flow, here, as in the rest of the body, the repair system in the vascular tissue of the skin is impaired.[3] As we saw earlier, many of the annoying skin changes with age, such as sagging, wrinkling, and spotting, come about because of the impaired repair systems. An extreme consequence in the bedridden is the occurrence of decubitus ulcers, aka bedsores.

Many of the changes I just described in the vascular system are due to the formation of—get ready—glycated proteins in the membranes of the blood vessels. Sugars in the blood and inside your cells contribute a lot to this process. Fructose—yes, that same high-fructose corn syrup in all our sticky sweet beverages is one of the worst offenders. Want a cheap easy way to keep your skin looking younger? Yes, cut down the sugar in your diet.

Aerobic exercise, anything from running marathons to thirty-minute brisk walks, also reduces the age-related decline in the vascular system.[4] This benefit may be simply from increased blood flow, though I discuss other benefits in the next chapter.

Sweat Glands. We also lose sweat glands as we age, and they don't work as well either. What happens? You sweat less, and your ability to cool down is impaired. Sebaceous glands, also found in the dermis, produce an oily or waxy secretion, called **sebum**, to lubricate and waterproof the skin and hair. Weirdly, although the number of these glands stays constant, they get bigger but produce less sebum with age. The diminished sweat and sebum production contribute to dry, rough skin. And, as we all know, dry skin can be itchy. Start with fragile skin, add scratching, and you have an equation for cracks and breaks in the skin.

Hair and Nails. Hair and nails are both produced by cells found in the skin. The changes you notice in the nails of older people—thickening and grooving—are another piece of fallout from reduced blood flow, this time to the nail bed. This slows nail growth, and they become thicker and more prone to breakage. As nails age, they can become vertically grooved or ridged, probably because of the skin's increasing inability to retain moisture, although it can also be due to a lack of certain vitamins or poor nutrition. Buffing the ridges may seem like a good idea, but that can cause the nail to split, which can increase the risk of infection.

Hair **follicles**, the cells at the root of the hair, like many other skin cells, become less active with age. And they don't regenerate as fast as they used to, causing hair to thin. Hair on the body is lost from the edges inward; in other words, you lose hair on the extremities before on the trunk. If you're male and your mother's father was bald, good chance you may lose your hair, too. This is called male pattern baldness. Male balding patterns start at the top of the head and progress downward. Females can experience it, too, in which case it's called female pattern hair loss, as they typically lose some but not all hair. By age fifty, pattern baldness affects half the male population and a quarter of the women. Other genetic factors are at play here, some of which I will mention in the final section of this chapter.

The hairline recedes in 80 percent of older women and 100 percent of older men. Why does it happen? Read on to the section on hormones and aging, and you'll find out. While hair is lost on top of the head, eyebrows, ear and nose hairs grow longer and coarser. Hormones cause this, too.

Pigment production also declines in the root cells of hairs. The result? Gray and, eventually, white hair. For most of us, at least half of all body hair has turned gray by age fifty.

WHAT ABOUT HORMONES?

Although reduced blood flow is the immediate cause of many of the unpleasant changes in the skin described above, hormones are another underlying cause. So, I will give you a lot of information about so-called **steroid hormones** (because they all get their start from cholesterol, called a steroid compound by chemists) and what they do in the skin. Their effects are seen throughout the body, so we will keep coming back to them in later sections.

Let's start with the hormonal effects of **estrogen**, which, contrary to popular belief, is not just a female hormone. (Nor is there a single form of estrogen; women have three common types.) Although this hormone is high in premenopausal women, where it's made in the ovaries, it's also found in males and made in many different tissues. Interestingly, in females, estrogens are produced by converting the male hormones (**androgens**) into estrogens. Androgens are made in the body by tweaking the molecular structure of cholesterol, which gives rise to all the **steroid hormone** families (e.g., cortisol, thyroid, growth hormone, vitamin D, etc.). Cholesterol has a bad rap because of its possible role in heart disease, but it is the building block for these hormones and an essential part of the wrapping or **membrane** of every single one of our cells. Because it's so important, we can manufacture all the cholesterol the body needs, and our liver and most other cells do just that.

As we know, aging skin is drier, rougher, and less able to retain moisture. Estrogens contribute to these changes because they affect skin thickness, wrinkle formation, and skin moisture. How? One action of estrogens is to stimulate the production of a compound called **hyaluronic acid (HA)**, which helps to keep skin hydrated. HA in the skin has the sponge-like ability to absorb large quantities of water—more than one thousand times its weight—and to combine with collagen and elastin. These so-called hydrated molecules support the structure of the skin, contribute to its elasticity, and provide the fullness in skin that prevents the appearance of wrinkles and fine lines. Age-related hormonal declines, as well as exposure to the sun and pollution, decrease the body's natural production of HA, resulting in reduced volume and the appearance of wrinkles.

Testosterone is the primary male sex hormone, although it, too, is produced in women from (of course) cholesterol. Testosterone is responsible for many of the characteristics of male skin such as coarser hair, thicker and oilier skin. In general, guys have a later onset for showing signs of skin aging because of testosterone.

At menopause, the abrupt drop in estrogen, one of the major female sex hormones, contributes to skin changes in women. Because male sex hormones, especially testosterone, are involved in skin sebum production, women may experience increased oiliness or even adult acne when the ratio between these two hormones becomes unbalanced, with testosterone getting a temporary upper hand. The effects of male sex hormones on skin are important in both sexes, and both can experience the effects of altered levels during aging.

During the transition into menopause (aka perimenopause), a woman's skin may appear flushed, red, and blotchy. Estrogens have anti-inflammatory properties, so the loss of these hormones can lead to increased inflammation, which can exacerbate certain conditions such as rosacea. **Rosacea** is a common skin condition in middle-aged women, especially those with fair hair and skin, causing redness and visible blood vessels in the face.

Remember, estrogens play a major role in maintaining the collagen and elastic network of the skin. Losing estrogens means losing dermal collagen production. So, skin thins, loses elasticity, and sets the stage for wrinkle formation. Estrogen loss also reduces the number of blood vessels in the skin, resulting in pale skin and fewer nutrients traveling to the skin. (I think I've gone on enough about changes in blood flow and all this skin damage.) So aging women get pale, thin, and dry skin. Because the drop in estrogen is sudden and more drastic than other hormones such as testosterone, you can also see an increase in characteristics such as increased facial hair caused by the relatively higher level of androgens.

The skin is not the only external feature that benefits from estrogens. Besides resulting in healthy, moist skin, estrogens can also make hair grow long and healthy. During pregnancy, when estrogen levels are high, women often experience hair growth. Plummeting postpartum and menopausal estrogen levels cause thinning, sometimes resulting in clinically significant hair loss.

In both sexes, **androgens** (male sex hormones) stimulate hair growth, but this effect varies in different parts of the body and has not been well-studied in women. In general, androgens stimulate beard growth but suppress scalp hair growth (as in pattern baldness), a weird duality known in the medical literature as the "**androgen paradox**."[5] Without getting too technical, here's what is going on: in the body, testosterone is converted by enzymes into another hormone, DHT. Different forms of these enzymes occur in scalp and facial hair root cells. Production of the enzyme in facial hair is turned up with aging whereas it declines in scalp hair. No one really knows why, but speculation involves declines in hair stem cells. A potential treatment is being developed into a drug that could affect those stem cells.[6]

And as women age, they become more insulin-resistant (I introduced the insulin system in chapter 3 and will come back to it in later chapters). This leads to a decrease in a protein produced by the liver called **sex hormone-binding globulin**, or **SHBG**. SHBG does what it says: it grabs the estrogens and testosterone that women make, and consequently they are less available to local tissues. Conversely, when SHBG drops, the hormone level in your bloodstream goes up. This is not a big deal in terms of estrogen, because it's going down with menopause anyway, but testosterone can become more available to your tissues and skin, and as discussed for men above, can increase facial hair growth. Yes, you get those hairs on your chinny chin chin.

While we're on the topic of steroid hormone effects on skin, we have to touch on thyroid hormones. The thyroid gland (a small butterfly-shaped gland just in front of the voice box) makes two hormones that affect a large number of systems, including the skin. Low **thyroid hormone (TH)** levels can cause scaling and thickening of the skin, making it rough and dry. Low TH can also cause eyebrow hair to fall out, scalp hair to become coarse and brittle, and nails to break easily. Too much TH produces the opposite effect in skin: the skin may be overly moist, often becoming red and flushed. Occasionally, a condition sometimes found during pregnancy occurs. This is characterized by brown patches on the face or other parts of the body that get lots of sun, such as the forearms and neck.

WHAT TO DO?

The first, and most obvious thing we should all be doing, from birth on, is using sunscreen. Broad spectrum screens protect against both UVA and UVB, both of which cause skin damage. SPF numbers refer to UVB protection, and numbers above thirty don't really offer that much more protection unless you are really sun sensitive. You should, however, reapply any sun protection that you use every few hours.

In women, research has shown improvements in skin elasticity, moisture, and skin thickness using either topical (skin cream) estrogen or **hormone replacement therapy (HRT)**. However, HRT does not always prove to be fully beneficial. For example, sun-damaged skin does not improve with estrogen treatment. And, an occasional side effect of HRT is increased pigmentation on cheeks—more age spots! The research on male skin and hormone therapy is even more sparse. Finally, be aware that there is a lot of unresolved controversy over the differing effects of bio-identical hormones (i.e., chemically identical to those produced by our body) and synthetic hormones (which are not chemically identical to ours).

Because collagen production is drastically affected by hormonal changes, we can combat this by using compounds that boost collagen production in the skin. Vitamin C has been shown to boost collagen production in skin. You have heard plenty by now about the vital role of collagen in skin. It occurs normally in both the dermis and epidermis (look back at figure 4.1), but as we get older, vitamin C levels fall. This vitamin also acts as an antioxidant in the skin, protecting it from free radical damage.

You can get some vitamin C from your food to migrate from the blood into the skin, but as you now know, aging has deleterious effects on the vascular system in the skin. The good news is that you can apply it topically, using creams or serums. The bad news is that getting it through the hard outer layer of the epidermis is not easy. If that outer layer is removed, say through laser treatments or chemical peels, then the route is open. But to get these treatments you have to go to a dermatologist or esthetician. In animal studies, using a low **pH** (below 4, this means it is somewhat acidic) preparation improved movement of the vitamin into the skin. In these same studies, the best absorption was found with a 20 percent vitamin C solution. Unfortunately, studies of these problems in people are only limited. Another problem with vitamin C is that it breaks down rapidly. Getting it in a combination with vitamin E helps to stabilize it.

Peptides (these are like proteins but smaller; one commercially available product is palmitoyl pentapeptide) can penetrate the skin and activate cells to increase production of collagen and other compounds increasing elasticity. A few studies have shown these to have anti-wrinkling effects, probably because of their role in increasing collagen production.[7]

Retinoids, including retinol, part of the vitamin A family, slow collagen loss and pigmentation changes. The most common, which are applied topically, are retinol, tretinoin, adapalene, tazarotene, alitretinoin, and bexarotene. These drugs (the most effective being tretinoin) act on genes that produce collagen and control inflammation. Thus, the retinoids can be useful against a variety of age-related skin damage ranging from sun damage to inflammatory conditions such as rosacea (facial redness) and melisma (patches of discolored skin).

Supplements. Research has increased into the effects of nutrients and vitamins, so-called **nutriceuticals**, as natural tools to reduce glycation. Naturally occurring antioxidants such as vitamin C, vitamin E, niacin, pyridoxal, and selenium have been proposed, although the evidence is somewhat preliminary. I talk more about general effects of nutraceuticals in chapter 10.

Drink your tea! A compound found in teas (EGCG), known for its antioxidant properties, adds collagen and improves skin condition in mice treated with a relatively high dose. A typical cup of green tea contains 100–150 mg of tea **polyphenols** (the generic name for a health-promoting compound found in plants), and about half consists of EGCG. (More on this and other compounds in foods in chapter 10.) The mice with the best response got 20 mg/ kg or about 2 gm for a 120-pound person. I would have to drink about forty cups of tea to get that amount.

Antioxidants. The body has a built-in antioxidant mechanism controlled by a molecule called **Nrf2**. Nrf2 is activated by a compound found in many cruciferous veggies (broccoli, cauliflower, Brussels sprouts), but especially broccoli sprouts. Been seeing these in the health food stores lately? Nrf2 reduces glycation. Another reason to eat your cruciferous veggies. A diet rich in healthy fats, such as omega-3s found in salmon and nuts, will also augment your natural antioxidant and anti-inflammatory processes.

Remember the role that sugar plays in sticking proteins together (glycation). Glycated compounds can be visualized in the skin under certain types of fluorescent light. Expect to see this in your dermatology and esthetician offices for assessing the effect of antiaging cosmetic products.

Nitric oxide (NO) is a gas produced within the body and acts on different tissues to regulate immune and inflammatory responses. Specifically, NO protects cells against the damaging effects of UV exposure and oxidation damage and turns off many of the inflammation pathways that your body produces (read more about this in chapter 5). Because it's a gas, it's been difficult to introduce it into the body in an amount similar to what you would produce on your own. A recent clinical trial showed that a topical ointment could release NO into skin cells, which then reduced infection and inflammation.[8] I think we'll hear more about this in the future. In the meantime, eat your beets and kale to get materials that your body uses to make NO.

Interventional Treatments. Dermal fillers containing hyaluronic acid can be injected into the skin in the area of wrinkles to help restore the skin's natural appearance. HA can also be injected into joints, where it acts as a cushion and thus reduces arthritic pain (but read the caveats for this application in chapter 6 on the skeletal system). Although the injections can act as a temporary an-tiaging treatment for skin, no good evidence indicates that putting it on your skin will have any effect other than moisturizing.

Superficial treatments such as exfoliation and moisturizers provide symp-tomatic relief for aging skin in both men and women. Extrinsic aging factors are inescapable, so sun protection is key. This is particularly important in aged skin, as it is thinner and allows even more penetration by damaging UV rays.

Corrective treatments for hair loss range from steroids to surgery, in which small patches of skin containing hair follicles are removed from the back and sides of the head and transplanted to those areas where hair loss is apparent. Sadly, these approaches don't restore hair to its original, youthful fullness. But don't give up hope if you are losing hair or have lost it. New results from stem cell studies of skin have identified some of the molecular signals that tell skin cells to grow hair. In mice, researchers transplanted small clumps of skin grown from cells that were treated with the signal molecules, and vigorous natural hair growth resulted.[9]

Senolytics. Remember the senescent cells (SC) I introduced in the previ-ous chapter? These are essentially cells that have gone rogue. One thing these cells do is to quit dividing. Cell division is a process designed to make new youthful copies of damaged cells. The replacements can then continue to perform the functions of the parent cells. Senescent cells don't do this and, consequently, damage tissue when they linger and grow in number, as is the case with age. And here's the insidious thing about SC. These cells produce compounds that cause neighboring cells to become senescent. Kind of like the bad apple that spoils the whole batch. In the skin, senescent cells prob-ably cause many of the issues associated with skin aging, such as wrinkles, thinning skin, and skin cancers.

Now you might be asking, can we do something to get rid of these things? The short answer is, "Yes." I wrote about several biotech companies that have developed drugs called senolytics (meaning senescent-killing) in the previous chapter. These are similar conceptually to the new generation of drugs that target cancer cells, killing them and leading to complete remissions in some cases. The problem with making senolytics available in the near future is that they are classified by the FDA as drugs and, therefore, have to go through a long, costly approval process.

One company is marketing a topical treatment that selectively destroys senescent cells in skin. Because their product is a topical cream (i.e., applied to the skin) and claims to rejuvenate skin, it goes through a cosmetic regulatory process rather than the FDA procedure certifying drugs. Cosmetics must meet FDA guidelines, but these are not nearly as strict as for drugs. Basically, the company has to provide data showing that their product will not damage DNA or skin or eye cells.

I want to stress that I'm not endorsing this product. In my opinion, it represents a novel approach to dealing with the underlying causes of aging and merits explanation. The active ingredient is an antimicrobial peptide (AMP). Briefly, AMPs are small molecules all living creatures make that function as part of the immune system response to potential pathogens. In other words, they have a protective effect. In skin, AMP help repair skin injuries.

The researchers started by screening 200 AMP for their ability to kill senescent cells. They identified four that did this in skin cells grown in a lab setting. Then, they did a clever thing and modified the structure of those four to get two peptides that worked even better to get rid of senescent cells in cultured skin. (Growing skin in the lab is a technique that has been perfected over the past twenty years and now is so routine that when people need large skin grafts, scientists often take a small biopsy from the person and in a few weeks can grow large sheets of their own skin.)

To test the effect of the AMP in people, they started with different aged skin samples, from newborns to those over fifty, and grew the skin in the lab. Next, they determined the biological age of each sample, using the epigenetic clock method described in the previous chapter. Then they treated the skin cells with their product and found that it could turn back the clock on the older skin. In addition, they measured markers unique to senescent cells and found that treatment with their product decreased the numbers of these cells in treated samples.

Bottom line: it may be possible now to selectively eliminate senescent cells in the skin. And because these cells contribute to age-related degeneration throughout the body, this may be a feasible strategy to reduce some deleterious effects of age in the not-too-distant future.[10]

WHAT ABOUT MY GENES?

As is the case with every system I present in this book, many genes influence the characteristics of skin. Very few simple associations exist between single genes and complex systems such as skin. But as genetic testing becomes more sophisticated, and more people have their genomes tested, we are learning more about how individual genes can affect systems such as the skin. The list that follows is not exhaustive by any means, and will be out of date by the time this book has been published, but it illustrates how genes impact your skin and what you can learn by having your DNA tested. I describe the mechanism for how different forms of a single gene can affect a specific character, such as skin pigmentation, in chapters 3 and 9. You can find more information about any of the genes in the list below at the websites I include in the next note.

MC1R and *ASIP* are two genes that play a big role in producing freckles, sun sensitivity, and red hair, but they have relatively little effect on eye color. Of course, you probably know if you have freckles or red hair without DNA testing.

IRF4 is another gene affecting skin color. IRF4 is a switch that can be turned up or down by other genes. When it is turned down, melanin production drops, and you get sun sensitivity and blue eyes. Again, you know your eye color and sun sensitivity, but I mention this gene specifically because if you carry at least one copy of the form that reduces melanin, you can be at increased risk for some skin cancers.[11]

EDAR2 contains the instructions for a receptor (i.e., a protein in the cell membrane that recognizes and transmits signals to the cell). This protein is involved in the development of the skin. One of its variant forms is implicated in male pattern baldness.

AR is the gene for the androgen receptor. Androgen is a male hormone; one of its many functions is to promote and maintain hair growth so a receptor that loses function will result in less hair. This gene is located on the X chromosome. Males have only one copy of the X chromosome, so any gene located on the X will make its presence known, as opposed to the case in females, who have two copies of the X chromosome. In females, a low-functioning gene can be masked by the presence of an alternate form on the other X chromosome.

Keep in mind that many genes determine the normal function and appearance of the skin. The roles of most of these are poorly understood. For instance, you have at least thirty and, possibly, more than forty-five genes for different types of collagen depending on how you count them. Mutations in many of these genes are known to cause different diseases,[12] but the exact roles of other genes in normal skin variation are poorly understood.

CONCLUSION

As the outer layer to our bodies, the skin is a litmus test for our self-perception of age. As such, we value and wish to preserve it. Prevention is the best strategy for preservation, but as in all of our bodily systems, that only gets you so far. External fixes, as I've discussed here, provide some symptomatic relief. Good diet and supplements may help, too. Senescent cell therapies may go beyond this; the jury is still out. At this point, without resorting to more extreme methods, such as injections, laser treatments, or surgery, we can't turn back the clock.

ACRONYMS

DHT: An androgen your body creates from testosterone
EGCG: Antioxidant found in tea
HA: Hyaluronic Acid
HRT: Hormone replacement therapy
NO: Nitric oxide
Nrf2: A molecule produced by your body that stimulates antioxidant production
SHBG: Sex hormone-binding globulin
TH: Thyroid hormone
UV: Ultraviolet radiation

5

Muscles

OVERVIEW

We can move, read, play sports, lift light and heavy objects, all because of the wonderful musculoskeletal system—so named because muscles must attach to bones to move them. But that's not all that muscles do for us. Amazingly, muscles act as an **endocrine** organ; in other words, our muscles release chemicals that coordinate and control events in the rest of the body. Importantly for readers of this book, muscle mass is a good predictor of health span—in other words, the more muscle you bring with you as you age, the more likely you are to be healthy. In this chapter I will describe what happens to your muscles with age. I will also tell you what is known about why they decline and actions you can take to minimize this loss.

Your muscle strength peaks during your third decade and then starts to decline during middle age. By the age of eighty, expect to have lost about 50 percent of your peak muscle mass if you don't work to retain some (or approximately 5 percent per decade or 1.5 percent per year). What's important to keep in mind about this loss is that it is not just simple atrophy, but it results from a combination of factors, including reduced input from the nerves that control the muscles and changes in chemical signals in the body that affect muscle maintenance. This loss of muscle, and the downstream consequences, which I discuss in detail below, are not trivial. Together, they account for more disabilities and limitations in aging adults than any other disease or disorder. It follows that the best predictor of death in older men is muscle weakness.[1]

We tend to think of the main role of the **skeletal** (aka **voluntary**) muscles as moving our bones. This, in turn, moves us and objects that we are manipulating. Muscles also hold a reservoir of proteins and, working with the liver, control the concentrations of glucose and amino acids in the blood. As we age, there are changes in the ability of the muscle to contract. These changes are due to events in the nerve controlling the muscle, as well as within the muscle cell itself.[2] We'll come back to all of these matters shortly.

But that's not all that muscle does. Our muscle cells release chemicals called **myokines** (*myo-* for muscle and *-kine*, meaning an activator) that talk to our immune systems. This interplay helps to regulate the immune system. And, not surprisingly, the production of these important myokines decreases as we get older. This means it's even more important to preserve muscle mass with age.

A word of warning: To me, this is the most significant chapter because of the clear role muscle strength plays in health span. Consequently, I go into a lot of detail about some of the ways muscles contribute to our longevity and well-being. If the jargon gets too much, or you are simply not interested in the detail, stick to the beginning of each section and avoid the Deep Dives and Side Trips.

WHAT EXACTLY ARE MUSCLES?

Anatomy. Each skeletal muscle, out of a grand total of about seven hundred (depending on how you count them), consists of a bundle of long fibers running parallel to the long axis of the muscle. In figure 5.1 you can see the entire muscle on the left, eventually terminating in the slender tendon that connects it to bone. The next tube to the right is a group of individual single

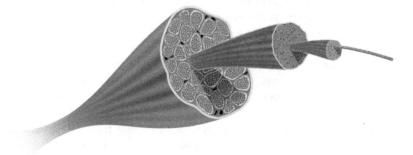

Figure 5.1. A single muscle cell, aka a myofiber. It is made up of myofibril bundles. The all-important mitochondria are scattered throughout the cell. The sarcolemma is just the membrane enclosing the whole muscle cell. © iStock / Aldona.

cells that act together. Continuing to the right is the single cell, often called a muscle fiber, or **myofiber**. Finally, inside each cell, the hairlike structure at the right side of the figure is the cable-like bundle of the **myofibril** containing the muscle proteins. These proteins do the work of contracting your muscles. When you send a message through a nerve telling a muscle to contract, two different proteins grab on to each other and shorten—thus contracting—all or part of the muscle. Imagine a line dance: everyone holding outstretched hands, then pulling their partners close. The line shortens like the muscle contracts.

When you use your muscles, forcing them to contract, the muscle cell experiences some stress, mainly due to the release of **free radicals** by the mitochondria, which are active during cellular work. This is a great example of the idea that some stress is good, in that this transient exposure to **oxidation** (a potentially damaging state due to reactive oxygen molecules, defined in chapter 3) triggers the body's defense and repair systems, resulting in muscle repair and growth.

One last point on these myofibers, the cells that make up our muscles: each one is built from the fusion of many precursor or **stem cells**, called **satellite cells** in muscle. Satellite cells tend to sit next to the blood vessel for the muscle, putting them in an optimal position to respond to signals from both the muscle itself and from events in the entire body. Satellite cells are activated by normal triggers, such as exercise, and by pathological conditions, such as injury and degenerative diseases. As you grew bigger during childhood, or gained muscle mass by working out, or recovered from injury, dormant satellite cells were activated and grew, eventually fusing, to produce new muscle cells. (The stem cells also make more of themselves when they are activated, so you always have some around.) Fused cells means that each cell has many nuclei, where the chromosomes are located, which means that the processes regulated by the genes there happen more readily. These muscle cells are called **terminally differentiated**; this means that they won't divide to produce more of themselves—we only get replacements from activated satellite cells. Satellite cells, like all stem cells, can produce more of themselves as well as the specialized cells that they regenerate. Sadly, satellite cell numbers diminish with age, falling from 8 percent of total muscle cell number in young adults to less than 1 percent after about seventy years of age. Someday stem cell therapies may be able to regenerate them.

WHAT HAPPENS IN MUSCLES AS WE AGE?

Aging causes a lot of physical changes in our bodies, but muscle loss is ubiquitous and potentially the cause of the most widespread damage as it results in frequent injuries of the elderly due to falls. As we get older, some muscle cells are inevitably lost, or, as implied above, simply not repaired. Without use, remaining muscles shrink, resulting in the loss of lean body mass and concomitant loss of strength, which gerontologists call **sarcopenia**.

During our youth, muscle mass and strength track together. Put another way, bigger muscles equal stronger muscles. With age, however, muscle mass and strength are not so closely linked. Although not many studies have looked specifically at this issue, here are some interesting findings. When muscle mass was estimated (I describe some of the methods for doing this in the box below), the strength/mass ratio declined dramatically with aging. In other words, as we age, we lose more strength than you would expect based on the amount of muscle you have. The implication of these studies is profound: the effects of aging on muscle are more complex than simple atrophy, and the aging effect is greater for strength than for the amount or mass of muscle present. No one knows exactly why, but some of the information I present in this chapter will give you some clues.[3]

Part of the muscle loss of sarcopenia is due to replacement of muscle tissue by fat and connective tissue (e.g., collagen). You probably have noticed this loss when looking at the hands of elderly people, which become thin and bony, with deepened spaces between the bones where muscle has not been replaced by much. In general, leg muscles atrophy more than upper body muscles. This may be due to arms being used more frequently in most people for day-to-day activities. A muscle such as the diaphragm, which remains active throughout life as we breathe, undergoes little change with aging. Given that muscle mass accounts for up to 60 percent of body mass, loss of this important metabolically active tissue can have profound consequences.

For most of us, the decline in skeletal muscle mass also contributes to the increase in the percent of body weight coming from fat, simply because we have less muscle in the total. This raises an important but somewhat obscure point: How is body composition measured? Ideally, we would like a perfect measurement of the amount of overall adiposity (i.e., fat), fat distribution (including visceral fat, which surrounds our internal organs, and fat infiltration into the muscle) and skeletal muscle. Then we could look at how all of these factors change with age. Unfortunately, all of the commonly used measures have some drawbacks, as I describe next.

A Deep Dive into Body Composition Measurement

Let's visit the various ways to determine body composition: the percentages of lean (i.e., muscle) and fat mass. First are the so-called **anthropometric measures** such as BMI (body weight, in kg, divided by body height, in meters, squared). But any simple measurement (e.g., weight or circumference—waist, arm, and calf have been used) is confounded by fat and doesn't correlate well with overall muscle mass because fat can ooze into muscle in unpredictable amounts.

The **bioelectrical impedance method** is based on the fact that body water (containing electrolytes) is a good conductor whereas fat tissue is not. Measurements are easy and noninvasive with the appropriate device, but muscle mass can't be measured directly; instead, it's estimated. The accuracy of the device depends on how much of the body is directly assessed: simply standing on scales sold for this purpose, which sends a current up one leg and down the other, is not very accurate.

Densitometry measures include underwater weighing and air displacement (a technique popularized by a product called the BodPod). All of these measures use weight to estimate body mass (no, not the same), and your body volume is then measured by displacement. As density equals mass/volume, then the proportion of fat and nonfat can be estimated. But because mass and weight differ, the estimate is just that.

Dual-Energy X-Ray Absorptiometry (DEXA) assesses bone, fat, and lean tissue. DEXA is often called the gold standard for body composition assessment. DEXA measures bone directly, then muscle and fat mass are calculated from formulas. This measure will be familiar to those of us struggling with loss of bone density—more on this in the next chapter.

Computed Tomography (CT) uses X-ray to make a series of cross-sectional images of the body from which tissue areas can be assessed. The estimate of muscle density using CT includes the fat both within the muscle and surrounding it. Thus, CT is the only method that can determine how much muscle is lost over time due to the gradual infiltration of fat. Because a large number of adjacent X-rays are used to create the image, the radiation dose can be the equivalent of hundreds of chest X-rays, making this test potentially less desirable.

Magnetic Resonance Imaging (MRI) can measure the composition of tissue, including its lipid content. A main advantage of MRI over CT is the lack of radiation exposure. This technique, like CT scans, is typically ordered by a physician and is pricey.

DEXA and CT studies estimate that the decline in skeletal muscle is less than 1 percent each year (to be exact, 0.64–1.29 percent per year for men, and 0.53–0.84 percent per year for women, over sixty years of age). Though these percentages seem low, they add up: averaging to 14 percent loss by the mid-sixties and 50 percent above age eighty. For specific muscles, the extent of mass loss may reach 20–30 percent for the limb muscles and up to 40 percent for the trunk muscles after age seventy. These numbers are staggering when you compare that loss to what we start with in our twenties.

Balance and Posture. Balance and posture are two critical functions that depend on working muscles. Balance is your ability to stand steadily, and posture is how your body parts line up properly in relation to one another. The falls and subsequent injuries that injure many in the aging population are a direct result of loss of these functions.

Sensors in muscles and **tendons** (which connect muscles to the bones they move) monitor activity. The sensors send that information to the brain. Our brains have presets as to how much contraction every muscle should maintain. Any deviation from that is a stretch, which requires an adjustment. The brain then sends instructions to the muscles to maintain balance, posture, and integrate movement.

A Deep Dive into Stretch Receptors

Specialized nerve fibers embedded in a unique region of your voluntary muscles, called the spindle, can detect stretch. A second region, the Golgi tendon organ, lies in the tendon that connects the muscle to the bone it pulls on. If the muscle is stretched, a signal is sent to the spinal cord, which, in turn, conveys it to the brain. In an example of a simple reflex, the spinal cord immediately sends a signal back to the muscle, telling the muscle to contract, to counteract the stretch. This keeps you in balance.

This back-and-forth between brain and muscle lets you respond to a changing environment to maintain balance and position. This control falls off with age for three reasons: first, the sensory feedback declines; second, reduction in muscle mass means fewer sensors in the muscles; and third, the brain is slowing down. So, as we age, we rely on visual information about the environment for balance, but our eyes get worse with age, too. As a result, postural sway increases with age, an effect seen more in women than in men. Finally, because fast-twitch fibers are lost disproportionately (more on this below), the ability to respond quickly to a challenge to balance means older adults fall more easily—an observation we are all too familiar with.[4]

Vascular System. One final contributor to sarcopenia comes from the age-related changes in the vascular system that I described in the previous chapter. It's happening here, too. The density of blood vessel capillaries in the muscles diminishes as we age, but our muscles still need the same amount of oxygen to contract. The cells that don't get enough oxygen and other nutrients are eventually lost.

WHAT IS THE ROLE OF EXERCISE
IN MINIMIZING SARCOPENIA?

Exercise. Exercise may be the best antiaging "drug" in your cabinet. Keeping the muscles active minimizes both loss of muscle mass and strength. You've heard the phrase, "Use it or lose it." This applies with interest to muscles. If you are less active, as are many residents of developed countries, particularly as they age, muscle cells aren't used, and thus don't initiate the process of repairing and rebuilding.

Keeping in mind that as the muscle cells don't divide to make more of themselves, our best option is to maintain the ones that we have. Given that we inevitably lose some, exercise will cause **hypertrophy** of existing fibers. In other words, the individual cells can get larger and thus stronger. This process requires building new proteins, so the building blocks of protein, amino acids, must be present in the diet. More on this later in this chapter.

Intense muscular workouts cause damage to the myofibrils, especially in areas where the protein filaments overlap, but the exact nature of this damage is not known. Yes, exercise damages the muscle cells, but they respond by fixing themselves and growing. When our muscles are young, new cells are produced during growth and repair processes when satellite cells are activated. As we age, we have fewer satellite cells (they've been used up over the years), and the ones that remain are less responsive to the signals that damaged muscle tissue send out. In both young and old muscle, the repair process requires time; resting after workouts is important.

Endurance and Power. Let's start talking about muscles by clarifying a few terms. First, **strength** refers to your maximum capacity to do some physical work, in the short term. You might be able to lift a fifty-pound box or weight easily whereas I may max out at twenty-five pounds. Endurance is the ability to do some physical work repeatedly over a longer period. To further complicate the discussion, we can talk about endurance itself in the short term. An example of this is doing a lot of repetitions of a strength-training exercise such as bench press or squat in the gym. Alternatively, endurance is probably more typically defined as long-term activity such as running or bicycling. I will come back to these two types of activities below.

A Deep Dive into Muscle Type

As you lose muscle mass, you lose strength but not necessarily endurance. Aging athletes are often better at endurance events, rather than events where bursts of speed or power are required. Endurance is more easily maintained with age because you lose fewer **type I muscle fibers** with age. Fibers are simply bundles of cells that work together as a unit. You can see these in figure 5.1. Type I—aka "slow-twitch"—muscle fibers fatigue more slowly than the "fast-twitch" **type II fibers**. Type I fibers provide muscle endurance. The slow-twitch type I muscle fibers have more mitochondria; and although they are smaller than the fast-twitch fibers, they get their oxygen and nutrients from a larger capillary bed. This combination explains their greater capacity for **aerobic metabolism** (i.e., they can continue to receive and use oxygen while they are working) and fatigue resistance, resulting in better endurance. The type I fibers produce less force compared to type II fibers, but they are able to maintain longer-term contractions, which accounts for their role in balance and postural control. These so-called slow-twitch fibers can hold a contraction longer (i.e., they fatigue more slowly) because they rely on aerobic metabolism, which uses mitochondria, to generate more energy. Fast-twitch type II muscles have a different metabolic system for using energy and, consequently, are much better at generating short bursts of strength or speed than slow-twitch muscles. But they run out of the oxygen and nutrients that fuel their contractions, and fatigue more quickly.

The fast-twitch, type II muscle fibers are further divided: type IIb produce the most force but fatigue extremely rapidly because they rely on **anaerobic metabolism** (i.e., not using oxygen or mitochondria, thus extracting only a fraction of the available energy from the fuel source); and type IIa are intermediate between the slow-twitch type I and true fast-twitch IIb. The type II fibers have fewer mitochondria and capillaries compared to slow-twitch fibers and fail faster. On the other hand, these larger-sized fibers are able to produce more force faster, an important consideration for power activities and rapid responses.

Just a few more words on muscle physiology: the slow fibers are the easiest to get going because they use the least energy, and our brains (which control every muscular contraction) are inherently stingy with energy costs. If you are lifting light weights, these type I fibers get called out first. Increasing the load on a muscle results in "orderly recruitment" such that the next most efficient fibers (type IIa) get called on next, and finally, the IIb. So, to maintain the fast fibers, which are the first to be lost with age, you have to work the muscle hard. So-called high intensity workouts do this effectively but clearly must be done with caution so as to avoid excessive damage (i.e., injury).[5]

Overview. To step back for a brief overview, the age-related decrease in muscle mass and strength we call sarcopenia is mainly caused by atrophy (i.e., shrinkage and eventual loss) of muscle fibers, especially the so-called fast-twitch fibers responsible for short-term maximal work (for the interested, specifically the type IIa). Much of the atrophy comes about because of a decline in protein synthesis, which I will tell you more about later in this chapter.

And, once the muscle fibers are lost, fatty tissue can barge in and replace it. More on this follows.[6]

Nervous Control of Muscles. Finally, to complete the mini-course in muscle physiology, we need to introduce the **motor unit**. This is a group of fibers of the same type, sharing a single nerve, the **motor neuron**, which is the control mechanism that tells the unit to contract. The fibers within this unit are typically spread throughout the body of a muscle. You can see two such motor units in figure 5.2, which illustrates how a single nerve fiber (aka neuron) branches to contact multiple fibers.

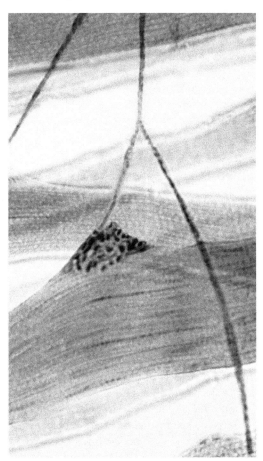

Figure 5.2.   Different nerves control different motor units. The nerves contact the muscle at the neuromuscular junction (NMJ). © Photodisc / Ed Reschke.

Slow-twitch units are small, containing about one hundred fibers. Fast-twitch units are much larger, with thousands of fibers per unit. Because the slow-twitch units are smaller, you have a lot more of them in a given muscle. When your brain sends a signal to a given unit, all the fibers in it will contract, at the same rate, with full force. The slow-twitch motor units are controlled by the smallest motor neurons. It turns out that the smallest neurons are the easiest to excite. This is another reason why the slow-twitch fibers are recruited first, for low-intensity activity such as standing or moving light weights.

As you start working the muscle harder, fast-twitch motor units will be recruited. To generate more force (e.g., to pick up a heavier load), you will have to recruit more units. As I mentioned above, when you start an exercise set, first the smaller, more-efficient slow-twitch units are called up. As these fatigue, and if they don't get time to recover, then the larger fast-twitch units are called in. So, if you work with a load that is too light, or stop before the fast-twitch fibers are recruited, they won't be worked. Alternatively, if you use a weight that is too heavy (say, 1–2 repetitions), all the motor units are needed just to lift it a few times. Then the fast-twitch units will fail first, and you don't work the intermediate speed fibers.

A Deep Dive into the Nervous Control of Muscle

The loss of type II fibers (aka fast-twitch) is due to several factors, like a lot of aging issues. First, one of many things that deteriorate with age is the number of so-called **neuromuscular junctions (NMJ)**. These are the places where the motor neuron that tells the muscle to contract connects to the muscle cell. The control center of the neuron lives in the spinal cord and sends the activating signal out along a thin fiber that splits into many smaller fibers, each of which ultimately ends in an NMJ.

In geriatric mice, fast-twitch fibers have lost more than twice as many NMJs as their slow-twitch counterparts. The damage in NMJs is complex and affects all of their constituent parts (e.g., the regions outside of as well as inside the muscle). As the muscle tries to repair the NMJ, sprouts from nerves from adjacent slow-twitch fibers connect to the damaged fast-twitch cell (remember, muscles have a lot more slow-twitch units). This sprouting is good, because it maintains control of the motor unit, but it converts the former fast-twitch to a slow-twitch fiber. Further, as motor neurons get older, they aren't as good at sprouting and reconnecting with nearby fibers that have lost their NMJ. Another thing that happens: the small slow-twitch fibers get larger with age, probably because fat infiltrates the fiber to replace muscle cells that are lost. Their increased size means you have less fine control of the unit. Finally, the type I (slow-twitch) fibers have more satellite cells than type II (fast-twitch) fibers. Recall that type I muscle fibers are recruited first, and thus, probably require more satellite cells to repair ongoing damage to muscle fibers. But as we age, the lower number of satellite cells in the fast-twitch fibers means these don't get repaired or replaced.[7]

Unlike mice, we aging humans lose motor neurons, probably because we live so much longer. In both aging rodents and people, fat and collagen (the protein of connective tissues; you'll remember it from chapter 4 as it is prevalent in skin) start creeping into the nerves as well as muscles. Initially, this slows the speed of the signal from the spinal cord to the muscle and eventually kills the motor neuron. If the neuron itself dies, of course the NMJ is lost. Unless the motor unit that was controlled by the defunct NMJ gets a new control from a sprout from a nearby neuron, the motor unit is lost. Several studies have found 25–50 percent loss of motor neurons between the ages of twenty-five and sixty. But this is usually not too noticeable until older ages (i.e., over seventy years) as there is a threshold for most people below which the muscle functions almost as well despite loss of motor units. In other words, you don't really notice that you can't pick up that New York City phone book quite as fast as you used to be able to. It's only when you're seventy and you've lost 50 percent of the motor units and you can't manage to pick it up at all that the loss is obvious. And the amount of loss varies from one muscle to another, with the slow-twitch losing less. Finally, the speed of the commands from the brain and spinal cord that tell the muscle to contract also slows with age.

Why bother telling you about these NMJs and their deterioration with age? It's currently not known whether the changes in the NMJ start the decline of muscle mass and strength (sarcopenia), or if their loss is a consequence. But it is important, because whatever starts the process will determine strategies and interventions aimed at delaying the onset of sarcopenia.[8]

Side Trip: Why Am I Getting More Muscle Cramps and Charley Horses?

Many of us find that as we age, we get annoying or painful muscle cramps, especially in the leg muscles, at night. When a voluntary muscle contracts without conscious control, it is called a spasm. If the spasm lasts for a long time, we call it a cramp. The muscle can actually bulge out and become visible during one of these cramps, which can last anywhere from a few seconds to a quarter of an hour or so, and the cramp can come back repeatedly until it finally relaxes. The cramp may involve a part of a muscle, the entire muscle, or several muscles that usually act together, such as those that flex adjacent fingers.

Researchers found that a rapid burst of activity in the motor neuron causes muscle cramps. By using anesthetic drugs (that block the signal from the nerve), they were able to distinguish between two possible explanations. First, the source of the inappropriate signals to cramping muscles might be motor neurons in the spinal cord. Alternatively, cramps might be due to spontaneous activity in the NMJ (remember, this is the point where the motor neuron contacts the muscle to tell it to contract). Because the drug, which shut down the signal from the nerve in the spinal cord, prevented the cramp, they concluded that some action in the spinal cord is causing these muscle cramps. What is going on? Scientists believe that **hyperexcitability** of the motor neuron produces contraction signals at inappropriate times, such as when you are trying to sleep. In other words, the nerve cell has been overstimulated and, like a tired toddler who gets cranky and irritable, acts up. What causes this? It may be due to fatigue from overexertion, dehydration (which can upset the internal balance of nerve and muscle cells), or some diseases.

If excessive muscle fatigue causes the hyperexcitability, one way to counteract it is by stretching the muscle. Skeletal, or voluntary, muscles have built-in monitors that tell them when the muscle is being stretched, as I described above. Too much stretch can damage a muscle, so these monitors guard against that. They do this by sending a message to the spinal cord, which then sends back a command to resist the stretch. You get a demonstration of this reflex when you are sitting on the table in your doctor's office, and she taps your knee with her hammer.

So how do you stretch a muscle if it intrinsically opposes stretching? Well, your muscles have a second reflex such that when you use one muscle, the opposing muscle (muscles that move the skeleton typically occur in pairs; when one contracts, the opposing muscle has to stretch) is blocked from contracting. So, when you contract one muscle, say the quadriceps on the front of the thigh, the reflex signals the hamstring on the back of the thigh to relax, allowing the hamstring to stretch. This is called "active stretching."

I have also had good luck with rolling the recalcitrant limb, in my case, the calf, on a firm foam roller. As you slowly roll a limb down the cylinder of a roller, the muscles are passively stretched. Much of your body weight presses on the back of the leg, where it contacts the roller. I think this simulates active stretching by unweighting the front of the leg.

Certain rare disorders can also cause the hyperexcitability; these are diagnosed by neurological symptoms. However, you can also affect the activity of your muscles by your hydration or electrolyte levels. This is because the signal between the nerve and the muscle is transmitted by electrolytes. In other words, too little or too much of these things can influence the signal intensity.

Levels of compounds such as calcium, potassium, sodium, can all affect neuromuscular activity. Likewise, hydration will indirectly affect the concentration of these materials—too little water in your blood will make them more concentrated and vice versa.[9]

Why Is All of This Happening? (A Deep Dive)

I gave you the bad news in the form of physiology (i.e., what is happening in and to your muscle cells). We have to go deeper, to the structures and molecules within the cells, to discuss processes that cause the age-related changes in the muscle. A bunch of reasons, sort of interconnected, account for muscle loss. These include inflammation, oxidation damage and related changes in mitochondria, hormonal changes, and programmed cell death (**apoptosis**). More obviously (or maybe not), changes in our behavior can also contribute significantly to muscle loss. Warning: This section gets somewhat technical, so you may want to skim, or skip entirely. You won't need this material to understand and benefit from the final section of my suggestions on how to minimize the sarcopenia process.

Inflammation. As I said in chapter 3, chronic, low-grade inflammation becomes more common as we age (cleverly named "**inflammaging**"). Certain **cytokines** (chemical signals released by the immune system cells that turn on other cells; see list below for more detail) are probably responsible for this so-called sterile inflammation—sterile, because we see no obvious cause such as infection or injury. When inflammation occurs as a response to infection, the cytokines cause tissue damage or death, which rids the body of the infection-causing organism. Sterile inflammation, on the other hand, just damages tissue and contributes to many of the maladaptive effects of aging.

A Deep Dive into the Inflammatory World of Cytokines

TNF-α: Tumor Necrosis Factor alpha is an inflammatory cytokine (i.e., causing inflammation) produced by the first responder immune cells during acute inflammation. It calls out a number of responses in targeted cells, leading to damage or cell death (apoptosis).

IL-1β: Interleukin 1-beta is another inflammatory cytokine produced by white blood cells, which are a subset of immune system cells. This cytokine is involved in a variety of cellular activities, including apoptosis. It also contributes to the pain associated with inflammation.

CRP: C-Reactive Protein is a blood protein whose levels rise in response to inflammation. Its job in the body is to attach to molecules found on the surface of dead or dying cells (and some types of bacteria). This binding then tells the immune system to destroy the cell. Many of us have had our CRP levels measured by blood tests. It's the go-to method for assessing inflammation.

IL-6: Interleukin 6 is an inflammatory cytokine produced by many cells (but first found in white blood cells called leucocytes, hence the name). IL-6 is also produced by fat cells and may be a reason why obese individuals have higher levels of CRP. IL-6 and TNF-α also block some of the tissue repair mechanisms initiated by growth factors such as IGF-1 (insulin-like growth factor, described in previous chapters; more to follow).

As you can see from the rogue's gallery in the cytokine dive, pain and cell death are part of the fallout we can expect from chronic inflammation. So how does this tie in with our aging muscles? By now you might expect high levels of these inflammatory cytokines, such as TNF-α and IL-6, to be associated with reduced muscle strength and mass, physical performance, and loss of mobility as we age. And you're correct: levels of these cytokines tend to increase with age. Muscle is very sensitive to cytokines such as TNF and IL-6, which promote protein breakdown, leading to sarcopenia.[10]

Inflammation is tightly linked to **apoptosis**, another pathway that can produce the cell loss of sarcopenia. Apoptosis is a program for cell suicide. The classic example of apoptosis is the removal of cells in the webbing between the fingers and toes during embryonic development.

During adult life, it can be advantageous to get rid of cells damaged by injury, oxidation damage, or transformation to cancer. Our cytokine friend TNF-α can induce apoptosis in muscle. Then, if too many muscle cells die, the muscle will shrink, contributing to sarcopenia.

Apoptosis and inflammation interact with a third mechanism involved in sarcopenia: **oxidation damage**, introduced in chapter 3. Under optimal conditions, there is a balance among oxidation, antioxidants, and cytokines. But too many free radicals (remember these, too, from chapter 3) coupled with too few cellular antioxidant defenses will cause oxidation damage in muscle, which can cause inflammation and its consequences.

Let's drill down a bit to get at the source of oxidation stress in muscle. Remember that muscles contract, which is a form of work, which requires energy. Where does the energy come from? The **mitochondria** take fuel, primarily in the form of glucose (though they can use other sources such as fats or proteins), and when oxygen is available, use it to generate the energy currency of the cell, **ATP**. As I explained in chapter 3, that oxygen can produce **ROS** (reactive oxygen species, aka free radicals), which in turn can produce oxidation damage. So, you would think that exercise would produce more

ROS than not exercising. However, the more you exercise, the more you train your muscles to turn up production of antioxidant defense systems. In other words, exercise itself is a great antioxidant supplement, probably the best one, as it is specific to your muscles. As I said earlier, exercise is a great example of **hormesis**, the situation where a little stress is a good thing.[11] And the levels of ROS produced during exercise can stimulate the muscle to perform better. That said, there haven't been many studies in older people on the potential benefits of antioxidants. Remember that our defense systems get weaker with age. Some researchers think antioxidants combined with exercise could be beneficial. But there is no agreement on this issue.

Finally, recall that as we lose muscle, something replaces it, and that something is often fat. Fat is a very interesting tissue, not just an inert layer of fat cells. These cells make many hormones as well as the cytokines, specifically IL-6, defined above.

A Deep Dive into the Anabolic Events in Muscle Cells

Muscle itself can make significant quantities of the cytokines described above. When they are produced in the muscle, they are called **myokines**. For example, when you exercise, your muscles release IL-6. Remember, this is a compound that stimulates inflammation. The more and harder you work, the more IL-6 is released, and this is true in spades as we get older. What, you say? Isn't exercise supposed to be good for me? Well, this illustrates the complexity of the inflammation story. When IL-6 is circulating in the blood, it stimulates the release of other compounds that inhibit the cytokines described above, as well as anti-inflammatory cytokines such as IL-10. IL-10 blocks the synthesis of many inflammatory cytokines. This process is a great example of hormesis: a little of a bad thing (the inflammatory IL-6) causes a beneficial result (turn down inflammation).

Muscle produces still more cytokines (remember, these are signals) that tell the muscle to grow and repair itself, and it also sends signals to other body cells. **Anabolism** refers to metabolic actions in the body that produce and maintain cells; the opposite effect (i.e., breakdown) is called **catabolism**. Anabolic compounds known as **growth factors** (more on this below), such as growth hormone (**GH**) and insulin-like growth factor-1 (**IGF-1**), control muscle cell survival, as well as normal growth during our early years. (There is more on this in chapter 3 if you want a refresher.) Most of us are familiar with anabolic steroids, which are growth factors, and are used, often illegally, to promote muscle **hypertrophy** (enlargement) because of their ability to stimulate muscle growth.

Your pituitary, a small gland at the base of the brain, releases growth hormone, which stimulates the liver to produce IGF-1. This, in turn, has many actions in the body, including muscle repair and growth.

In adults, when muscles are challenged or damaged, stem cells are recruited by growth factors and produce new muscle cells. IGF-1, for example, can act on many different targets such as stem cells, myofibers, muscle metabolism, protein synthesis and breakdown, and neuromuscular junctions (NMJs). Although IGF-1 and other growth factors such as growth hormones sound like candidates for reducing muscle loss with aging, the picture is complicated. Weirdly, too much of these factors actually inhibits muscle repair.[12]

Your skeletal muscles also produce growth factors essential to motor neuron survival. Remember, these are the nerve cells that tell the muscle to contract. These cytokines affect neurons differently during specific ages when those nerve cells produce the membrane pores (known as **receptors**) that allow the growth factors entry into the cell. As we age, our motor neurons make less of certain receptors and more of others, which may account for part of the counterintuitive IGF-1 story. In fact, the extent of sarcopenia correlates well with the drop in receptors for nerve growth factor.

Like fat, our muscles are not just passive targets but actively interact with the rest of the body. And this makes sense, given the beneficial effects of muscle on overall health. For example, when you work your muscles (exercise), they release the cytokines I described above, called **myokines**, which affect other muscles, as well as fat, liver, pancreas, bone, heart, immune, and brain cells.

Some of these myokines act on the immune system, helping to keep it active. As we age, the immune system doesn't work as well. Part of the problem is that it is less efficient at cleaning up signals such as inflammatory cytokines. These then accumulate, leading to the inflammaging underlying many age-related disorders. Muscle loss is another unwanted side effect of all this inflammation. Less muscle, less immune system regulation, and more inflammation: a vicious cycle. The way to break the loop is to keep as much muscle mass as possible.

A particularly interesting myokine is myostatin, which has the counterintuitive effect of inhibiting muscle growth. But this makes sense, in that you don't want your muscles to get too big. As in the three bears story, you want your muscles not too big, not too small, but just the right size. So, a dynamic interplay between muscle growth factors and inhibitors such as myostatin keeps muscle size in the appropriate range. Animals that don't produce myostatin (due to a mutation in its gene), or animals treated with drugs that block its effects have significantly larger muscles. The myostatin gene, and its role, were identified from studies of two breeds of cattle that were bred for large size and lean muscle mass. The Belgian Blue and Piedmontese cattle breeds[13] were found to lack myostatin, accounting for their size and musculature. I'll have more to say about myostatin and anabolic compounds below.

Another important myokine is called apelin. Of course, its levels decline with age but are boosted by exercise. Its effects read like a fountain of youth: stimulating production of new mitochondria, facilitating protein synthesis, and helping muscle stem cells to function.[14]

Our skeletal muscles suck up a large proportion of the sugar circulating in the blood. As we lose muscle, blood sugar levels can rise contributing to an age-related risk for type 2 diabetes. Conversely, exercise stabilizes blood sugar levels.[15]

Mitochondria. Recall from the introduction to this chapter that mitochondria are the energy generators for the cell. In young adults, 5–12 percent of the volume of muscle fibers, depending on muscle type (fast-twitch versus slow-twitch), is made up of mitochondria. For reasons that are not understood, the number of these organelles declines as muscle cells age.

Actively working muscles use mitochondria extensively. This means there is more opportunity for releasing the damaging ROS (reactive oxygen species, or free radicals). But it turns out that mitochondria release more of the damaging ROS when they are idle. When mitochondria are processing fuel at a high rate during exercise, antioxidant defense systems are turned on. Endurance exercise will also cause the muscle cells to produce more mitochondria and activate the systems that repair and replace them. Of course, this counters the age-related loss of these vital organelles, which in turn, counters muscle loss.

As mitochondria are damaged with age, they become "leaky," and some of their membrane material escapes into the cell, where it can trigger cellular suicide—contributing to muscle atrophy and sarcopenia. Ironically, mitochondria in older cells often lose this suicide pill, which further increases the damage to aging muscle by stimulating inflammation and oxidation damage.[16]

A Deep Dive into Mitochondrial Aging

Not many studies have looked at what happens to mitochondria specifically as we age. In one, young (twenty-one years) and older (seventy-five years) men were compared before and after aerobic exercise training for twelve weeks. Both groups showed similar increases in muscle mass and the proteins that regulate mitochondrial activities. The younger group did beat out their elders in VO_2 **max**, a measure of how much oxygen you take in while exercising.

When muscle biopsies were compared between young and old active men, a higher rate of muscle cell death was seen in the older muscles. This cell death results in the atrophy characteristic of sarcopenia and was caused by the "leakiness" of the mitochondria. Thus, the suicide signal was higher in the older subjects, but the mechanism that actually kills the mitochondria failed more often. This result suggests a possible fix, which I will discuss below.[17]

Remember the neuromuscular junctions (NMJs) where the nerve connects to muscle to start the contraction? Excessive amounts of ROS can contribute to the degeneration of the NMJ. Oxidation damage by ROS messes up the structure of the proteins that build the NMJ, kind of like bubble gum in your hair. In mice, when the cleanup process that removes damaged mitochondria (a type of **autophagy**, which you may recall from chapter 3) is improved, NMJ loss is reduced.[18]

WHAT TO DO? OR ARE THERE INTERVENTIONS THAT REDUCE OR REVERSE SARCOPENIA?

There are definitely factors in your environment under your control that can reduce muscle loss with aging. I introduced you to the role of exercise above, but just in case you still aren't convinced, I'll give you more evidence showing how it works to protect and retain muscle mass and the many metabolic benefits of lean muscle. What you eat is also important. I'll tell you about several aspects of your diet. First, how much protein and carbohydrate? And second, dietary or caloric restriction (DR and CR). Finally, I'll discuss the evidence for or against other supplements such as hormones and anabolic compounds.

Exercise. Literature on the antiaging benefits of exercise is vast. Virtually all agree that resistance (weight) training can slow and even reverse some of the muscle loss that comes with aging. Because of the changes in muscles described earlier (atrophy, fewer satellite cells, and reduced activity of these stem cells), we can maintain and build strength by augmenting the muscle cells we have. But we can't build new muscle cells like we could when we were young.[19]

Physical activity, or its lack, also impacts the mitochondria. A sedentary lifestyle will decrease the number and efficiency of mitochondria in your muscles, whereas exercise builds and maintains healthy mitochondria. One study of older people in Italy found a striking correlation between levels of a protein involved in shaping the mitochondria and a decrease in muscle mass and force in elderly subjects. Sedentary individuals had lower levels of this protein, but it remained high in the muscles of seniors who had exercised regularly throughout their lives, suggesting a way to assess mitochondrial quality during aging.[20]

We talk about exercise as either endurance (aerobic) or **resistance** (strength) training. Of course, there can be combinations, too. Endurance exercise is characterized by repeated low-force contractions over a relatively long time period (e.g., over twenty minutes). In contrast, strength training involves relatively few high-force contractions (less than 2–4 minutes of total work per muscle group). Studies with different outcomes abound, so the jury is still out on the relative benefits of these types of exercise and how much to do. That said, in order to build, and even maintain, muscle strength and mass, you must do some strength training. And this type of exercise has a slight advantage over endurance training for maintaining the important NMJ, which I discussed at great length a few pages earlier.

A Deep Dive into the Biochemistry of Exercise

Amazingly, these two types of exercise—endurance and resistance—stimulate different biochemical pathways in the muscle. Long-term muscle contractions, which are aerobic (oxygen-using), deplete the glucose reserves of the cell, triggering a series of reactions that result in an increase in production of **PGC-1α** (remember from chapter 3 that this is the chemical signal that initiates repair systems and development of new mitochondria). PGC acts within the muscle cell to counteract its age-related loss and weakness. On the other hand, resistance training, with higher force contractions, starts the cell down an alternative pathway. The result of this path is to increase protein synthesis, eventually increasing muscle mass. From this perspective, both types of exercise are important: endurance for inducing repair and maintenance systems and resistance for preserving muscle mass.[21]

Like everything, PGC-1α levels decline with age, but exercise ramps them up. In both trained and sedentary seventy-one-year-olds who worked out hard on a stationary bicycle, PGC-1α levels jumped. Surprisingly, the sedentary men had twice the increase. These findings clearly show that our aging muscles respond to exercise by increasing mitochondrial function.

Another study of healthy, non-exercising older adults (average age seventy) looked at the genes that were active in their muscles. Initially, they showed a gene-expression profile typical of poor mitochondrial function. But in just six months of resistance training, this profile completely switched to one similar to that seen in young adults. Exercise also improved their muscle function: the older adults were 59 percent weaker than the younger adults before training, and only 38 percent weaker afterward.[22]

Back to Exercise. Aerobic training has been shown to provide benefits for everything from cognitive function to heart health, but strangely, not a lot of studies have focused specifically on muscles. One recent study looked at the difference in motor units (MU, a measure of muscle mass introduced earlier in this chapter) by comparing three groups. The study included young (average

age twenty-five) and two groups of old males (average age sixty-five): inactive and master athletes. These master runners had maintained high levels of running their whole lives. The number of motor units (technically each MU is the muscle fiber and its motor neuron) in a running muscle, in the calf, was similar between the old masters and the young men, while the non-running old men had lost about 30 percent of that muscle. Importantly, when MU in non-running muscles were examined, the old masters were comparable to the inactive men. In other words, use it or lose it.[23]

I have to interject a small caveat. Exercise is not a total fountain of youth. Muscle strength and power do drop off even with consistent training. But you can maintain a higher level of strength and power with exercise. For instance, eighty-year-olds (of both sexes) who worked out with weights had equivalent strength to an untrained group of sixty-year-olds and were four times as strong as untrained individuals of the same age. Not a bad return: a twenty-year gain in terms of muscle retention.[24]

Finally, I want to emphasize that not all exercise is the same. During long-term (usually considered one to several hours) exercise at moderate intensity (e.g., brisk walking; 50–75 percent **VO$_2$ max**, a measure of your maximum aerobic capacity), mitochondria produce a small amount of ROS, which is readily removed by the antioxidant system. Long-term exercise stimulates production of more mitochondria and antioxidants while simultaneously decreasing levels of inflammatory cytokines. During high-intensity (80–100 percent VO$_2$ max; e.g., sprinting or heavy weights), short-term (several minutes to an hour) exercise, many more ROS are produced.

Before you grab the running shoes and head out, recall the idea of hormesis: that is, there is a beneficial amount of any stress such as exercise. Some studies have shown that excessive amounts of endurance training can actually decrease repair and sprouting in motor neurons in old rats. And they ran eight hours a day. Recent findings in people suggest that long bouts of high-intensity aerobic exercise in older individuals (over forty-five years) can be damaging to the heart. So, it may be that resistance rather than endurance exercise is better as we age. Or not. In just one month, mice that ran about four kilometers a day (that's a lot for a mouse) were able to reverse age-related damage to NMJs in the muscles that were exercised. Sadly, for us humans, the loss of motor neurons in the spinal cord does not seem to be prevented by any type of exercise. However, resistance training does cause beneficial changes in muscle and nerve function that can compensate for those losses. This benefit appears to occur because when motor neurons are activated during exercise, they increase production and transport of growth factors that extend their life spans.[25]

You can get more bang for your buck in the resistance workouts by using some tricks. I mentioned high-intensity workouts previously. Another method is blood-flow-restricted exercise. This reduces blood flow to the muscle and restricts the venous return by putting a cuff around the portion of the muscle closest to the heart. This limits oxygen in the muscle and prevents it from getting rid of wastes, thus stressing the muscle. Combining blood flow restriction with low weights increases the rate of muscle protein synthesis and increases muscle mass (hypertrophy). Better still, satellite cell numbers are increased by this type of exercise. This method was pioneered by Dr. Yoshiaki Sato at the University of Tokyo, culminating in the patented KAATSU system, and has since been expanded to include various devices. Although it is generally a safe and effective training regimen because the low weights cause less injury, there have been reports of injuries. As with any exercise program, best to get expert advice and instruction.[26]

Muscle lengthening contraction (**LC**, also known as **eccentric** exercise) similarly causes release of large amounts of ROS. The problems associated with LC start with the stretch response in the muscle cells, which I explained above. In LC, you make your muscle contract (work) while simultaneously asking it to elongate. Try running downhill, or lowering a weight from a bent arm, and you'll feel the eccentric contraction. Some myofibers can't resist the stretch of the LC very well, and their membranes are damaged, stimulating the release of inflammatory cytokines. What's more, the signals produced by these ROS inhibit PGC-1α and the normal spike induced in it by exercise. (Recall that PGC-1α mediates the repair systems of the cell.) This means that LC exercise should be minimized, particularly under heavy load. That said, light loading can be a beneficial rehabilitation method. This is especially true as we get older, and our muscles are more easily injured and thus subject to inflammation.[27]

Alternatives to Exercise. By now you get it that exercise is the best way to combat sarcopenia. What to do if you can't (or won't) exercise regularly? As you probably know by now, many of the benefits of exercise come from the stress it causes to the muscle, which then turns on repair systems. But what if you can stress muscles in other ways? Electrical stimulation is one such way.

Neuromuscular electrical stimulation (**NMES**) applies electric current from surface electrodes to trigger muscle contractions. This technique has been used successfully to stimulate muscle growth in athletes, children, and patients with various diseases. In older individuals (study groups ranged in age from sixty-five to eighty-five), NMES increased strength assessed by various parameters such as muscle force, balance, fiber size, and even satellite cell number.[28]

Low-level electric current has been used to affect nerve activity in brain regions involved in standing and walking. This type of stimulation (called transcranial, meaning directly into the brain) has been shown to improve standing and walking in healthy older adults. In fact, this intervention may benefit both cognitive and motor skills.[29]

Another beneficial factor is "heat stress." Heat is known to stress cells and turn on various repair systems. In mice placed in heated chambers at 40°C, for thirty minutes a day (think mouse saunas), sarcopenia was reduced or even reversed after four weeks. This effect was most pronounced in slow-twitch muscle, which makes sense as these muscles rely more on the oxygen-based metabolism controlled by mitochondria.[30] This effect may explain the reduced mortality seen in Finnish men who frequented saunas regularly. More on this in chapter 9.

How Much Protein? Part of the reason for the age-related muscle loss (sarcopenia), which is the focus of this chapter, is an imbalance between muscle protein synthesis (**MPS**) and breakdown rates (**MPB**). Some of the preceding pages have explained the reasons for decreased MPS and increased degradation. Of course, it's the protein in your muscles, specifically two types called actin and myosin, that do the work of contracting the whole muscle (e.g., a bicep or a tricep). If you don't use your muscle, then synthesis or building (MPS) drops off so much that this factor alone can explain the age-related wasting without any breakdown thrown in.

How do we synthesize muscle protein? The accepted logic is that you have to eat a lot of protein—many people say animal protein—to build muscle. In fact, our bodies can synthesize most **amino acids**—the building blocks of protein—from smaller constituents available in almost all foods. We do need to get some amino acids, called essential amino acids (**EAA**) from dietary sources. Then, inside the muscle cells, genetic instructions are followed for building specific types of muscle fiber (think fast- and slow-twitch). The fibers themselves are built of chains of the actin and myosin proteins (refer back to figure 5.1 to see these).

OK, back to the muscle loss story: in healthy, active individuals, muscles are continually being broken down and rebuilt. This process is called turnover, and it emphasizes the balance between breakdown and synthesis. Turnover doesn't change so much with aging as does the ability to build muscle using protein from food. Physiologists call this inability **anabolic resistance**. The "resistance" to incorporating EAAs into new protein is a major cause of muscle loss due to both aging and physical inactivity. I think of it as your muscle cells getting progressively worse at being able to pull the protein building blocks out of the blood. Growth factors such as IGF-1 facilitate the process of getting the building blocks, whereas cytokines such as IL-6 block it. And remember that IGF-1 is a growth factor whose release is stimulated by high protein and caloric intake. To put it another way: to keep muscle mass as high as possible, we need EAAs from protein in our diets, along with physical activity, and as little breakdown (MPB) as possible.

Let's look at some numbers. If you've fasted overnight, eating fifteen grams of protein (about as much as in two large or three small eggs, or one moderate scoop of protein powder) will double the rate of MPS (muscle protein synthesis). The protein will also decrease the breakdown slightly, about 25–30 percent. Moderate to severe exercise of just about any type will increase MPS substantially and MPB moderately in the fasted state, but eating a high-protein meal after the workout will further increase post-exercise MPS and decrease MPB. Bottom line: eating protein after exercise not only maintains but also helps build the muscle. The optimal timing for eating the protein is not known. Different studies have given different results, but it seems that a window of several hours after exercise is reasonable.

As you age, the anabolic response (i.e., using dietary protein to build muscle mass as described above) to exercise and protein consumption decreases. If physical activity declines also, as it does in many aging adults, muscles waste away noticeably, often replaced by adipose tissue (aka fat). Let me say that again: your ability to build muscle protein (MPS) following amino acid intake declines with age. But we can sidestep this problem by being smart about eating.

First, be aware that larger amounts of protein (more than twenty grams) at each meal can stimulate the synthesis of muscle protein. Remember that age-related decline in MPS? One way around it is simply to eat more protein. But don't stop reading here and start eating more protein because how much you should eat has a sweet spot, and if you eat too much, that might be bad for you in the long run. I'll come back to this point shortly.

Second, eating an easily digestible protein such as whey, a common component of many protein powders, can further stimulate MPS. The most important EAA for jump-starting MPS is **leucine**, though other similar amino acids called branched chain amino acids are also important. These amino acids activate the **mTOR** pathway in the cell, culminating in protein synthesis. I introduced this growth path in chapter 3 and discuss it again in chapters 9 and 10. Some research suggests that leucine supplementation, particularly during or after strenuous workouts, but not before, will stimulate muscle synthesis.

By timing your workouts and your protein intake, you can take advantage of the coupling between muscle loading (use that results in breakdown, MPB) and buildup (MPS). Several studies comparing young (twenty years) and older (fifty years) athletes have shown that exercise before a meal containing more than twenty grams of good quality protein results in a larger proportion of the amino acids being used for MPS. And more good news: resistance exercise (weight training was studied) can enhance the sensitivity of the MPS responses to amino acid for days after the workout.[31]

Finally, you don't really need to start worrying about the anabolic resistance part of the equation before about age fifty. At earlier ages, your muscle cells are still pretty good at grabbing the EAAs out of the blood and using them. But remember the leucine signaling effect? The longer that signal, like a green light for cellular growth, is on, the greater the chances that you may be overstimulating cancer cells. Recent research in mice (where the diet can be controlled in experiments) and humans (where researchers must collect data on large groups over a period of years) shows that too much protein, especially animal protein, earlier in life resulted in big increases in cancer and diabetes later in life.[32] I have to give my typical caveat about these long-term, observational studies in humans: they rely on questionnaires and lump together people of lots of different age groups, so take them with a grain or two of salt.

Nonetheless, the studies in mice and cells growing in the lab are suggestive that high protein intake, while stimulating muscle synthesis, can have long-term deleterious results. So, what is too much protein? Current suggestions are: less for younger people (0.5–0.8 gm/kg of body weight), but higher for older (post-fifty) (.8–1.8 gm/kg of body weight).[33] Note the variability from the studies, so experiment on yourself. And if you engage in a lot of the kind of exercise such as weight training that builds muscle, you will need slightly more.

Translate you say? Well, if you are a 150-pound guy in your forties, sixty grams of protein may be your upper limit. If you're a 115-pound little old lady like me, I should get about the same. Another translation: four ounces of chicken breast (about a cup of chopped meat) gives you about thirty-five grams of protein. Many websites can tell you exactly how much protein is found in any given food.

What about Carbohydrates? A few final words about diet. Recall from earlier chapters the damaging effects of blood sugar (glycation). The same damaging effect occurs in muscle protein (as well as the collagen components of muscles). This damage occurs regardless of age, but as you saw in the preceding section, muscle remodeling is diminished as we age, so the glycated proteins hang around. In rodents and human muscle cells grown in culture, age increases the number of affected proteins. And they don't function like they should, so this will contribute to sarcopenia.[34]

When you cut back on carbs, you reduce glucose levels. This increases mitochondrial activity, which, in turn, increases ROS release. These ROS act as a mild stressor, or hormesis. The ROS signal turns on an adaptive response, namely antioxidant release. Interestingly, taking antioxidant supplements inhibits the ROS signal and prevents the adaptive response. Exercising when your muscles have a low level of stored glucose enhances the adaptations your muscles make to endurance exercise. Things like PGC-1α, mitochondrial enzyme levels, fat burning, and anti-inflammatory compounds all rise as a result.[35]

Of course, hormesis is all about dosage. Too little is bad, too much is bad. So, with respect to carb intake, how low should you go? Everyone is different, so there is no simple answer. Experiment on yourself, monitor how you feel after exercise following different types of meals. Keep a journal. My suggestion? Keep your carb intake, especially processed carbs and simple sugars, as low as you can. Read labels and avoid added sugars.

Caloric or Dietary Restriction (CR). Many studies, in animals and humans, have shown CR to have a beneficial effect. CR, which I described in the introduction and address in great detail in chapter 9, mitigates many aging effects, including muscle loss. In rats, CR virtually eliminated losses in muscle mass, force, and oxygen delivery between young and old rats, in part because the function of the mitochondria of the CR rats was preserved.[36]

How does this work? Remember that the mitochondria, key energy-producing structures essential to muscles, can be damaged as we age. If the cell can't get rid of them, they can release compounds that cause muscle cell death. This, in turn, can cause muscle loss. The process by which the cells get rid of damaged mitochondria, called **mitophagy** (which literally means eating mitochondria), is impaired with age, but this is reversed by CR in rats and humans.[37]

A Deep Dive into CR

If you want to delve a bit deeper, here we go. When you exercise, calcium is released inside the muscle. This is the chemical signal that tells the fibers inside the muscle cell to pull against each other, producing the contraction. Not surprisingly, the cell has built-in monitors, like the carbon monoxide monitors many people have in their homes, to keep track of calcium levels. When calcium levels are high, as during exercise, this sends a signal turning up the PGC-1α system (which I described earlier; briefly, this system supports repair and maintenance). Then, cellular defenses against oxidation damage, inflammation, and other repair systems such as mitophagy are turned on.[38]

If you need another reason to appreciate the wide-ranging effects of CR, here it is. In mice, both exercise and CR had beneficial effects. Exercise acts only on the muscles that are used, but CR affects all the muscles. And only the CR reduced the loss of the motor neurons in the spinal cord.[39]

Hormones. We all know that our sex hormone levels decline as we get older. But does this affect our muscles? The answer is a resounding "Yes." Remember that the female hormones are estrogens and progestins; the male versions are androgens, of which testosterone is the best known. Interestingly, estrogen is produced in the body by modifying testosterone. I'll describe some of the data showing the relationship between these hormones and sarcopenia. Eventually, I'll get around to what to do about it.

In healthy men, testosterone levels drop off at a rate of about 1 percent per year after age thirty. In women, testosterone decreases between twenty and forty-five years of age. In both sexes, but especially in men, the testosterone loss is associated with decreasing muscle mass and strength. This relationship shouldn't surprise us, given that testosterone is the main hormone stimulating protein synthesis in skeletal muscle and promoting muscle repair by satellite cell activation (the muscle stem cells).

Testosterone produces a plethora of effects because it binds to a receptor protein, one of those gates in the cell membrane that takes the hormone inside. Once in the cell, it turns on a bunch of different genes, depending on the cell type where this is happening. In addition to its role in maintaining and repairing muscle, testosterone is involved in sperm production, testicular function, hair growth, bone density, libido, and secondary sexual characteristics. The decline in testosterone levels is correlated with mortality in older men. Sarcopenia leads to skeletal frailty, which is linked to often-fatal falls. Testosterone deficiency is also associated with diabetes and metabolic syndrome. This last is a cluster of conditions that occur together. These conditions include increased blood pressure, high blood sugar, excess body fat around the waist, and abnormal cholesterol or triglyceride levels. When you have three or more of these symptoms, you have an increased risk of heart disease, stroke, and type 2 diabetes.

Recent studies have showed that androgen replacement therapy increases muscle mass in both men and women sixty-five years of age or older, depending on how they received the hormone and how long they took it. Specifically, testosterone causes a dose dependent (the more you take, the bigger the effect) increase in satellite cell number, and in both the number of muscle fibers and their size, though the increase in strength was less striking. But before you run out and beg your doctor for a prescription, be aware that the data on testosterone is a bit spotty. Early studies found a number of adverse side effects, including cardiovascular damage, elevated hemoglobin levels, prostate enlargement, and increased risk of prostate cancer. More recent results, though still mixed, give testosterone a boost in the fight against sarcopenia, especially in light of the fact that testosterone also increases bone mineral density and bone strength.

In aging women, androgen deficiencies are associated with loss of muscle mass, as well as changes in sexual function, cognitive function, emotions, and bone density. After menopause, testosterone drops to about 15 percent of pre-menopause levels; this level can continue to decline in the following years. Thus, there may be a therapeutic role for testosterone replacement among menopausal and postmenopausal women, although blood levels of the hormone should be monitored so that the lowest effective dose of testosterone can be used.

Estrogen levels also drop precipitously at menopause, as I discuss at more length in the following chapter. Estrogen has diverse beneficial effects on muscle: reducing inflammatory responses, combating oxidation damage, activating satellite cells to repair damaged tissue, and increasing satellite cell numbers. Estrogen also has antioxidant effects in muscle cells. Hormone replacement therapy delays age-related muscle loss and accumulation of fat in skeletal muscle. Postmenopausal women who used hormone replacement had a small but consistent increase in muscle strength compared to those not taking the drugs.[40]

A new class of drugs, the selective androgen receptor modulators (SARMs), currently in clinical trials, have been shown to bind to the androgen receptor and act specifically in muscle without adverse effects on the prostate in men or masculinizing effects in women.[41]

Both skeletal muscle and satellite cells contain receptors for both estrogen and androgens. The action of the hormone within these cells (i.e., maintaining or repairing myofibers and activating satellite cells) is mediated by binding the hormone to its receptor. So, it makes sense that hormone replacement therapy (HRT) would increase muscle mass and maintenance. HRT in both sexes has other effects, which I will expand on in chapter 10.

Another effect of HRT emerged from the large MYOAGE study, a nineteen-country study funded by the European Union from 2009 to 2013. Postmenopausal women using HRT showed higher levels of IGF-1, which, you may recall, activates protein synthesis and slows breakdown. Of course, too much IGF-1, like too much of most biologically active substances, can be a bad thing.[42]

The immune system is also affected by these hormones. This is yet another explanation for the sex differences in muscle loss seen with aging. Low levels of estrogen in women correlate with increases in the cytokines described in the sidebar above. Interestingly, cytokines are mainly produced by fat tissue, which increases in many postmenopausal women. Cytokines such as IL-6 decrease the response of muscles to IGF-1, further contributing to sarcopenia.[43]

A final factor contributing to sarcopenia is the programmed cell death called apoptosis. Under some circumstances, apoptosis is beneficial. But, if the regulation of apoptosis goes awry, then maladaptive tissue loss can occur. And it looks like this is going on in our muscles as we age—the thermostat gets turned up on apoptosis both in the myofibers and the satellite cells. Both androgens and estrogens have been shown to regulate apoptosis through different pathways, further emphasizing the importance of these hormones in maintaining muscle through the life span.[44]

Vitamin D. Vitamin D is a strange nutrient, neither fish nor fowl. Technically it's not a vitamin, as all mammals can theoretically synthesize enough of our daily requirement in skin cells (I talked about this earlier in chapter 4) from the action of sunlight on cholesterol. As if that's not confusing enough, the compound that is made in the skin or taken as a supplement (few foods contain it) must then be converted (in the liver and kidneys) to the active form. Although two similar compounds are produced in this way, I'll just call them vitamin D as the technical terms are each about as long as this sentence.

The main role of vitamin D is in maintaining calcium and phosphorus at their optimal levels in the body, and thus it is paramount in healthy bone maintenance. It is also central to normal immune function and cellular actions dependent on calcium and phosphorus. Vitamin D is a steroid hormone much like the androgens and estrogens, acting in a similar way: binding to its receptor and activating genes in the nucleus, thus eliciting different effects in different cell types.

Because motor neurons rely on calcium to translate the contraction signal to their muscle targets, it makes sense that vitamin D would play a role in maintaining muscle as we age. In fact, studies have found a strong correlation between blood levels of vitamin D and muscle strength and physical performance.[45] There doesn't seem to be any down sides to supplementing with a reasonable amount of the vitamin: 1,000–5,000 mg/day, but I do revisit this issue in the next chapter. It's probably not a bad idea to have your vitamin D level checked before buying the larger quantity.

Not surprisingly, vitamin D acts synergistically with other interventions that promote and maintain muscle growth. Resistance exercise and protein supplementation, in combination with vitamin D, increased muscle growth in the elderly.[46]

Growth Hormone and Insulin-Like Growth Factor 1. I introduced you to these acronyms (GH and IGF-1) in chapter 3 in the section on inflammation and discuss them a lot more in chapter 9. Briefly, GH does a lot more besides making you grow as a child. Throughout your life, it regulates cell reproduction/division and repair and, therefore, anabolic or building aspects of metabolism. GH coordinates these actions by causing the release of IGF-1, which is made in the liver. IGF-1 circulates through the body and affects metabolism in virtually all our cells, specifically acting to stimulate anabolic (buildup) pathways. IGF-1 is the primary instigator of muscle repair and growth. Its central role is due to its multifaceted effects: it stimulates satellite cell reproduction and muscle protein synthesis, it inhibits muscle protein breakdown, and inhibits inflammation. In another example of the insidious effect of **inflammaging**, the more inflammatory cyotokines we release as we age, the less IGF-1 we produce.

The levels of both GH and IGF-1 decrease with age in adults, when we also see a decline in the pathways that build and maintain muscles. Daily GH production drops by approximately 15 percent per decade after the age of thirty, with a parallel decline in IGF-1 secretion. Although this drop does contribute to sarcopenia, the decline in these growth factors may actually reduce cancer risk as both GH and IGF-1 are potent stimulators of runaway cell growth, which can lead to cancer.[47]

In a large study of aging adults, lower IGF-1 was associated with the risk of sarcopenia, especially in women. The authors thought this connection was due primarily to the prominent role IGF-1 plays in controlling re-innervation of muscle fibers that have lost their motor neuron connection (the NMJ).[48]

Early trials of GH supplementation gave positive results in terms of increasing muscle (assessed as lean body mass). After longer periods (over a year), negative side effects (joint and muscle pain, edema, carpal tunnel syndrome, and hyperglycemia) emerged. These findings cast doubt on the efficacy of GH for treating sarcopenia. A recent study in rats, which looked more closely at the effects of different doses, found that lower doses did not produce the adverse effects and did result in numerous positive outcomes ranging from increased muscle mass and strength, antioxidant levels, and mitochondrial production.[49] I expect we'll see more human trials soon.

Creatine. This is another substance your body produces that declines with age. Creatine is a compound that you can get from your diet, mainly from meat and fish. The body also produces it, mainly in the liver and kidneys. It is a big player in muscle strength and performance because of its action in muscle cells. Here, it rescues ATP when this essential energy player becomes depleted.

If you want more detail, here it is. Creatine forms a chemical called phosphocreatine, which acts like a battery because it stores something called phosphate. When you work a muscle hard, it burns through its ATP, its energy source, rapidly, often in less than ten seconds. To rebuild the ATP, you need to add phosphate. This is where the creatine comes to the rescue. The phosphocreatine releases a phosphate group and adds it to an ADP (which has two phosphate groups) to form ATP to give you additional power.

Creatine supplementation for sport performance was popularized in the 1992 Olympics when several athletes, in different sports, reported using it to enhance their training. Since then, it has become popular with the general public, both for athletic performance and simply to increase muscle mass. Creatine also has a number of other effects, such as lowering plasma triglyceride (aka fat in the blood) and total cholesterol levels, and a trend toward lower fasting blood glucose levels.

Supplementation typically produces a 10–15 percent increase in strength and a 1–3 percent increase in muscle mass in the first few months of resistance exercise training. The effects of supplementation are typically highest in people with the lowest level of creatine. That said, numerous studies report increases in muscle mass, performance, and metabolic effects in people of all ages supplementing with creatine.

Researchers have tested creatine in doses as high as twenty grams per day in humans with no ill effects. Virtually all of the published research has been done with creatine monohydrate powder dissolved in liquid. The main documented side effect is weight gain, in part because you gain muscle mass.[50] However, increasing creatine in your muscles can cause them to pull water from the rest of your body. If you supplement with creatine, you should be conscious of drinking extra water to prevent dehydration. In a few people, creatine causes nausea and stomach cramps.

PGC-1α. I know, another horrible acronym. The full term is even worse. I introduced this creature in chapter 3 and reintroduced it earlier in this chapter. Because it's easy to forget what these terms mean, basically, it keeps your mitochondria alive and well. And, of course, you know how important that is. Given everything I've said about this compound, you might think that interventions to increase its level in muscle would be a promising avenue for slowing and reversing sarcopenia. Unfortunately, no drugs that stimulate PGC-1α activity specifically in muscle have been found. And too much PGC-1α causes detrimental effects in muscle, heart, and other tissues. A healthy and active lifestyle featuring exercise and good nutrition remains the best option for maximizing your PGC-1α production.[51]

Myokines. What about myostatin? Remember that this myokine (a signal produced by muscle cells whose lack makes those cattle breeds bigger) inhibits muscle growth. Maybe if we could turn it down or off, our muscles could keep growing as we age. This suggestion is not just speculative, as there is a lot of circumstantial evidence that myostatin plays a big role in sarcopenia, most likely by inhibiting the muscle stem cells.

Early studies showed that removing myostatin did increase muscle mass, but it also reduced the aerobic capacity of the muscle by reducing the number and efficacy of mitochondria and cutting the density of the capillary bed supplying the muscle. Well, what if we figured out a way to reverse the negative side effects? Turns out there is such a miracle drug, called AICAR. This drug has been tested in mice and seems to mimic the beneficial effects of exercise in muscles. Now, remember that we are not mice, and that studies on humans have shown some, but not all, overlap with mouse research. So, the good news is that in old mice whose myostatin production is turned off, AICAR does increase PGC-1α and exercise capacity. In the control animals with normal myostatin levels, AICAR did nothing. Bottom line: this is a promising area of research, but nothing may come of it for years.[52]

Parabiosis. Another promising line of research that may not deliver in time for my aging muscles is **parabiosis**. Not exactly a household term, this is a treatment tested in rodents in which the circulatory system of young and old animals is joined. The old animals get the blood of the young ones running through their veins. It may not be a fountain of youth, but close. Geriatric mice and rats look and act younger after a short time.

Significantly for this chapter, parabiosis with young mice enhanced the regeneration of muscle in old partners. The regeneration came from activation of stem cells from the old animals, not those from the younger ones. This suggests that there are signals in young animals that can work on us older individuals to bring our dormant stem cells back online. Lots of research right now. Stay tuned.

WHAT ABOUT MY GENES?

A lot of extremely debilitating diseases are caused by mutations in genes that encode vital components of muscle—for example, the muscular dystrophies. Our knowledge of the genetic control of normal, or enhanced functioning, is much scantier.

The first gene I can tell you about relating to muscle function is called *ACTN3*. This gene codes for a protein called α-actinin-3. Let's just call it ACTN. This protein is found in fast-twitch fibers. Remember, these are the cells that produce fast, powerful contractions in activities such as sprinting and weight lifting. Like many genes, *ACTN3* has several different forms. One form produces a functional ACTN protein, whereas the other, mutant form produces a nonfunctional protein. Amazingly, if you have two copies of the mutant gene, you don't have a disease. This is very different from most of the genetic diseases I referred to above, in which two copies of the mutant gene will give you the disease.

Even more interesting is the fact that about one-fourth of the world's population has two copies of the nonfunctional gene. You've probably heard about this gene, which does contribute to muscle power generation. But unlike what you may have heard, it only contributes a small amount, maybe less than 5 percent. So, it's not a big deal for sprinting or power lifting, as some folks have suggested, unless you are an Olympic athlete where 5 percent can be a big deal. Several studies have found that most sprint or power athletes at that level have one or, more often, two copies of ACTN3. On the other hand, having two copies of the nonfunctional ACTN3 may actually enhance your endurance.[53]

Another gene that I discussed earlier in this chapter is called *MSTN*. Remember that myostatin inhibits muscle growth, so if you have one form of this gene that doesn't do its job as well as the normal inhibitor, you will have bigger, stronger muscles. We all have paired chromosomes, meaning that for each gene, we get two copies that can be the same, or different, from each other. People with two copies of the form associated with lower inhibition will have bigger and stronger muscles than people with one copy, who in turn will have bigger, stronger muscles than those with no copy of that form.

The third gene that has been shown to affect performance is called *ACE*. This gene directs production of an enzyme that, in turn, produces a hormone that influences blood pressure. You may have heard of blood pressure drugs called *ACE* inhibitors. These drugs act by blocking the action of the enzyme. Like many other genes, *ACE* has several variants. One of them, let's call it #1, lowers *ACE* activity. For reasons that are not understood, this variant is found frequently in elite endurance athletes such as distance runners, rowers, and mountaineers. The other form of the *ACE* gene, let's call it #2, increases *ACE* activity and is associated with power and strength performance. *ACE* probably functions in many ways in the body besides its role in maintaining blood pressure and may affect muscle efficiency through mechanisms that have not yet been identified. Interestingly, one adaptation of indigenous peoples living at high altitudes in Ecuador is the #1 form. In a high-altitude environment, this form causes the lungs to work harder to extract oxygen.[54]

CONCLUSION

Lots of things are happening in your muscles as you age—and the process starts way before you notice it. Despite a fantastic amount of research progress in the past decade uncovering the roles of cytokines, hormones, antioxidants, and metabolic compounds, few pharmacologic fixes have emerged. The best options for maintaining muscle mass and function are still the simplest and have the fewest adverse side effects: exercise and caloric restriction. I will revisit these topics, with more details, in chapter 9.

ACRONYMS

ATP: Adenosine triphosphate, the energy carrier used by your cells

BMI: Body mass index

CT: Computerized tomography, an imaging technique

DEXA: Dual-Energy X-Ray Absorptiometry

DR: Dietary restriction (sometimes caloric restriction, CR)

EAA: Essential amino acids

GH: Growth hormone

HRT: Hormone replacement therapy

IGF-1: Insulin-like growth factor-1

IL-6: Interleukin 6, a molecule produced by the immune system causing inflammation

IL-10: Interleukin 10, also produced by the immune system, but turns down inflammation

LC: Muscle lengthening contraction

MPB: Muscle protein breakdown

MPS: Muscle protein synthesis

MRI: Magnetic Resonance Imaging

MU: Motor unit

NMES: Neuromuscular electrical stimulation

NMJ: Neuromuscular junction

PGC-1α: Peroxisome proliferator-activated receptor gamma coactivator 1-alpha, a master switch regulating many energy pathways in the cell

ROS: Reactive oxygen species

SARMs: Selective androgen receptor modulators

TNF-α: Tumor Necrosis Factor alpha, an inflammatory molecule produced by the body

Type I: Often known as slow-twitch fibers, these are aerobic, capable of long contraction

Type II: Often known as fast-twitch fibers, these are mostly anaerobic, exhaust rapidly

VO$_2$ max: Maximal oxygen consumption (V for volume, O$_2$ for oxygen) measures your cardiovascular fitness

6

Skeleton

Your bones provide attachment points for the muscles we talked about in the previous chapter. When a muscle contracts, it pulls the bone it's attached to in the direction of the contraction (figure 6.1). Together, the musculoskeletal system allows us to stand, walk, dance, and so much more. And, like the rest of the body, it is a dynamic system, constantly changing. In this chapter I'll give you an overview of what bones are (their anatomy), how they are maintained (their physiology), what to expect of them during the aging process, and a few suggestions about how to delay or reverse age-related bone loss.

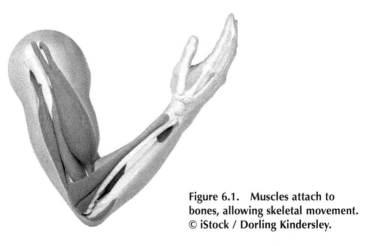

Figure 6.1. Muscles attach to bones, allowing skeletal movement. © iStock / Dorling Kindersley.

OVERVIEW

Your skeleton is made up of 206 bones, though you were born with a few more that fused later in life. And some of us have a few more or less but usually that doesn't cause problems. We call bone an organ because as a living, complex tissue it has many functions. Bones support and protect various organs (think ribs and skull), produce blood cells in the marrow, store calcium and other minerals, provide rigidity and support for the body, and allow motion (as we saw in the previous chapter). Bones come in a variety of shapes and sizes and have a complex internal and external structure. Like the rest of our bodies, bones and their connection points, the joints, are affected by the aging process. As with muscle, these changes can have a significant effect on our quality of life.

Bone is constantly being broken down and rebuilt. In other words, our skeleton is a dynamic environment. This process is like a homeowner who is constantly remodeling the house by tearing out older parts and replacing them. In fact, the process of active bone changes is called remodeling. By constantly monitoring and replacing damaged sections, the repair system of the body can keep our bones in top condition. Bone quality depends on the balance between formation, done by a cell called an **osteoblast**, and bone absorption, done by **osteoclasts**. Throughout our lives, bone resorption and formation are coupled processes. Formation outstrips absorption until late adolescence, equalizes through the twenties, but begins to reverse after our third decade. That means we are losing bone from our thirties on.

WHAT ARE BONES?

Anatomy. Before I tell you more about what happens in that bone-building reversal that starts at thirty, I have to tell you a little about bone anatomy. Your bones are made up of organic tissue (stuff your body makes) and a hard, mineral, inorganic substance made mostly of compounds containing calcium and phosphate. The organic tissue of bone is made up of different types of cells and the materials they produce.

Osteoblasts make other cells called **osteocytes**; together these form the organic bone tissue and build the inorganic parts. **Osteoclasts** break down and reabsorb bone tissue. The exterior surface of your bones is a smooth layer made of flattened osteocytes, kind of like the epidermal cells at the surface of your skin. The center of the bone is a honeycomb of the inorganic stuff, but it also contains marrow, nerves, blood vessels, and organic connective tissue such as cartilage.

The hard outer part of the bone is called **compact** bone. Most of the weight of your skeleton is compact bone. The rigidity of this part of the bone is important, because it doesn't bend and supports our weight and the loads we put on our skeletons. It also protects the softer center portion of bone. Deeper inside the bone we find a spongy type of tissue called **cancellous** bone. This bone is a honeycomb of open spaces interspersed with marrow (where blood cells are produced) and blood vessels. Because this part of the bone is so open, it makes up less than 20 percent of the weight of the skeleton but most of the volume. The relative softness of this part of the bone is important because it provides some elasticity to bones. Yes, although it sounds counterintuitive, it's important for bones to be able to bend slightly; otherwise, they would snap when loaded.

Physiology of Bones. Like other tissues, our bones are constantly being built up and broken down; scientists call this process remodeling. Existing bone is broken down by osteoclasts ("clasts" for short), residue removed by macrophages (clean-up cells), and then new bone built by osteoblasts ("blasts"). About 10 percent of your skeleton is replaced in this way each year. Why, you ask, do our bodies take the time and energy to do this? Well, there are several reasons. First, other parts of the body need calcium, so breaking down bone releases calcium to the blood, where it can travel to the places that need it such as nerve and muscle cells. Second, remodeling repairs damage from everyday stresses. Repeated stress on the bones, such as weight-bearing exercise, causes the bones to thicken at the points where they are loaded. Finally, the size and shape of the skeleton changes over our lifetimes.

The cells we met above (blasts and clasts) are responsible for remodeling. They are influenced by specific signals, which act like volume controls, to enhance or inhibit the process. These cells also release chemicals influencing each other; this ensures local control. For example, reabsorption by osteoclasts is inhibited by a hormone called **calcitonin**. Calcitonin is released from your thyroid gland and attaches to receptors on osteoclasts to turn down their activity. Calcitonin lowers blood calcium and phosphorus through this inhibition, because then the clasts don't break down bone to release these minerals. Osteoblasts are not directly affected by calcitonin; but because the two cell types affect each other's activities, eventually the drop in osteoclast action will decrease osteoblast activity. Then, because hormones typically occur in pairs with opposing effects, **parathyroid hormone**—released by the parathyroid glands—will get turned up to stimulate osteoclasts, which will increase blood calcium levels.

It's important to keep in mind that the balance between the two hormones described above occurs in a perfect world. This relationship is an example of

homeostasis, or balance in the body. As we age, the controls on homeostasis get messed up. One thing that often happens is that the parathyroid gland goes a little crazy. As you now know, this will turn up the bone-absorbing actions of the clasts.

The bone-building activity of blasts is turned up by growth hormone (from the pituitary), some thyroid hormones, and the sex hormones. To make the story even more complicated, vitamin D, parathyroid hormone, and **cytokines** (remember, these are chemicals released by some cells that act on other cells) released by osteocytes also stimulate the blasts. The vitamin D story merits telling, both because of its illustration of homeostasis (your body keeping things stable) and its supposed role in treating **osteoporosis** (excessive bone loss that occurs with age or disease; more on this later).

As you may recall from the previous chapters, vitamin D is really a hormone that acts by entering cells and turning on certain genes—these will vary depending on which cell the vitamin gets into. Some of these genes control absorption of calcium in the gut. Other genes get turned on in bone, kidney, and parathyroid tissues to regulate calcium balance.

You can begin to see how vitamin D contributes to maintaining bone health by promoting calcium absorption from our food, by increasing osteoclast numbers leading to bone reabsorption, by keeping calcium at a level sufficient for bone building, and by controlling other hormone levels such as parathyroid. I will return to this important substance when I introduce actions you can take to promote bone health.

WHAT HAPPENS TO BONE AS WE AGE?

Around the age of thirty, bone absorption starts to surpass bone formation. From this age on, the loss of bony tissue is progressive. Cancellous (spongy) bone loss starts first and consistently outpaces compact bone loss, though that occurs, too. You can see that loss by comparing the two panels in figure 6.2. Imagine what happens when a tree begins to die from the inside out: it looks healthy on the outside but not on the inside. Consequently, it's liable to break in the smallest snowstorm or windstorm. Remember that the cancellous tissue on the inside of the bone provides elasticity. Much of the elasticity of this part of the bone stems from long fibers of collagen. These act much like vertical beams that support tall buildings. This collagen can be disrupted and weakened by **AGEs** (advanced glycation end products; remember how sugars can glob proteins together? If not, see chapter 4). When it's lost, even though the hard outer shell remains, fractures are more likely. Unfortunately, most

HEALTHY BONE   **OSTEOPOROSIS**

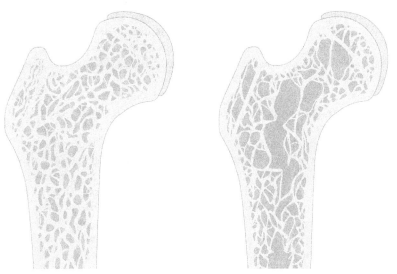

Figure 6.2. Healthy bone and osteoporotic bone. © DigitalVision Vectors / wetcake.

measures of bone density rely on methods that only examine the outer layer of compact bone.

By eighty, men will have lost an average of 27 percent of the less dense cancellous bone, whereas women will have lost an average of 43 percent. A similar disparity in compact bone loss is seen between the sexes. This bone loss in women accelerates greatly at perimenopause and even more after menopause. Although men don't experience a menopause, declining testosterone production can cause bone loss. When bone loss reaches these extreme values, we call it osteoporosis; lesser amounts are termed **osteopenia**. Osteoporosis is a very real condition with serious consequences in terms of higher fracture risk. Osteopenia, on the other hand, simply tells you that you are at risk for possibly developing osteoporosis in the future. Numerous websites discuss the risk factors and treatments for osteoporosis; the National Institutes of Health hosts an excellent one. And the University of Sheffield in the United Kingdom has developed a simple online tool allowing you to estimate your level of bone loss if you have a bone density measurement.[1]

Clearly something is happening in women: in the United States, more than 70 percent of all fractures occur in women, with most of these (90 percent) in white women. Interestingly, African Americans and Hispanics account for only 4 percent each of total fractures, despite comprising almost 30 percent of women. Putting these points together, estrogen seems likely to be involved. And this is absolutely the case, as has been shown in numerous studies of both animals and humans. Testosterone plays a role as well, but to keep things simple, I'll focus on the dominant role of estrogen. This hormone influences bone health in both sexes, but the relative contribution of estrogen in men is uncertain.

So, let's look a little deeper at the cells involved in bone formation and absorption. This process is really crazy, and a little complicated, so bear with me. The osteoblasts (think b—blast—for bone building), along with some other cells, produce a substance, let's call it **RL**, that binds to a **receptor** called **R**. Remember that receptors are kind of like locks embedded in the outer layer of cells. R sticks out of the surface of the blasts. When RL attaches to R, it's like turning a key in a lock, and the osteoblast is activated to release a bunch of different things, including cytokines (remember these cell-activating things from the previous chapter), which tell the osteoclasts to start breaking down bone. Yes, I know it's crazy. The blasts actually tell the clasts to break down bone. But recall from my discussion of physiology that breakdown and buildup are two sides of the homeostasis coin, both occurring simultaneously. The former just gets out of hand with age.

Here's where it gets complicated. The blasts also make something called **OPG** that is kind of a dummy, nonworking version of R. So, when lots of OPG is around, RL attaches to it instead of to R. Then, the blasts don't release the signal telling the clasts to break down bone. The final piece of the story is that estrogen turns down the production of RL by blasts and turns up their manufacture of OPG. So, when estrogen is present, the situation is pretty stable. And this takes place in both men and women, though to a much greater degree in women.[2]

Parathyroid hormone acts in a similar way, by binding to osteoblasts. Once the hormone attaches to the blast cell, it makes more RL and less OPG. This means more RL can attach R, which, as I told you earlier, stimulates clasts to remove bone. Then, you get more bone reabsorption. In some older women, parathyroid hormone levels go up with age. It's not clear how much this affects bone loss. This hormone level might be going up simply because we get less calcium out of our food. Remember, the job of this hormone is to keep blood level of calcium stable.

Blasts also release a hormone called **osteocalcin**. Let's call it **OSC** for short. OSC turns up blast activity, thereby increasing bone building. OSC also regulates mineral deposits in bone, the stuff that makes your bones hard. Another interesting feature of OSC is that it is released from your bones when you engage in aerobic exercise. This OSC tells the working muscles, in the case of aerobic exercise the slow-twitch variety, to take more nutrients such as glucose and fatty acids out of the blood, so you burn those calories. The OSC also encourages the mitochondria to make more ATP. In a positive feedback loop, OSC causes the release of the inflammatory molecule **IL-6** (which I introduced in the previous chapter). IL-6, in turn, talks to bone, telling it to release more OSC. Of course, OSC production declines with age, and we see decreased endurance. Speculation is that OSC supplements could reverse the age-related decline, but we have no experimental evidence yet.[3]

Finally, **senescent cells** (recall from chapter 3 that these cells can no longer divide and start releasing chemicals that promote inflammation in their vicinity) in your immune system ramp up the activity of osteoclasts. This action, which leads to bone loss, probably aggravates the symptoms of osteoporosis and rheumatoid arthritis.[4]

Back to the bones: A lot of softer cancellous bone is found in the vertebrae, wrist, and hip. Consequently, as we age and lose this bone, we are at increased risk of fractures in all of those areas. Bone loss also accounts for the height decrease commonly seen with increasing age. As much as 1–6 inches (2.5–15 centimeters) can be lost.

As bone contains most of the calcium in the body, increasing bone loss decreases your total calcium level. Because this is a building block of bone, the loss of calcium means it's harder to build new bone. This causes a positive feedback cycle in which bone is lost, causing more bone loss. Eventually we end up with osteoporosis.

WHAT TO DO?

New Measures of Bone Density. The traditional measure of bone density relies on imaging by dual X-ray absorption (DXA; I described this in the previous chapter). DXA can provide an accurate measure of bone mineral density, the amount of the hard, inorganic, rigid material in the bone. Clinicians like this term, but it's simpler to say bone density, so that's how I will refer to this attribute of bone. Although bone density is supposedly the most important factor in determining fracture risk, the elasticity of the inner matrix also contributes to protection from fractures. Consider this statistic: almost two-thirds of older individuals who break bones don't have the low bone density that defines osteoporosis. What's going on? Probably, the changes in bone remodeling in the matrix contribute to this disturbing finding. Other contributing factors include age-related muscle loss (you heard plenty about this in the previous chapter), as well as changes in the nervous system that affect balance and vision. But let's stick with the bone story here.

Until recently, we had no way to measure density of the inner, cancellous bone. Some new methods make this measurement feasible. Combining information from these techniques, such as micro CT scans or high-resolution MRI, could allow a more targeted strategy for treating osteoporotic bone loss.[5]

Calcium. If we could turn back the clock, we could go back to our teen years when bone was being added and do all the right things. Because that's not possible, what can we do later in life? Let's start with the building block of bone. The recommended daily intake (RDI) of calcium for women over fifty is 1,200 mg/day and 1,000 for men. But, as we get older, the digestive system gets worse at absorbing calcium from foods, so the RDI increases to 1,300 mg/day for women and 1,200 for men after age seventy.[6]

These suggestions are not without controversy. A recent review examined more than fifty studies looking at the effects of calcium supplementation on fractures in individuals over the age of fifty. Amazingly, very few randomized clinical trials look at the efficacy of calcium supplementation. By combining the results from both randomized and other studies, the authors concluded that little evidence shows that calcium intake is correlated with decreased risk of fractures. People taking a high dose of 1,700 mg/day had a small reduction in risk. Before you start taking these mega-doses of calcium, consider this: the researchers reported that this amount can produce cardiovascular risks and gastrointestinal side effects such as constipation, which cause many people to stop taking the supplements.[7] And remember that although calcium is part of both the outer and inner layer of bone, more is in the outer compact layer, which is less critical in terms of minimizing the fractures that occur with osteoporosis.

Vitamin D. This important micronutrient ensures healthy levels of calcium in your blood by instructing your intestinal cells to absorb calcium from your diet. In addition, vitamin D acts directly on osteoblasts and clasts to direct bone growth and remodeling. Consequently, many scientists and physicians advocate vitamin D supplementation, but a comparison of multiple studies found little agreement. Remember that we can't make our own vitamin D, and most foods don't contain much, if any. The body will synthesize it if you get out in the sun. So, if you never get out in the sun, you might need more vitamin D than suggested here, as it is produced in skin cells exposed to sun.

Maybe it's the combination of calcium and vitamin D that is important to supplement. Well, a recent study that looked at results from thirty-three clinical trials with more than fifty thousand subjects found no significant effect of supplementation on fracture reduction.[8] But these studies that combine results have some statistical problems, which I discussed in the introduction, and I use caution in interpreting them.

Unfortunately, experts can't agree on what the blood level of the vitamin should be. The National Institute for Medicine recently suggested a level of 20 ng/ml for the active form of the vitamin in the blood. This was based on studies showing an elevated risk of fracture in (white) women and men with levels less than that. If that sounds reasonable to you, then the dietary guidelines from the Food and Nutrition Board at the Institute of Medicine of The National Academies (a very prestigious group of scientists) may be appropriate: a minimum of 600 IU (i.e., international units) vitamin D for adults 51–70 years of age, and 1,800 IU for adults seventy-one years of age and older is recommended.

In a recent presentation at the meeting of the Endocrine Society, a new and more accurate method of measuring vitamin D in the blood showed that in postmenopausal women, the supplementation required to get to 20 ng/ml in the blood is closer to 400 IU.[9] If you're feeling confused, you're not alone. For many people, a little over-supplementation has no downside. To reach toxic levels, you'd have to take massive amounts for months. This is because all the vitamin D you get from food, pills, and sunlight has to be converted in your body to the active form; of course, your body will try to regulate it closely. That said, in some people the regulation doesn't work well. Too much of the vitamin can result in high blood levels of calcium, which can produce a variety of unpleasant symptoms, such as nausea and vomiting, weakness, and frequent urination.

Hormone Therapy. Both estrogen and progesterone act to prevent bone loss as well as stimulating bone formation, as I described earlier. Studies in both the United States and Europe showed that postmenopausal women taking estrogen, either alone or in combination with progesterone—the combination is typically called hormone replacement therapy, or HRT—had a significant reduction, as much as 50 percent in rate of hip fracture.[10]

Even the Women's Health Initiative (WHI), whose methodology I criticized in chapter 1, confirmed the reduced rate of fractures. The only drawback to the use of estrogen, or HRT, for dealing with the danger of osteoporotic fractures is the necessity to continue taking it proactively. Best-case scenario is to begin shortly after menopause and then keep taking it. Unfortunately, the protective effect of estrogen is lost when its use is discontinued.[11]

Similarly, HRT improved bone density. One major study that showed this was the postmenopausal estrogen/progestin interventions (PEPI) trial, a three-year, randomized clinical trial (remember that these are considered to be the "gold standard" of tests for drug or treatment efficacy). Some 875 healthy women took different combinations of HRT or no drug. All combinations of estrogen and progesterone significantly improved bone density.[12]

Testosterone may also protect against bone loss. One study contrasted standard HRT with estrogen/progesterone plus testosterone. Both treatments decreased bone loss and increased spine and hip bone mineral density. The addition of testosterone further increased hip bone density.[13]

Drug Therapy. I won't get into a discussion of the various drugs (e.g., bis-phosphates such as Fosamax) as these have been marketed for years, and the pros and cons are well known. A new class of drugs, being marketed aggressively by the pharmaceutical industry, has a very different type of action. Because you may be unfamiliar with the term **monoclonal antibody (MA)**, which is what these new drugs (e.g., romosozumab) are, let me explain.

As you may know, one way the immune system can fight foreign invaders is to produce proteins called antibodies. An antibody recognizes a very specific piece of a second molecule. This piece is called an **antigen**. Monoclonal antibodies are produced in a test tube to respond to a known antigen, which the MA will then attach to. This binding blocks the ability of the second molecule to do what it would normally do. When the second molecule is part of a foreign invader, the antibody will inactivate it. In the case of an MA used as a drug, the MA will block the normal activity of some process in the body.

We have many examples of MA as drugs. Typically, they have fewer side effects than older medications that have broader actions. That's good. But the actions of the antigen-containing molecule are not always known, so MA can also have off-target effects. For example, the new osteoporosis MA—romosozumab—may cause a slight increase in heart attacks.[14] Bottom line: if you decide to go the drug route, examine the side effects carefully. If you have a family history increasing your risk to an apparently low-risk side effect, that may be a red flag for you.

Collagen Supplementation. Animal studies of osteoporotic bone loss are tricky because most animals don't go through menopause. But scientists can fake it by removing the ovaries of study rodents. In one study of female rats, supplementation with high-dose **hydrolyzed collagen (HC)**—basically gelatin that's been partially broken down—improved bone weight and strength, even compared to rats that had not had their ovaries removed. I'm always skeptical about the body's ability to absorb oral protein; after all, the acid environment of the stomach breaks down proteins. But in the case of collagen, there are reasons my skepticism seems (mostly) unwarranted. First, hydrolyzed collagen has already been broken down and is more likely to be absorbed, and then used, in bones and joints. Second, animal studies have shown that it is absorbable. The HC was labeled with radioactivity and then fed to rats. In these animals, 15–25 percent of the HC did end up in bones and joints. Although these studies don't tell us much about a relevant dose or duration over which HC should be taken to strengthen bones, the results are promising. And HC is pretty benign stuff to put into your body. (Read the section on HC supplementation for arthritis below.)[15]

Exercise. The use it or lose it rule applies to your bones, too. This means you have to load your skeleton. In other words, to maintain your bones you must do weight-bearing exercises, forcing you to work against gravity. Some examples of weight-bearing exercises include weight training, walking, hiking, jogging, climbing stairs, tennis, and dancing. Examples of exercises that are not weight-bearing are swimming and bicycling.

I'll tell you more about why this happens below, and why it's ever more important as we age, but just to convince you, if you need convincing, here are a few examples. Astronauts lose up to 2 percent of their bone density each month they are in low gravity. On the other extreme, professional tennis players have one-third more bone in the arm that slams the ball than the arm that tosses it into the air.

Physical activity stresses the skeleton for many reasons. Most obviously, muscles are pulling on the bones, and gravity is putting additional load on them. What types of loading lead to increased bone density? First, the load has to be intermittent, like you would experience during walking, running, or weight training. You can't just sit around in a high gravity chamber to build bones.

While you are standing, walking, running, and so forth, your bones are experiencing pulls from the attached muscles that actually deform the shape of the bone somewhat. Remember, the bone has a lot of relatively soft tissue that is somewhat elastic. When bone is loaded and responds by deforming, the cells respond by increasing the bone-building part of the remodeling system. It's still a mystery to scientists as to the exact stimulus that tells the bone cells to build. Of course, too much load or deformation could overload the elastic capacity of a bone, resulting in injury or fracture.[16]

As you exercise, blood flow is increased to exercising muscles, which stimulates your vascular (circulatory) system. And why would this matter for my bone health? First, one unrecognized aspect of the skeleton is the large amount of vascular tissue—blood vessels—there. The blood vessels in bone are necessary for nearly all skeletal functions, including development, general homeostasis (i.e., keeping a steady state), and repair. A large part of your overall blood flow, between 10 percent and 15 percent, goes to your skeleton. Back to the exercise link: loading your bones in weight-bearing exercise stimulates their growth, in part by increasing blood flow. Conversely, unloading (sitting on the couch) decreases your bone mass. And even a few days of unloading decreases the blood flow to bones. Bottom line: exercise maintains bone health in a variety of ways.[17]

Finally, recall the earlier discussion of osteoporosis. Though you may think of this as injury to the skeleton, it's actually a disorder of your metabolism. Consequently, blood flow to your bones can play a big part in the development of this condition. One study, of more than two thousand women sixty-five or older, showed that bone loss correlated with decreased blood flow, especially in the hip. This, and other studies, suggest that interventions that increase the health of the vascular system can help fight osteoporosis. In fact, this may be one way in which vitamin D and hormone replacement act against bone loss.[18]

Recently, researchers have identified another kind of signal to tell your bones that they are being loaded and thus to build themselves up. Studies in sheep and rats have shown that high-frequency, low-magnitude mechanical stimulation (LMMS) improves both the amount of bone and its density. Amazingly, the magnitude of the stimulation—a vibration—doesn't matter; the frequency, or speed, is key. This type of stimulation could be especially beneficial to the frail elderly or individuals recovering from injury or disease because the strains delivered by the machines are much lower than those experienced during exercise. Early clinical trial results using LMMS show promise in both postmenopausal women and disabled children.[19]

Blood flow restriction exercise, which I introduced in the chapter on muscles, has also been shown to increase bone mass, though unfortunately few studies have been done in women.[20]

Role of Diet. Remember that as sarcopenia develops with age, muscle tissue is slowly replaced by fat and fibrous tissue? Well, something similar occurs in bones. Normal marrow tissue is slowly replaced by fat cells as we age. But it's not a simple relationship. Consider this fact: obese people typically have higher bone density (they carry more load on their bones) but are more prone to fractures. No one knows exactly why. One thought is that the stem cells that are the source of new bone tissue can become co-opted by increasing amounts of fat in the marrow where the stem cells are found. Once the bone stem cell transforms to a fat cell, it will never be able to produce more bone.

In mice, where researchers can tweak diet and exercise to look at what happens to bones, here's what they found. First, high-fat diets increased fatty tissue in the marrow, but in short-term studies (less than three months), diet didn't affect either type of bone (compact or cancellous). When some of the mice from each diet were put on running wheels, the amount of fat decreased and bone volume stayed high.

WHAT ARE JOINTS, AND WHAT
HAPPENS TO THEM AS WE AGE?

The joints are articulations, or connections, between bones. They are designed to provide different amounts of movement. Some joints, such as the knee, move smoothly under heavy load while simultaneously allowing large range of motion. Others, such as the sutures connecting the skull bones, don't move at all after they fuse during childhood.

Anatomy. Anatomists classify joints in a bewildering variety of terms. I won't burden you with these; if you're interested, you can read about them on Wikipedia. In this section, I will introduce you to a few that are especially affected by age.

As we age, many of us develop stiffness and pain in the **synovial** joints. These include the knees, wrists, elbows, and hips. This type of joint allows free movement—as opposed to a direct connection of the bones—often through a wide range of motion. A membrane lining the joint surfaces secretes a lubricating fluid called synovial fluid (figure 6.3). As we get older, we make less

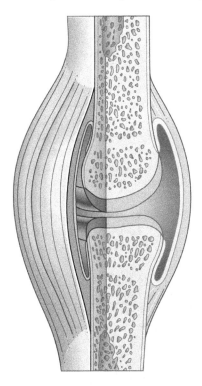

Figure 6.3. The knee, a synovial joint. Note how the fluid (dark layer at bone ends) synovial fluid cushions and protects the surfaces of the two bones meeting there. © iStock / Dorling Kindersley.

synovial fluid. In addition, the membrane can become damaged, as can the articular (moving) surfaces of the bones making up the joint, and the **cartilage** that is also present in the joint. Cartilage is a tough, rubbery tissue that covers bones at joints, as well as building certain structures such as your nose, outer ears, and part of the rib cage. Cartilage, like bone, is produced by cells living in the joint, called **chondrocytes**.

The cartilage—called articular cartilage—that covers the joint surfaces reduces friction and acts as a shock absorber. This cartilage wears down over time, allowing the bones to touch. This doesn't feel good. The ligaments holding the bones in place also wear, like old rubber bands, losing their elasticity. Together, all these changes reduce the range of movement in affected joints.

The spine is also greatly affected by aging. The joints between adjacent processes of the vertebrae are called facet joints. These joints are designed to allow flexion (bending) and extension (straightening and lengthening) and to limit rotation. Each facet joint has a different design, so different parts of the spine have different amounts of mobility.

The spine also has a second type of joint, which you perhaps have never considered as a joint, the discs. The discs, located between adjacent vertebrae, are cushions between the bones, but they also hold the bones together, allowing limited movement. The shock absorption role in the spine is crucial but, unfortunately, the discs degenerate sooner than any other connective tissue in the body, often leading to back pain.

Arthritis. Arthritis simply means inflammation of the joint, although the term can include a variety of joint-related conditions. **Osteoarthritis (OA)** is the most common type of arthritis and the most common cause of disability as we age. OA results in progressive loss of the cartilage in the joint. This process often begins with injury or alignment problems but is aggravated by age. Other risk factors for OA include obesity and genetics. As the population has aged and gotten heavier, the frequency and effects of OA have risen dramatically.[21]

As cartilage is damaged, it becomes the target of inflammation. Remember that inflammation is a normal part of the healing process, but it can get out of control, especially as we age. Damage to cartilage reduces its ability to protect the joint, leading to more damage and further inflammation. This vicious cycle creates a chronic inflammatory condition.

Some of the usual suspects in inflammation are at play in joint damage. AGEs (advanced glycation end-products—remember these from previous chapters) make your cartilage cells more brittle and likely to tear. ROS (reactive oxygen species, ditto) inhibit growth signals and augment messages from the surroundings that tear down cartilage. Lower levels of GH (growth hormone) further decrease the ability of the cartilage cells to repair themselves. So, you end up with fewer healthy chondrocytes and more senescent cells. And these bad guys, of course, contribute to more inflammation, completing the vicious cycle of joint deterioration.

The obvious symptom is joint pain, which can be confirmed diagnostically (though probably unnecessarily) by X-ray. OA is the most common reason for joint replacement, and we all know people who have had this surgery, or have experienced it ourselves. There are other options; read on.

Disc Degeneration. After forty, more than 60 percent of us show evidence of disc degeneration, though not everyone feels it. Briefly, each disc is made of a tough outer fibrous rim, surrounding the gooey center, kind of like a jelly donut. The gel is the shock absorber. In addition, it is also a pressure equalizer. Think about lifting a box to your right side. Your spine will experience an unequal load, but the gel in the disc will ooze from that side to the other, equalizing the weight distribution. As we age, this gel dehydrates, causing the disc to shrink. You have surely seen the extreme end result of this process, which, if uncorrected, causes the extreme curvature of the upper spine called a dowager's hump.

Not only does disk shrinkage cause us to lose height, but it also makes the disc drier, thinner, and more delicate. This increases the risk of tearing and consequent herniation. Herniation just means that the outer portion of the disk has a tear, and the jelly in the middle bulges out. This leak can put pressure on nearby nerves, causing pain or numbness in the affected arm or leg. However, not everyone with a herniated disk suffers these symptoms.

The pressure can cause pain, as does the inflammation caused by leakage of the gel from the center of the disc. Remember that inflammation is the body's response to injury, but it can also cause pain due to the swelling that is produced by increased blood flow to the injured area and the release of cytokines (which I described in detail in the previous chapter).

At the same time, bony outgrowths called **osteophytes** can grow on the vertebrae. When osteophytes develop on the articulating surfaces of joints, the smooth, articular cartilage becomes bumpy and ridged. The cartilage also thickens and loses its elasticity. All of these changes contribute to the loss of normal flexion and extension of the lower back, further accenting a stooped posture. This affects the neck, as you jut your head forward and tilt it up to see normally. Finally, all of these changes affect the center of gravity, slowing your gait, which also becomes shorter, more cautious, and wider.

WHAT TO DO?

Presently, the FDA has not approved therapies to treat the underlying disease process of OA. Consequently, many people suffer the symptoms until they finally have the joint replaced when the damage has become severe. Nonsteroidal anti-inflammatory drugs (NSAIDs such as ibuprofen) or injections (see below) can reduce pain and alleviate stiffness, but these options don't change the progression of the disease.

Collagen Supplementation. Because collagen is a big component of cartilage as well as bone, maybe oral HC could alleviate osteoarthritis. A small randomized clinical trial (thirty people 35–65 years of age with severe knee pain) showed that taking 5 gm of HC twice a day for thirteen weeks significantly reduced knee pain. The researchers used both bovine (cow) and pig-derived collagen; they were equally effective. Importantly, the study also looked at blood levels of various indexes such as blood sugar, cholesterol, and so forth, and found that taking HC did not affect any of these.[22]

Steroid Injections. **Steroids** are a class of drugs with a variety of applications, including anti-inflammatory effects, thus their use in treating OA. Although they relieve symptoms, long-term use is associated with a lot of deleterious side effects and can actually damage the tissues they are used to treat.

HA Injections. **Hyaluronic acid (HA)** is nature's lubricant. HA is the major lubricating compound in synovial joint fluid, where it also helps to hold the fluid in place by thickening it. It is also an important part of cartilage, because it helps the tissue stay elastic by holding water. As we age, we lose HA in joints and cartilage. One therapy to reverse this is the injection of HA-based compounds (often called viscosupplements). But do they work?

A large review of numerous clinical trials found that HA produced significant improvements in pain, function, and stiffness, lasting up to four months. Although most trials accept people of different ages, it seems that older individuals (over sixty-five years) responded similarly. And different formulations of HA (from different manufacturers) performed equally well.[23]

Stem Cells. More and more people are turning to stem cell injections for OA. Although long-term results are lacking, many studies have shown that in the short term this treatment works pretty well for OA of hip and knee.[24] In mice, stem cells even reverse osteoporosis.[25]

Before we get into the treatments, let's talk more specifically about just what stem cells are and what they can do. Imagine a ball at the top of a pointy mountain. It can roll down and end up anywhere. The stem cells in an embryo are like that ball—they can end up anywhere in the body and then give rise to all of our adult cell types. Because most of these embryonic stem cells are obtained from aborted fetuses, their use is restricted by law in the United States.

But our adult bodies have stem cells, too, just not as many and not as amazingly versatile as those from an embryo. Whenever you have an injury, or even when you finish a hard workout, damaged tissue has to be repaired. Stem cells come to your rescue. As we get older, we just have fewer of them, and they don't work as well. As we all know, kids heal faster than adults.[26]

You probably don't have to think too hard to recall a time you've injured yourself. I fall pretty often, running down steep trails, but, fortunately, my worst outcomes have been bruises or skinned knees. Those cuts and abrasions send a signal to your blood calling for help. The first step is to get more blood flow there. This brings immune cells to pick off any bacteria that may have sneaked in. The immune cells also signal local stem cells to get to work. They begin dividing to make more cells to fill in the holes. Then, the stem cells also release "growth factors" that take off the brakes on cell division and activate more stem cells. In just a day or so, these little cell factories have scabbed over the scrapes and grown new skin.

So, these things sound like magic, right? Who wouldn't sign up to get shot up with these amazing cells to heal all kinds of problems?

Several caveats are in order. First, be aware that injected stem cells come from different sources. Ideally, these would be taken from your body, cultured in a lab, to increase their number, then reinjected into you where needed. (No one yet knows how to infuse stem cells into the blood intravenously with an address on them for delivery to various areas in the body.) Most research studies have used this method, called **autologous** stem cells; "auto-" refers to self. Other sources of stem cells include umbilical cord, placenta, liposuction, or bone marrow donors. All of these are collectively termed **allogeneic** sources, because "allo-" means other (i.e., from someone else). Placental cells are promising, because a placenta has so many of them, but a problem for this and some other sources such as fat is to purify the type (e.g., cartilage-producing) you want.

Studies of stem cell therapy for OA mainly use a type of stem cell called **MSC**, which comes from bone marrow. MSCs are like stealth cells, because they can avoid the attention of the immune system, which would otherwise result in rejection. Thus, allogeneic MSCs may be an alternative to autologous MSCs.[27] Most of the clinics in the United States that inject stem cells for OA use allogeneic MSCs. But it's important to keep in mind that most studies of stem cells in OA have used autologous cells. Interestingly, one recent study that injected allogeneic MSCs into older people found remarkable improvements in physical performance and reductions in inflammation. And I'm talking about overall improvements, not just in a single targeted joint.[28]

MSCs can be purified easily from a bone marrow collection (yes, they put a big long needle into a bone, often your hip, and collect some marrow) and these cells grow rapidly in lab cultures. Although this method is readily adaptable for clinical trials, it is not suited for commercial application as it takes too long and would be prohibitively expensive. MSC from other sources, such as liposuctions, umbilical cord blood, and placenta, all share the ability to evade the immune response. Because allogeneic MSC are easily stored, they have clear value for commercial use. One potential disadvantage is that their long-term effects are not known.

Researchers have found big differences in responses to MSC from different donors and even different bones in the same donor. Other factors that affect the result of stem cell treatment are the material in which they are mixed, the way they are infused, and the number of cells that are infused. Clinical trials are underway to investigate all of these points, but we have no clear-cut answers yet.[29]

Chondrocyte Cells. A similar therapy uses cartilage cells taken from your own joint (i.e., autologous cells). Vericel[30] developed this commercially available treatment, called MACI (for matrix-applied autologous cultured injected **chondrocytes**; these are the cells that produce cartilage). Your surgeon takes a biopsy sample from the damaged cartilage in your knee (this is the only joint the company has a product for) and sends it to the lab, where they grow the cartilage cells (chondrocytes). When they have enough, the cells are layered on a membrane, which is built of pig collagen, and engineered to be the same size as the missing cartilage from your knee. Then you go back to surgery to have the MACI implanted into your knee. This is the first FDA-approved product to grow cells on scaffolds using healthy cartilage tissue from the patient's own knee. A five-year follow-up study showed consistently better results with MACI than from microfracture surgery. **Microfracturing** is a somewhat controversial treatment developed in the 1990s to try to get cartilage to repair itself by drilling tiny holes through the cartilage and into the bone. Although results were mixed, it had a decent success rate in young people. However, the results with MACI are so good that it has replaced microfracture as the most common treatment for cartilage damage in the knee (but see my disclaimer in the note).[31]

Alternative Therapies. Novel treatments are in the R&D pipeline. One targets the so-called **extracellular matrix (ECM)**, which is where the materials in the synovial fluid and cartilage are made. Another focuses on **senescent cells (SCs)**, many of which are found in the damaged cartilage of OA. (If you've forgotten about SCs, you can go back to chapter 3 to refresh your memory.) In mice, it's possible to selectively kill SCs in animals with serious OA and restore a healthy, pain-free joint.[32] Another promising line of research currently in pre-clinical trials shows that by inhibiting or blocking the chemical signals that inflammation produces, the damage of OA can be stopped and even reversed.[33]

But these are in clinical trials now; results and actual treatments will not be available for several years.

Surgery. According to a recent report from Johns Hopkins Medical University, about 500,000 Americans have surgery each year just for low back problems, costing more than $11 billion. So-called structural conditions are the best candidates for surgery. These include nerve damage, spinal tumors or deformity, trauma, and spinal stenosis, a narrowing of the spinal column. Surgery can also treat herniated or "ruptured" disks, but it is often unnecessary. Remember that disc changes occur with age, often causing these "leaks" in the discs. So, many of us have herniated disks with no symptoms at all. And many people with back pain from this type of disc degeneration recover within a few months without surgery.[34]

As I said in chapter 1, I don't address current medical practices, but given the controversial nature of outcomes of back surgeries, I would suggest that anyone considering surgery for degenerative conditions do research and consider the statistics, or rather, lack of them. Many people who have surgery (20–50 percent by various estimates) don't get relief. Conversely, many people who don't have surgery recover on their own. A Canadian expert on back mechanics noted that when he prescribed the same amount of rest to patients as they would have required following a surgical procedure, 95 percent reported relief of their symptoms.[35]

WHAT ABOUT MY GENES?

Genes play an important role in the development, maintenance, and composition of the skeleton, like all of our body parts. Unfortunately, the exact roles of many of these genes have yet to be identified. Numerous studies, both mapping genes for these characteristics of the skeleton and meta-analyses of their results, point to the existence of many genes, each contributing a small effect to bone health. With the continued collaboration between large-scale genome projects such as 23andMe and various national databases (e.g., NCBI, the National Center for Biotechnology Information), I anticipate this hole in our understanding of the genes controlling bone health will start to fill.

That said, we have hints that some alleles (these are the varied forms of a given gene) can contribute to some of the conditions discussed in this chapter. For example, an allele of a collagen gene found much more frequently in Caucasians than Asians may explain some of the higher risk for osteoporosis in the former group. Another risk allele for osteoporosis has been found to affect the activity of osteoblasts (the bone building cells). As scientists learn how these alleles act, they can develop therapies to reduce risk or enhance protection.

Bottom line: All of the physiological systems involved in bone and joint maintenance have genetic controls, in addition to environmental inputs. Variants (i.e., different alleles) in any of the genes influencing the system (e.g., bone building or bone resorption) can result in more or less risk for age-related problems.

CONCLUSION

We have a lot of promising new approaches for bone and joint repair. Unfortunately, maintaining these body parts in a youthful state is more difficult. Diet and exercise are good starts, but even taking these preventive steps won't necessarily protect you from the bone loss of osteoporosis or the joint deterioration of arthritis. The possibility of stem cell rejuvenation is on the horizon. I predict exponential growth of studies and technical advances in the coming decade.

ACRONYMS

AGEs: Advanced glycation end products

CT: Computerized tomography scans, a type of X-ray

DXA: Dual X-ray absorption

ECM: Extracellular matrix

FDA: Federal Food and Drug Administration, which approves all drugs in the United States

GH: Growth hormone

HC: Hydrolyzed collagen

HA: Hyaluronic acid, nature's lubricant

HRT: Hormone replacement therapy

IL-6: An inflammatory molecule

IU: International Unit, a way of measuring doses of vitamins

LMMS: High-frequency, low-magnitude mechanical stimulation

MA: Monoclonal antibody, an immune system molecule that has a single target

MSC: A type of stem cell that comes from bone marrow

MRI: Magnetic resonance imaging, a high-resolution image that shows soft tissue

OA: Osteoarthritis

RL: A substance that binds to a receptor called **R** to activate an osteoblast

OPG: A nonworking version of R that removes RL so it won't activate the osteoblast signal that starts the osteoclasts on their bone-breaking actions

OSC: Osteocalcin turns up blast activity, thereby increasing bone building

SC: Senescent cells

WHI: Women's Health Initiative, a large study of hormone effects on various aspects of women's health

7

Cardiovascular System

Your cardiovascular (CV) system consists of the heart, blood vessels, and about five liters of blood constantly moving through the system. It's a plumbing system with a pump—the heart—about the size of your fist and a bunch of pipes of various sizes. Except the pipes aren't passive tubes, and the pump has a lot of settings. The heart is the hardest-working muscle in the body. Even when you are calmly sitting or even sleeping, it's pumping more than five liters (about five quarts) of blood through the body every minute.

Just as in all of our body's systems, the CV system experiences normal aging. Some of these events include slight slowdown in heart rate, maybe abnormal rhythms to the beats, and loss of some of the muscle of the heart (recall sarcopenia). Many parts of the system stiffen as we get older as the elastic proteins age and are replaced by less stretchy fibrous connective tissue. This replacement causes stiffening of the valves connecting the chambers of the heart and many of the blood vessel walls.

Many of us develop high blood pressure (**hypertension**, defined clinically as a pressure greater than 130/80) as we tick off the years. About eighty-five million Americans are thought to have hypertension. Some increase is due to the stiffening of the artery walls (more on this below), but other factors contribute. For example, a special kind of nerve cell in your blood vessel walls monitors blood pressure and sends that information to the brain. Then, the brain can talk back to the muscles in the wall to change the pressure. Sometimes it's necessary to change the blood pressure—for example, when a part of the body needs more blood flow. These nerve cells lose sensitivity with aging, which can explain our decreased ability to regulate blood pressure. For instance, when you get up suddenly, you may feel dizzy because the pressure in the arteries to the brain doesn't adjust as well as it once did.

A Deep Dive into Blood Pressure

The pressure of the blood pushing against the vessel wall is known as **blood pressure (BP)**. We've all had it measured. BP often changes, as I mentioned in the preceding paragraph. Some hormones, as well as those signals from the brain, affect the rate and strength of heart contractions. Stronger contractions and increased heart rate will increase blood pressure. Blood vessels can also affect blood pressure. When a vessel contracts, the diameter is decreased. This contraction, called vasoconstriction, is controlled by hormones and brain signals, and increases the blood pressure and decreases the blood flow in the constricted region. Think about water going through a pipe. If you use a smaller pipe, less water will get through, but because more is trying to get through, the pressure in the smaller pipe will be higher. The amount of blood in the body also affects blood pressure. A higher blood volume raises blood pressure by increasing the amount of blood pumped by each heartbeat. Finally, thicker, more viscous blood (from dehydration or clotting disorders) can also raise blood pressure.

Other changes in the system, such as **cardiovascular diseases (CVD)**, are pathological and the main cause of serious illness and death in modern society. CVD are diseases involving the heart or blood vessels, or both. They comprise a large group of disorders, including hypertension, coronary heart disease, stroke, and congestive heart failure. CVD has ranked as the number one cause of death in the United States every year since 1900. Nearly twenty-six hundred Americans die of CVD each day—roughly one person every thirty-four seconds. The American Heart Association emphasizes this problem, projecting that, by 2030, 40 percent of U.S. adults will have at least one form of CVD, medical costs of CVD will triple, and these increases will be due to aging of the population.[1]

Below, I will present the mechanisms that underlie many of these age-related pathologies and potential strategies to address the cellular and biochemical causes. I won't address specific pathologies. We have a lot of different CVDs, which can present differently in different people, making their diagnosis and treatment an individual decision. Neither will I discuss the dietary cholesterol/ saturated fat hypothesis. There are plenty of good books and articles on this topic, which is peripheral to the age-related effects I am focusing on.

WHAT IS THE CARDIOVASCULAR
SYSTEM AND WHAT DOES IT DO?

The main job of the cardiovascular system is to transport oxygen, nutrients, hormones, and waste products. These substances are carried in the blood, which, weirdly enough, is a liquid connective tissue. Blood is made up of red blood cells, white blood cells, platelets, and liquid plasma. The CV system also has a protective role. White blood cells, part of your immune system, clean up dead and dying cells and fight pathogens in the blood. Platelets and red blood cells seal wounds to keep pathogens from entering the body and essential fluids from leaking out. The blood also carries antibodies and other compounds produced by the immune system. Finally, the CV system is essential in our ability to maintain a constant internal environment. For example, blood vessels help to stabilize body temperature by controlling the blood flow to the skin. Other factors maintained by active changes in the composition of the blood include its acidity, or pH, and the concentration of various substances such as sugar and oxygen.

Anatomy. We have three major types of blood vessels: **arteries**, **capillaries**, and **veins**. The size of blood vessels determines the amount of blood that moves through the center, called the **lumen**, where the blood flows. Around the lumen is the wall of the vessel, which may be thin in the case of capillaries or very thick in the case of arteries.

If you think about how water flows through pipes, where a bigger diameter means water can move faster, you can get an idea of how blood moves through the vessels. In the big vessels, it moves pretty fast and has more pressure. In the tiny ones, it oozes along with very little oomph. All the vessels are lined with a thin, smooth lining called **endothelium** that keeps blood cells inside of the blood vessels and helps prevent blood from clotting. The endothelium lines the entire circulatory system. We'll revisit the endothelium shortly as it has a major role in the CV system.

Arteries are blood vessels that carry blood away from the heart. Blood carried by arteries is usually saturated with oxygen, having just come from the lungs. Arteries experience the highest blood pressure in the body as blood is being pumped out of the heart by a lot of force. To withstand this pressure, the arterial walls are thicker, more elastic, and more muscular than those of other vessels. The largest arteries, which are closest to the heart, have the most elastic tissue so they can passively stretch and relax with each heartbeat. Smaller arteries have more muscular walls.

The **smooth muscles** here can contract or expand to control how much blood moves through that particular part of the system. This is how the body controls how much blood flows to different parts of the body under different circumstances. For example, after you eat, your intestine requires more blood to move the digested nutrients to the tissues where they will be used or stored. So, the vessels supplying the intestines open up, and a lot of other vessels close down. Smooth muscles are not controlled voluntarily; rather, they respond to nerves from our autonomic (involuntary) nervous system, as well as hormones and other chemical signals.

Arterioles are narrower arteries that branch off from arteries and carry blood to capillaries. They experience lower blood pressures and, consequently, have thinner walls than arteries.

Capillaries are the smallest and thinnest blood vessels in the body and also the most numerous. They infiltrate virtually all tissues of the body and border the edges of the few tissues that don't get a direct blood supply. If you're curious, these tissues are things like the cornea in the eye, some layers in the skin, and connective tissues such as tendons and ligaments. Capillaries connect to arterioles on one end and **venules** on the other. Capillary walls are made of a thin layer of endothelium. This means there is very little separation between the blood and the tissues. The endothelium acts like a filter to keep blood cells inside while allowing liquids, dissolved gases, and other compounds to diffuse into or out of tissues.

The heart, which is the pump responsible for pushing the blood through all those blood vessels, is a sophisticated device. It has two sides. The right side connects to the lungs, where carbon dioxide is dumped out and oxygen picked up. The left side connects to the body. Each side has two chambers, an upper, smaller, receiving area called the **atrium** and a lower, larger, pumping chamber called the **ventricle**.

During one heartbeat, aka a **cardiac cycle**, blood first enters each atrium and some passively flows into its connected ventricle, through a one-way valve. This flow gets the ventricle partially filled. Then, the atria contract, pushing as much blood as possible into the ventricles. This is the LUB of the LUB-DUB sound of a heartbeat. Now, the ventricles are almost full and experience high pressure. Then, they contract and push blood out of the heart and into the arteries. When the ventricles are contracted, and pressure in the heart is maximal, the heart is in **systole**. After the ventricles contract, they relax—this portion of the cycle is called **diastole**—and the passive filling starts again. Remember, these are the two numbers in your blood pressure, which is recorded as systole (higher)/diastole (lower).

The heart generates its own rhythm of beats because of specialized cells, called **pacemaker cells**, that produce electrical signals. If these are damaged, or stop working, an artificial pacemaker can be inserted to take over the job of sending out those signals.

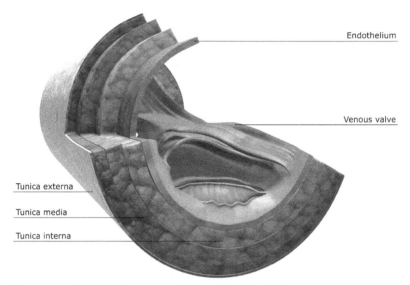

Figure 7.1. **Endothelial structure.** © iStock / MedicalRF.com.

WHAT HAPPENS AS WE AGE?

Heart Aging. Age is the main risk factor for the development of cardiovascular disease (CVD). More than 10 percent of Americans seventy years or older develop heart failure. Heart failure means that the heart isn't pumping as well as it should be and can't supply the cells with enough blood. More than 90 percent of Americans eighty years and older have symptoms of arterial disease, typically narrowing of arteries, which predisposes to CVD. Symptoms include fatigue and shortness of breath and sometimes coughing. The most serious and life-threatening effect of arterial disease is a heart attack, known in the medical jargon as a myocardial infarction (MI), literally meaning death of the heart muscle.

A similar proportion of the elderly develop **atrial fibrillation**: 4 percent of people ages 60–70 years, rising to 10–17 percent in the 80+ elderly.[2] Atrial fibrillation means that the upper chambers (the atria) lose their rhythmic beats and start contracting chaotically and irregularly—out of coordination with the lower ventricles. Symptoms can include heart palpitations (when you feel weird rhythms or skipped beats), shortness of breath, and weakness.

Structurally, the most obvious event that occurs as we age is the increased thickness of the walls of the left ventricle. This is the heart chamber that does the most work, as its job is to pump oxygenated blood to the entire body. The increased thickness, known as **hypertrophy**, means there is less room for blood inside the ventricle, so the heart has to work even harder to maintain delivery to the body. The atria, too, enlarge with age.

Functionally, a few things occur in the heart as we age. First, the filling of the ventricles during diastole, when the atria are contracting, slows down. This means the atria have to work harder, and as a result, they become enlarged. This problem in diastole is worse in people with atrial fibrillations. Problems involving systole, when the ventricles contract, cause a decline in the maximum heart rate and amount of blood pumped out of the ventricle during exercise. This decline can eventually lead to heart failure. In about half of all cases of heart failure, however, there is no systolic dysfunction. This type is called heart failure with **preserved ejection fraction** (**PEF**, because the amount of blood pumped out from the ventricles has not decreased). PEF is especially common in the elderly, and because it is poorly understood, there are no good therapies. Some evidence shows that the endothelial cells lining the vessels of the heart are affected in PEF.[3] More on this below.

Second, we lose pacemaker cells. Because these cells create the regular rhythm of heart beats, their loss can result in heart palpitations, dizziness, and fatigue. Also, typical changes in aging muscle (e.g., replacement of muscle cells with connective tissue, which I discussed in chapter 5) can interrupt the electrical connections among pacemaker cells. Just as in any electrical circuit, if the wiring is disturbed, the circuit will malfunction. The result? Screwy heartbeat patterns called **arrhythmias**, the most common being atrial fibrillations.

If we look at heart cells, the most obvious change in the aging organ is the development of fibrous tissue, a kind of scar tissue. The process is called **fibrosis**. Why do we get this buildup in our hearts? Immune system cells are attracted to damaged tissue. The initial cause of the damage is not well understood. Some recent research has shown that as we age, the cells lining blood vessels release inflammatory cytokines (signals that tell the immune system there has been damage, possibly long-term **oxidation damage**; more on this follows). The first immune cells to arrive attempt repairs. The next wave of immune cells is specialized to produce inflammation, which can be beneficial in some settings, but in the heart and blood vessels, this hinders regeneration and promotes fibrosis. Of course, this latter group of cells comes to predominate as we age, leading to the phenomenon of **inflammaging**, which I discussed earlier. It is now well accepted that this inflammation is one of the mechanisms underlying cardiac conversion of muscle to fibrous tissue. Less muscle means the heart has to work harder, and so it grows, culminating in even more hypertrophy.

Remember from chapter 4 that **collagen** is like a molecular scaffolding outside the cells that helps to hold them in place. Collagen and its sibling, **elastin**, are strong and, especially in the case of elastin, elastic, substances that not only hold cells in place, but also allow them to expand and contract during normal activity. This is obviously important in the case of a tissue such as the heart muscle that expands and contracts with each beat. These beneficial proteins are replaced with not-so-elastic fibrous materials as our hearts age, a process called remodeling. Atrial fibrillation results from fiber deposition in the atria.[4] In people with heart disease, higher blood levels of the types of fibrous proteins found in the heart are good predictors of the seriousness of their cardiac problem.

Another change in hearts of the elderly is deposits of **amyloids**. Amyloids are globs of proteins that have become stuck together. Not surprisingly, when proteins that are normally arranged in a symmetric or other functional shape become clumped, they don't work as they should and may cause problems.

Amyloids form when quality control (QC) systems in cells miss proteins that are the wrong shape. Because proteins are big, complicated things with critical 3-D structure—think Lego architecture—it's easy for mistakes to slip into their assembly. The QC systems are good but miss occasionally. These abnormal proteins can then clump together and form the globs that can interfere with normal cell function. Amyloids are best known for their role in Alzheimer's disease, but they contribute to other pathological conditions, including heart disease.

Amyloid deposits can be found in both the atria and ventricles, although the specific proteins that are clumped vary depending on location. Atrial amyloids are more common and, not surprisingly, contribute to the development of atrial fibrillation.

As you now know, changes in the structure and function of cells and organs ultimately stems from events within cells. Let's tour some of the cellular events in the heart to find the explanation for the pathologies contributing to heart disease.

A Deep Dive into Cardiac and Smooth Muscle Cell Mitochondria

Given the constant activity of our hearts, it's obvious that cardiac cells require a lot of energy, mainly supplied by their **mitochondria**, one of many subcellular structures called **organelles** (introduced in chapter 3). As in other tissues, as our heart cells get older, our mitochondria don't work as well. This decline is due to a number of interrelated factors we've encountered before.

First, we have to go back to **oxidation damage** and **reactive oxygen species (ROS)**. ROS are inevitably produced in the mitochondria because of the way these structures process the fuel from food. Surprisingly, mitochondria are remarkably sensitive to the ROS they produce themselves. Oxidative damage lowers their activity and further increases ROS production. Despite innate defenses against these ROS, over the course of our lifetimes, some mitochondria will be damaged. Unfortunately, the damaged ones can proliferate, and the mitochondrial population of a cell can come to consist of suboptimal mitochondria, much like bad neighborhoods can develop. Not only do the damaged organelles generate less energy, but they also release more ROS and accumulate more damage in a vicious cycle. Finally, the cellular cleanup process of **autophagy** (introduced in chapter 3), which could get rid of the damaged mitochondria, doesn't work as well as we age.

Risk factors for cardiovascular disease, such as hypertension, high cholesterol, diabetes, and cigarette smoking, all contribute to oxidative stress in the vessel walls by increasing ROS production. As ROS levels go up, they inevitably exceed our innate antioxidant defense systems.[5]

ROS can and do damage the DNA of the mitochondria. When smooth muscle cells from human blood vessels (I'll tell you more about these shortly) are mixed with ROS in the lab, their mitochondria develop some of the damages seen in these organelles from people with CV disease. Not only do these cells produce lower levels of ATP, but they are also more likely to suffer large structural changes that result in **cellular senescence** (introduced in chapter 3) and cell death.[6]

If DNA repair is not working, the mitochondria can't fix themselves. Then genes in these critical organelles are altered, not for the better. The result? The proteins these genes produce don't work as they should, and the mitochondria don't produce the energy they would normally.

Calcium Pumping. Mitochondria are not the only structures affected by ROS in the heart tissue. An important protein that can be damaged by ROS in muscles is the calcium pump, which moves calcium molecules around in the muscle cell. The movement of calcium into a muscle cell causes it to contract. An important corollary is that in order for muscles to relax, the calcium must be pumped back out. This pumping takes energy in the form of ATP. Damaged mitochondria produce less ATP, meaning the muscle cells take longer to do that pumping, and, of course, a damaged pump doesn't work as well. Remember that changes in diastole prolong the relaxation phase of the cardiac cycle, making it less efficient. Damage to the calcium pump is a major source of this problem.

Arterial Dysfunction. The main player driving the increase in CVD risk with aging is **arterial dysfunction**. This just means that the ability of the arteries to assess and respond to changing needs in their neighborhood declines. Here's why.

As we get older, our arteries change in two ways that contribute to the risk for CVD. These two events are connected, as you will see in the following section. One is stiffening of the large elastic arteries, especially the aorta and carotid arteries, which supply the head and brain with blood. These arteries are designed to expand as blood is pumped out of the heart and then recoil. This recoil is basically like a compressed spring that passively assists the heart in pushing the blood out to tissues and cells. As the arteries stiffen with aging, pressure in them increases. The left ventricle (the pumping chamber) has to work harder pushing blood into the less-elastic arteries, causing cardiac hypertrophy, which you know is a fancy way of saying the heart becomes enlarged. Finally, tissues in organs with a lot of blood flow (e.g., brain and kidney) are damaged when blood slams into them with additional force.

The second important change with aging is **endothelial dysfunction**. Remember that the endothelium is the layer between the blood in the **lumen** (open space in the middle) of the artery and the outside wall of the artery. This single layer of cells, which you can see in figure 7.2, is a stage where many important events take place. These include movement of oxygen and carbon dioxide into and out of the blood, a similar exchange of nutrient and waste, as well as water and hormones.

Scientists used to think that this layer in the artery acted like a sieve, passively filtering material that was allowed to pass between the blood and the underlying tissues. Now we know that an additional and critical role of the endothelium is to synthesize and release many biologically active molecules that influence the function and health of arteries and the surrounding tissues. Arguably, the most important of these molecules is the gas **nitric oxide (NO)**, which has several actions. First, it causes vessels to dilate (expand). Second, NO has anti-inflammatory effects. Third, it supports cell growth and thus repair of vessels. Finally, NO prevents unwanted clotting. Thus, endothelial dysfunction means the normal, healthy structure and function of this tissue are disturbed. This dysfunction is usually due to reduced production of NO.

Endothelial dysfunction is a main risk factor for **atherosclerosis**, aka "hardening of the arteries," which is a predictor of CVD risk. More specifically, atherosclerosis—*athero* means something soft and gooey, and *sclerosis* means hardening—results from the buildup of **plaque**, a gunky mix of vascular and immune system cells, lipids, cholesterol, calcium, and waste from dead cells. Remember the cellular senescence that damaged mitochondria can cause? That's where some of those dead vascular cells come from. We start gunking up our arteries, and it's the arteries supplying the heart that are especially significant here, early in life. Maybe by the time you're thirty, and definitely in your forties, you have this stuff.

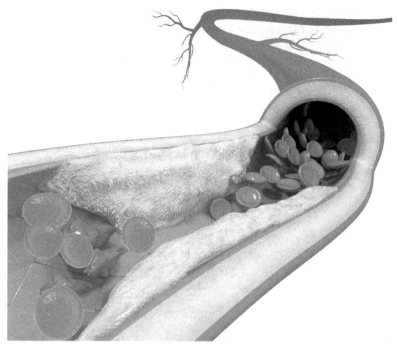

Figure 7.2. Plaque accumulation narrows an artery. © Science Photo Library / PIXOLOGICSTUDIO.

Atherosclerosis technically refers to the deposition of plaque in medium and large arteries. Arteriosclerosis, on the other hand, refers to changes in the medial layer of smaller arteries (you can see this in figure 7.2). However, the two terms are often used interchangeably.

When the endothelium is damaged, say by ROS or inflammation, your immune cells build a kind of scab over the affected area. This is the beginning of plaque. Cholesterol plays an important role here, so we'll come back to plaque and atherosclerosis shortly.

Chronic stress makes the whole process worse. The hormones that our bodies release when in a fight-or-flight situation increase blood pressure and change blood chemistry in ways that increase vessel damage and generate plaque.[7]

Endothelial dysfunction is also a suspect in many of the common diseases of aging, including cognitive impairments, Alzheimer's disease, insulin resistance, and sarcopenia.[8]

Cholesterol. This supposed bad actor also increases with age. People often forget that cholesterol is necessary to life, because it is an essential component of the membrane that surrounds each and every one of our cells. Too much of it, particularly one specific type, the LDL, contributes to CVD. Be forewarned: the relationship between LDL and heart disease is complex and not completely understood. I will just scrape the surface and refer you to more detailed sources if you want to dig deeper.

First a little nomenclature. LDL refers to low-density lipoprotein. No wonder we say LDL. Recall that cholesterol is a lipid. This means that it, like fats, won't dissolve in water. Visualize a salad dressing of oil and vinegar—the watery vinegar won't mix with the fatty oil. The body has to wrap cholesterol, and other fats, in protein wrappers to move them through the watery environment of the blood; these wraps are called lipoproteins.

Before we start talking about its transport, let's consider where the cholesterol comes from. Because it's essential to all animals, just about every one of our cells can make it. This means that you can eat a completely vegan diet, with no animal products, and not suffer a lack of cholesterol. Most of us, however, get some from diet and some we manufacture. Regardless of the source, most of it eventually ends up in the liver, where it is packaged into an LDL **particle**. In other words, one big protein-wrapped carrier transports a bunch of cholesterol. Current thinking is that it's better to count these particles than to measure the total amount of cholesterol they carry to get an idea of the risk the LDL may pose.

Without getting too complicated, several subtypes of LDL all carry cholesterol that can be delivered to body cells that need it. These cells take in the cholesterol by way of a **receptor**, like a special gate that only opens for the LDL particle.

Problems arise if a lot of LDL is circulating in the blood. Then delivery is refused by the body cells, and the LDL stay in the blood longer. LDL are particularly susceptible to **oxidation** damage. Once damaged, they are more likely to, in turn, damage the vascular **endothelium**, which you just read about. In a nasty positive feedback loop, once the endothelium is damaged, LDL particles can more readily cross into the inner layer of the vessel wall. Here, LDL are picked up by immune system cells called **macrophages**. This term literally means "big eaters," and these cells do just that. They are the vacuum cleaners of the body, taking in foreign cells and waste material, which are then broken down. Alternatively, the waste is stockpiled if they can't easily be degraded. All those earlier-mentioned risk factors for increased ROS production, such as smoking and hypertension, also contribute to a more permeable endothelial membrane more easily invaded by LDL and macrophages.

One reason we get more LDL as we age is that we make fewer of the LDL receptors that remove it from the blood. The main reason we make fewer receptors is that we make less bile acid. This stuff is made by the liver from cholesterol and is transported to the intestine, where it helps digest fats. Adding insult to injury, our LDL goes up as we age, and our ability to eat fat and digest it easily goes down. But I digress; back to cholesterol. The liver is using less of it for bile acids. The liver also makes the LDL receptors. Being a thrifty organ, the liver cuts back on its production of receptors, much like you would cut back on your driving if you no longer commuted to work.

And if that's not enough, as we age, we see changes in the microbiome, the many species of helpful and some not-so-helpful bacteria in the gut. Although the microbiome still remains something of a black box, the roles of many species are becoming clear. Some of these species can affect your level of cholesterol. Remember the bile acid I just introduced you to? Some of it is broken down by your gut bacteria into a form that is then excreted. Your liver, which is like an orchestra conductor and monitors levels of all kinds of substances in the body, responds by using some cholesterol to make more bile acids. This response, in turn, lowers your blood cholesterol. But it seems that as we age, the bacteria responsible for this neat trick decline in abundance, meaning that cholesterol in the blood rises.[9]

WHAT MECHANISMS ARE CAUSING ALL OF THIS?

If we want to know how to avoid or remedy those changes in artery function, we must know what causes them. Most of these mechanisms are things I've told you about in earlier chapters, so this should be old hat.

Stiffening. Increased stiffness comes as the structure of the arterial wall changes. These changes include replacement of muscle (look at figure 7.1 above; this happens in the medial layer) with collagen and calcium, breakage of elastic proteins (like what happens in the skin; this occurs in the medial layer shown in the figure), and our old friend, the advanced **glycation** end products (**AGEs**). Of course, you recall these molecules produced by sugar in the blood reacting with various proteins to stick them together. And not surprisingly, AGE formation is aggravated by oxidative stress caused by increased **ROS**. And, of course, plaque contributes, too.

Endothelial Dysfunction. To assess how well your vascular endothelial layer is functioning in humans, researchers measure how much a vessel dilates (opens up) when it is stimulated. This measurement is called **endothelium-dependent dilation (EDD)**: the bigger the EDD, the better the endothelial function (and vice versa). A related point is that arteries that maintain good EDD despite being gunked up with plaque can still expand more readily, somewhat mitigating the narrowing effect of plaque buildup.

A downside to this expansion is that these compensatory enlargements can produce small aneurysms. You can see this bulging in figure 7.3. These bubble-like expansions of the artery mean there is no narrowing of the internal diameter, so blood flow is unimpeded. Unfortunately, the expanded area has a weaker wall that, when excessively enlarged, is prone to rupture.

The body has a few ways to dilate arteries (EDD), but they all involve the enzyme that produces **NO (nitric oxide)** in endothelial cells. NO that is released by these cells travels into the muscle cells (in the medial layer; see figure 7.2), causing them to relax. This dilates the artery and, consequently, blood flow increases. Declining vascular NO is the major cause of endothelial dysfunction found in CV disease. Not surprisingly, **ROS** from damaged mitochondria reduce NO production. In a recent study from my hometown of Boulder, Colorado, twenty healthy men and women ages 60–79 took an antioxidant that specifically targets mitochondria (Mito-Q, which I describe in chapter 10). Within six weeks, age-related changes in their blood vessels reversed, giving them EDD of adults fifteen to twenty years younger.[10]

Normal vessel   Aneurysm

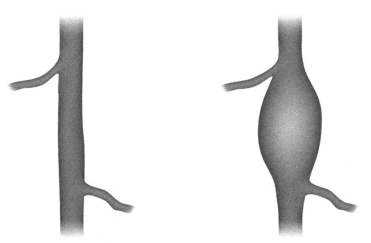

Figure 7.3.   Enlarged section of artery (aneurism). © VERONIKA ZAKHAROVA/ SCIENCE PHOTO LIBRARY.

Oxidative Stress. Endothelial dysfunction in both animals and humans is linked to oxidative stress in the artery. What causes this? There are two mechanisms, both of which are promising areas for remediation. First, high levels of ROS (reactive oxygen species) and reduced (or even unchanged) levels of your normal antioxidant defenses. Increased ROS react with NO and the enzyme that makes it, sucking it out of the artery cells. This drop in NO means less dilation, and thus less blood flow, and all the downstream bad stuff that endothelial dysfunction means.

Inflammation. Inflammation and oxidative stress reinforce one another, so it's not surprising that chronic low-grade inflammation occurs as our vessels age. Inflammation, as discussed in earlier chapters, is a normal part of your immune system, but it gets out of hand as we get older, resulting in this chronic "inflammaging" phenomenon (introduced in chapter 3). The immune system responds to inflammation by producing **cytokines** (for a refresher, you can go back to the sidebar explaining these things in chapter 5; they are basically messengers released by cells that call on other cells to respond), which can either increase or diminish inflammation. Naturally, the cytokines produced by aging blood vessels are the ones that increase inflammation.

Other Immune System Responses. Another function of your immune system is to patrol the body looking for foreign invaders, such as bacteria or damaged cells. The patrol units of the immune system are specialized cells. People love to make the analogy between the immune system and a military force. In that metaphor, some immune cells would be like a small stealth patrol attracted to the vascular endothelium, where they can wiggle through that layer of the vessel to investigate the underlying cells. In the process of infiltrating the vessel wall, they can irritate the cells there. Of course, likelihood of this rises as we age. It might be because the infiltration rate increases with age. Alternatively, more immune system cells may get into the vessel wall. If you think of these immune cells as soldiers on patrol, you can imagine the older ones being careless, or a larger patrol being needed. It's not known which process causes the inflammation. Regardless, as I discuss in detail below, regular aerobic exercise inhibits the inflammatory response produced by the circulating immune cells. Exercise also reduces many of the other vascular aging mechanisms.

Senescent Cells. As I've discussed before, senescent cells accumulate as we age, and their maladaptive signals can disrupt organs such as the heart. These cells, which have survived past their normal life span, cause chronic inflammation, buildup of unwanted collagen (that fibrosis I talked about earlier in this chapter), and other age-related problems. In the CV system, senescent cells in the endothelial layer accumulate calcium, which contributes to stiffening of arteries and hypertension. In the vessels, when those immune cells become senescent, they produce plaque that narrows and weakens blood vessel walls. The combination of these two processes—high blood pressure and weakened blood vessels—causes a large portion of the death toll from CVD. And in the heart, chronic inflammation contributes to the changes I described above that replace the all-important muscle with connective tissue.[11]

Back to Plaque—A Deep Dive[12]

All of the above processes act together, probably in different proportions and sequence in different people, to produce plaque. This is a major player in CVD, so if you want to know more about how it's formed and what it can do, read on.

As you now know, damage to the internal wall of the artery will stimulate the immune cell response. These cells are like a road crew patching a pothole. Often the initiating event is the migration of LDL cholesterol particles into the smooth muscle layer. And the smaller particles have an easier time getting in. Thus, the significant role of these smaller, so-called Lp(a) particles in heart disease.

Once in there, LDL can sustain oxidation damage by ROS (I discussed these "reactive oxygen species" in detail in chapter 3). When LDL is damaged by oxidation (e.g., from mitochondrial malfunction), the immune system sends cells called macrophage. Macrophage literally means "big eater"; these are the cleanup cells of the immune system. These cells build a patch over the damage, which starts the formation of plaque. But the oxidized LDL also triggers a change in the smooth muscle layer of the artery, causing it to become more like a bone cell. This cellular change means that the endothelial layer becomes increasingly loaded with calcium, causing it to become stiff—yes, like bones.

The macrophages that respond to the damage due to ROS become engorged with cholesterol from LDL that they have "eaten." Consequently, they develop a fluffy appearance, hence their "technical" name: foam cells. Foam cells stick to damaged areas of the vessel lining—the endothelial layer—adding to the growing plaque. The macrophages then begin to release compounds that cause more inflammation. A vicious cycle results.

A lot of the stuff inside the growing plaque deposit is cholesterol that has been taken up by foam cells. Remember that cholesterol is a gooey substance without much stable structure. Thus, the plaque can also be gooey. Your immune system recognizes this and builds a cap to keep it from leaking into the blood. This patch on the plaque can come in one of two varieties.

In so-called vulnerable plaque, the outer cap is not very sturdy and can break off as passing blood, especially with higher blood pressure, erodes it. The released fatty core can be dislodged, allowing it to travel through the circulatory system as a clot. When a clot gets stuck in a smaller vessel, it obstructs blood supply. If this happens in the heart, you have a heart attack. If it happens in the brain, you have a stroke. You get the picture. If that's not enough, the accumulation of all that gunk in and on the vessel wall narrows the lumen, which, of course, restricts blood flow. This restriction results in higher systolic blood pressure and lower diastolic pressure, and the associated problems in the heart I discussed earlier.

The second type of plaque, "stable plaque," has—you guessed it—a thicker cap. Yes, resistant to breakage and clot release, but this comes at a cost. Because it's thicker, it narrows the artery more with the concomitant reduction in blood flow.

The so-called good cholesterol, HDL, actually removes the oxidized cholesterol from the artery walls. In addition, HDL reduces the amount of calcium deposited in the vessel wall, making the artery less stiff.

Paradoxically, statins, used to decrease LDL cholesterol, also increase the deposition of calcium in plaque. No one knows why this happens, but it is well accepted that statins are protective against CVD. Researchers speculate that more calcium makes the plaque more stable, thus less likely to break free to cause heart attacks.

Another paradoxical effect of statins is that, although the drug doesn't have the same effect on lowering cholesterol in everyone, most people taking these drugs do show health benefits. It turns out that some statins improve the ability of the aging immune system to locate harmful bugs. At least some of the benefits from statins may be due to this unexpected finding.

A new test, the coronary artery calcium test (CAC), is a type of X-ray that measures the amount of calcium in the arteries of the heart. The CAC score is a relatively good, though not perfect, predictor of future heart disease. If you have stuck with me so far, you probably understand why.

Brain and Central Nervous System. All of these vascular effects are especially significant in the brain, which requires a constant supply of oxygen and nutrients. Consequently, the brain's vasculature is equipped with special control mechanisms that regulate blood supply. When nerve cells are working and require additional blood flow, they send signals to the blood vessels. The vascular endothelial cells and muscles then respond, with a temporary increase in flow, tightly linked to the nerve cell activity level. This coordinated response breaks down in conditions such as hypertension, Alzheimer's, and stroke. Consequently, the active nerve cells don't get the blood they need, causing more tissue damage. The signaling breakdown between the brain's needs and the blood vessels' responses is due mainly to oxidation damage by ROS in the vessels.[13] I'll go into more detail below on the source of these ROS and potential therapies.

Dementia and other brain disorders are aggravated by a "perfect storm" of events in the cardiovascular system. As the brain's capillary system deteriorates with age, it is less able to deliver sufficient nutrients and oxygen to cells. Heart failure worsens this condition. When increased blood pressure is added to the mix, cells can be damaged or killed. In the brain, this cluster of events causes many tiny, silent strokes, each destroying a minuscule section of brain tissue—but it adds up over time.

EXERCISE AND CVD

Aerobic Exercise. Doing only resistance exercise (i.e., weight lifting) doesn't improve the health of your arteries, though it provides many other benefits that I described in chapter 5. In some studies, resistance exercise has even increased the stiffness measured in the carotid artery, which is the large artery carrying blood to the brain. Simply adding aerobic exercise offsets the negative effects of resistance exercise on this stiffness. Some studies have shown that the effect of aerobic exercise is limited to the large elastic arteries (aorta and carotid) but doesn't affect stiffness in smaller vessels. This is an active area of ongoing research.

Want some specifics? Let's start with animal studies. In rodents (rats and mice), like humans, sedentary old animals have stiffer carotid arteries than young control animals. The age-related stiffening was associated with two changes in the makeup of the arterial wall. First, more collagen (fibrous tissue) was laid down in the outer layer. You can look back at figure 7.1 to refresh your memory as to the vessel structure. Second, **elastin**, the protein that keeps tissue supple and elastic, was lost from the middle layer of the carotid artery. These changes, in turn, led to higher amounts of signaling **cytokines** released by the vessel wall, which stimulated more collagen synthesis—in other words, a vicious cycle.[14]

The way researchers look at aerobic exercise in laboratory rats and mice is to give them running wheels. Rats and other rodents love these things. When older animals were given access to a wheel, they jumped on, and this aerobic activity reversed the carotid stiffening seen in controls not given running wheels. Specifically, collagen (and other stiffening components) was reduced. The dilation of their blood vessels, mediated by NO, returned to the level seen in young control animals. Oxidation damage of collagen by immune system cells was also reduced. Wow! Aerobic exercise is like the fountain of youth in mice!

In older human men, when blood flow was stimulated to assess EDD (recall this term for vessel dilation), sedentary subjects showed smaller increases than young controls. Remember, more dilation is good, as it means your vessels readily expand to accommodate changes in blood flow. By comparison, EDD was the same in young men and older men who regularly exercised aerobically. The researchers found that twelve weeks of brisk walking in previously sedentary older men was sufficient to restore a younger EDD level. When arterial stiffness and blood pressure were measured, the same beneficial results of exercise were seen in the older men.[15]

In women, the role of regular aerobic exercise, on both endothelial function and arterial stiffness, is not as clear-cut. When sedentary postmenopausal women were compared with active postmenopausal women (both groups had low levels of estrogen), arterial dilation showed no difference. Remember that dilation indicates the ability of the artery to expand and carry more blood. The same program of brisk walking that, in men, increased artery dilation, did not do so in postmenopausal women in some studies. When estrogen replacement therapy was added to the experiment, the blood flow measure increased following aerobic exercise training in women who received estrogen but not in the control group that did not get the hormone. This finding supports the role of hormone replacement in combating age-related changes in women, but it was a small study.[16]

Oxidation Damage. So, what's going on in these endothelial cells to cause the age-related changes that can be reversed by exercise? As we get older, you may recall, our antioxidant defenses decline, and we may even produce more of the damaging **ROS** (reactive oxygen species). And, yes, this has been shown to take place in the arteries. It's not understood why our antioxidant defenses decline as we age. Regardless, higher levels of ROS decrease the efficacy of **NO**. The ROS react with the NO that's released from the endothelial cells, removing the NO and its beneficial effect. Then, to add insult to injury, the fallout from that removal inhibits the production of NO and simultaneously increases ROS production. But regular aerobic exercise prevents and even reverses oxidation damage measured in the arteries of both mice and people. In mice, where it's possible to do more extensive biopsies, **mitochondria** (the power plants of the cells) produced more ROS as the animals aged, but this was reversed in old mice who ran on a wheel.

Going back to our mitochondria, recall that these crucial organelles accumulate damage as we age, much like cars that aren't serviced regularly. Both resistance and aerobic exercise affect these little guys in two ways. First, in people and animals that engage in these activities, their mitochondria reproduce more, increasing the number of functional organelles. Second, exercise gets rid of mitochondria with damaged DNA. This cleanup has several important effects: improved energy production and fewer numbers of dying or senescent cells. Guess what? This means less plaque, less atherosclerosis, and less CV disease.

Role of Inflammation and the Immune System. In old mice, like older humans, immune cells increasingly creep into the vessel walls, as I discussed earlier when describing plaque formation. When old mice are given running wheels, those cells disappear. This suggests that aerobic exercise suppresses either the ability or the inclination of the immune cells to get inside the arterial wall. Fewer immune cells means that they send out fewer cytokine signals that stimulate inflammation. Less inflammation, of course, means better arterial function.

Heart Cell Regeneration. In a study done in mice, researchers found that exercise stimulated the heart to make new muscle cells, both under normal conditions and after a heart attack. The human heart is really bad at regenerating itself. Young people can renew around 1 percent of their heart muscle cells every year, and that rate decreases with age. Losing cardiac muscle is linked to heart failure, so anything that increases muscle cell formation can prevent CVD.[17]

WHAT TO DO (BESIDES EXERCISE)?

Antioxidants. Given the preceding discussion of the role of oxidation damage in vascular and heart tissues, you might think, why not just take high doses of antioxidants? But remember that taking these compounds can limit your internal production of them, which can be finely tuned to the places and times needed. And it is important to recognize that ROS have some useful roles in cells, so inappropriate use of antioxidants may be harmful. That said, the place where most ROS are generated, and have the most potential to do harm, is in the mitochondria. In the last decade, a large amount of work has been devoted to developing antioxidants targeted specifically at the mitochondria. Studies of mitochondria in test tubes showed that some of these drugs protect mitochondria from the harmful effects of excess ROS, such as mutations in the mitochondrial DNA and membrane damage.[18]

Preliminary work in mice showed that mitochondrial-specific antioxidants improved EDD (dilation) in old sedentary mice but had no effect on young animals or on old wheel-running mice. Similarly, injections of vitamin C, which is a potent antioxidant when administered at high doses, selectively restored EDD in older sedentary men, while young controls and active older men were unaffected. In healthy, estrogen-deficient postmenopausal women, high-dose vitamin C improved carotid artery stiffness in sedentary subjects to levels found in aerobically trained women. These results further support the role of ROS in endothelial dysfunction in sedentary individuals. Exercise (and estrogen in older women) reduces the ROS damage to endothelial function. So, targeted antioxidants can help, but keep the caveats about their side effects in mind.[19]

One of these mitochondrial-specific antioxidants, MitoQ, has been shown to decrease cardiac hypertrophy and atherosclerosis in mice. Several preliminary clinical trials in people have been done. In one recent study, EDD improved by more than 40 percent in people taking MitoQ. This is another area of ongoing research, and I return to this specific compound in chapter 10.[20]

Anti-inflammatory Drugs. Oxidation damage stimulates inflammation and vice versa, so we should expect the inflammaging that develops with age in the vasculature. Just as in the muscles, inflammatory **cytokines** (I listed them in chapter 5), increase over time in arteries from experimental animals and autopsied human tissue. When some of these cytokines are blocked experimentally in mice, using a drug called sodium salicylate, oxidation damage is reduced, and dilation (EDD) increases to levels seen in young mice. In people, the drug reduced the cytokine in the endothelial cells of older, sedentary men but had no effect in young control males or older, active men. The arterial dilation in the sedentary men treated with sodium salicylate also improved.[21]

Eat Chocolate. No, I'm not joking. A meta-analysis (where researchers looked at seven studies, pooling the results) of chocolate consumption and cardiac disorders suggests that "higher" levels of the yummy stuff are protective against a variety of cardiovascular (CV) pathologies, including stroke, heart attack, and CV disease. This type of analysis has a lot of limitations, which I've railed against in earlier chapters. Unfortunately, because most of the studies this group looked at did not quantify the amount of chocolate that was eaten, I can't tell you how much chocolate you should eat. That said (somewhat tongue in cheek), these data are intriguing, given that dark chocolate is known to have antioxidant properties and, in moderation, would not add too many calories.[22]

Senolytics. Those senescent cells that accumulate in our blood vessels and accelerate the aging process are cells that have stopped dividing and instigate inflammation. Like the bad apple in the barrel . . . They contribute to numerous age-related disorders, including heart failure, diabetes, and atherosclerotic diseases. Conversely, when these bad actors are removed or suppressed in experimental animals, many features of aging are reversed. **Senolytics** are drugs targeting senescent cells. Several clinical trials of these drugs are currently in process. One promising drug combination joins the cancer drug dasatinib with a natural, over-the-counter anti-inflammatory called quercetin. Dasatinib eliminated senescent human fat cells, while quercetin was more effective against senescent human endothelial cells. A combination of the two (D+Q) was most effective overall. So far, only D + Q has been assessed in the clinical setting, and none of the current clinical trials are testing whether senolytic drugs can inhibit cardiovascular disorders. But, in mice and rats, targeting and removing senescent cells stopped the progression of vascular disease. I discuss these in more detail in chapter 10, and recall the unusual development of one such as a cosmetic, described in chapter 4.

A related strategy involves suppressing the development of senescent cells in the first place. To explain the proposed approaches, I have to give you some background on a protein called **sirtuin** (**SIRT1** for short). SIRT1 does a lot in our cells because it activates other proteins, essentially having its fingers in a lot of pies. Two of its known effects are to activate **autophagy** (the cellular cleanup process), linking SIRT1 to caloric restriction (CR), and to inhibit chronic inflammation, presumably by inhibiting cellular senescence. In mice, increasing SIRT1 levels reversed arterial stiffness and extended life span. Resveratrol, which is the agent in red wine claimed to inhibit aging in mice, activates SIRT1. Resveratrol is a maybe, and you would have to take a lot of it in pill form to get the effects shown in mice. The activity of SIRT depends on **NAD⁺**, an all-important mediator in cells that I introduced in chapter 3, which tends to decrease in all our cells with age. In vascular cells grown in the lab, increasing NAD⁺ levels decreased the number of senescent cells, while decreasing NAD⁺ caused an increase in their number.[23] I'll come back to NAD⁺ shortly. And for more detail, hold your breath for chapter 10.

Clearly, we don't have much evidence yet in people, but these results are promising, not just for CV disease, but many age-related disorders that have been linked to senescent cells.[24]

Minoxidil. Minoxidil (aka Rogaine) is sold over the counter to stimulate hair growth. In a different formulation, oral minoxidil is sometimes prescribed for high blood pressure that has not responded to other medications. The drug may have this effect by increasing elastin production. In studies in mice and rats, minoxidil induced elastin formation, lowered blood pressure, and increased arterial diameter. In older animals, age-related stiffening and decreased diameter were reversed. What's more, these changes persisted for weeks after the drug was no longer in the bloodstream. Nothing yet in humans, although early studies of the drug showed it was safe for balding patients with CVD.[25]

Rapamycin. Remember that master regulator of cell growth, **mTOR** (introduced in chapter 3)? People have had the idea that if you turn down mTOR with drugs such as rapamycin, this will mimic the inhibitory effect of caloric restriction on growth. Although rapamycin appears to extend life span by inhibiting cancer, some studies have looked at heart disease. Most of these studies have been done in rodents, which, like humans, develop symptoms of CVD with age. When mice were fed rapamycin, a number of those symptoms improved in old mice: EDD improved, arterial ROS levels and stiffness both decreased.[26] I return to this drug in chapter 10.

The one approved application of rapamycin (aka sirolimus) in CVD is the use of stents coated with this drug. A stent is a tube that is inserted into a blood vessel, typically an artery, to keep it open. Several large clinical studies have shown that patients treated with coated stents have lower rates of hardening arteries, compared to bare-metal stents, resulting in more successful outcomes.[27]

NAD+ Stimulants. Remember that NAD+ is an important signal that, in addition to regulating SIRT1, tells the cell to produce more antioxidants. The production of NAD+, like many other helpful compounds in the body, falls off with age. Several compounds that can augment NAD+ levels are being tested for their effects in various systems. One of these, NMN, is a building block of NAD+ currently being investigated for its effect on numerous age-related pathologies. In aging mice, NMN reversed many of the arterial and endothelial dysfunctions described above. When cells from aortas were grown with NMN, their NAD+ and antioxidant levels increased. Another building block of NAD+ is called NR. In several small trials, this vitamin has been shown to be safe and to increase NAD+ levels. It is currently available and sold as Niagen.[28] More on all of these in chapter 10.

Stem Cells. Cardiovascular disease can deprive heart tissue of oxygen, killing the cardiac muscle cells. This, in turn, triggers a disaster cascade: formation of scar tissue, compensatory increases in blood flow and pressure, and increased stress on remaining heart cells. The heart eventually fails. Restoring damaged heart muscle tissue, through repair or regeneration via stem cells, is an exciting new avenue of research.

A number of stem cell types, including embryonic stem (ES) cells, cardiac stem cells (found only in the heart), muscle stem cells, adult bone marrow cells, and others have been tested in rodents with promising results. A few small studies have also been carried out in humans, usually in patients undergoing open-heart surgery. The results of these tests showed that stem cells injected into the circulation or directly into the injured heart tissue improve cardiac function. Although much more research is needed, these preliminary clinical experiments show how stem cells may one day be used to repair damaged heart tissue, thereby reducing the burden of cardiovascular disease.[29]

One vascular disease in people has been treated with stem cells in a long-term study, which has been ongoing for more than five years. Angitis-induced critical limb ischemia (call it AICLI) is caused by inflammation of blood vessels in the arms or legs that creates blockages in the limb arteries. Serious cases result in amputation and even death in some instances. About 20 percent of patients can't tolerate the surgical reconstruction that can treat AICLI. In a small study, twenty-seven of these patients were treated with injections of stem cells. Some 90 percent survived without limb loss, and 65 percent were able to resume a normal life. These results are promising for the use of stem cells in other vascular disorders.[30]

Multivitamin Supplement? Unlike the paragraphs above where I describe positive results, here I tell you that there is not much evidence for taking a multivitamin supplement specifically to reduce your risk of heart disease. Six large studies, including the long-term Physicians Health Study II, all showed the same results: the supplement doesn't do this. What does contribute to heart health and longevity, and is probably cheaper than supplements, is a diet high in fruit and vegetables. Specifically, to reduce risk of heart attacks and strokes, aim for at least 600 gm (just over a pound) per day.[31]

Diet. Many books have been written about heart-healthy diets, and I won't attempt to recapitulate them here. Remember, my goal in this book is to present new research that has not been widely publicized. That said, I do recommend Michael Gregor's monumental tome on the beneficial effects of foods on a variety of health issues including CVD. Gregor has pulled together a phenomenal amount of research on this issue and collated it in an accessible manner. Be forewarned, however: his agenda is to convert the reader to a plant-based diet. His dietary recommendations for CVD fall into the low-fat camp, which not all researchers accept. Although numerous studies have linked high consumption of animal protein with higher death rates, this is a controversial area, and new studies emerge almost weekly. Gregor promotes a range of nutritional fixes for various conditions, not all of which have good supporting evidence, so you have to sort the wheat from the chaff by looking at his extensive references.[32] As always, keep in mind that nutritional studies in humans are almost completely observational. As I described in the introduction, these studies have some serious problems, especially if they have not been replicated or if the number of people in the study is small, both of which tend to be true for many nutrition studies.

Finally, feed your microbiome. We don't know much at this time about which species interactions are best for our heart and other systems, but preliminary evidence clearly indicates a protective role for some species. Probiotic foods such as yogurts and other fermented items, which contain live bacteria, as well as prebiotics, such as garlic, onions, and legumes, which are preferentially metabolized by your gut bacteria, are one way to offset the decline in protective bacteria that occurs with age.[33] More on this important topic in the final two chapters.

Alcohol? Drinking has long been linked to modest gains in heart health, though this conclusion has been tinged with controversy. Several recent, large studies do support the finding that moderate drinking can provide benefits to the cardiac system. Keep in mind that these studies are observational (remember that from chapter 1?), meaning that they identify trends but not necessarily the causes of the observations. It's possible that the health effects come from other lifestyle factors common among moderate drinkers, such as a strong social network. And, many people who identify as teetotalers abstain for a variety of health conditions. Including them in studies could skew the results to make people who don't drink look unhealthier and to link drinking to health benefits.

Given those caveats, what are the benefits? In the large British CALIBER study, the researchers found that nondrinkers were at increased risk for eight of the twelve heart ailments examined, compared to moderate drinkers. These conditions include the most common cardiac events, such as heart attack, stroke, and sudden heart-related death. Nondrinkers had a 33 percent higher risk of angina—a condition in which the heart doesn't get enough blood flow—and a 56 percent higher risk of dying unexpectedly from heart disease, compared to people who drank a glass or two of alcohol a day. But moderate drinking did not protect against four less-common heart problems that blocked blood flow to the brain, causing milder strokes and bleeding in the brain.[34]

The CALIBER study was unique in that "nondrinkers" were separated into categories to differentiate people who never drank from those who quit drinking (who may have been heavy drinkers in the past, so may have a higher risk of heart problems). Past studies that pooled these groups made risk to non-drinkers look higher. Drinking too much, of course, negates these benefits and increases the risk of heart problems.

But these results shouldn't tempt people who don't drink to start to gain protection from heart disease. Drinking alcohol can cause liver disease, and some studies suggest that it contributes to breast cancers. Safer ways to reduce cardiac risk factors, include quitting smoking, exercising regularly, and eating a healthy diet. These are all commonsense recommendations also endorsed by a recent worldwide study that the Gates Foundation supported. These researchers examined a very different population than the British group followed, and they used a "meta-analysis," which combines previous study results; you know by now my opinion of these analyses. Nonetheless, their conclusion that alcohol use contributes to "all-cause mortality" (i.e., death for any reason) is a sobering one.[35]

Environmental Triggers. A few cautionary words are in order at this point. Many events can contribute to loosening the plaque in arteries, causing it to detach and result in a heart attack. Statistically, heart attacks are more common during colder temperatures and early mornings. The importance of sleep is highlighted by a gigantic unregulated experiment done on all of us—about 1.5 billion people—living with daylight saving time. In spring, when we lose just one hour of sleep, heart attacks increase by 25 percent in the next few days. Conversely, in the fall, that one extra hour is protective, reducing coronary events by 20 percent.

Upper respiratory infections, including influenza and pneumonia, also put people at greater risk for heart attacks. Finally, the risk for a fatal heart attack goes up during and immediately after exercise, especially in individuals who are not very physically fit. This is why you always see the caveat about checking with your doctor before beginning an exercise program. The risk associated with exercise is worsened by air pollution, especially particulate air pollution. Of course, emotional stress can also precipitate coronary events such as heart attacks, but the connection between these events is less well-studied.

WHAT ABOUT MY GENES?

To start, there is evidence for both protective and damaging roles in the CV system for many genes. And researchers are constantly discovering new ones. Consequently, the list that follows is very preliminary, but current evidence does support these genes. That said, remember that many lifestyle factors, such as sleep and diet, will affect the action of your genes. In other words, you may carry some **risk alleles** (the form of the gene that can put you at risk of CVD), but your lifestyle choices can affect that risk. Remember, I discussed the action of these forms of genes in chapter 3.

CETP. This gene encodes a protein that transfers cholesterol from HDL to LDL. This is not a good thing, as LDL can infiltrate blood vessel walls, leading to atherosclerosis and heart disease. Alleles that reduce the typical activity of the protein (i.e., LDL to HDL) are, therefore, protective. Several of these have been identified and confirmed in human studies, leading to the development of a drug to inhibit CETP activity, which may decrease LDL.[36] Other changes to this gene make LDL particles larger, which makes it harder for them to burrow into artery walls. Larger particles are, therefore, protective against artery disease.

NPC1L1. This gene determines the action of the "doorway" that moves cholesterol out of the gut and into the circulation. Reducing the activity of this gene will, therefore, reduce LDL and risk for vessel damage. In addition to affecting baseline LDL level, mutations in this gene can also affect one's response to some cholesterol-lowering drugs that act by blocking the doorway.[37]

ApoE. There are three common alleles of ApoE. The proteins produced by these alleles are called ApoE2, ApoE3 (which is the most common in the United States), and ApoE4. Having one or two copies of the ApoE4 allele puts you at increased risk for a variety of conditions, including atherosclerosis, Alzheimer's disease, and multiple sclerosis, in addition to accelerating telomere shortening.[38] The E2 allele is somewhat protective, and the common E3 allele appears neutral for these risks. One uncommon allele, ApoE5, seems to increase the risk of heart attacks.[38]

HMGCoA. This gene encodes a major enzyme in cholesterol synthesis, the one blocked by statins. Statins, of course, are the main drugs currently prescribed to lower cholesterol and protect against heart disease. Interestingly, the enzyme and its gene were not known until after statins were discovered, when research turned to understanding why the drugs worked. Several forms of this gene reduce CVD risk by lowering LDL levels. These protective alleles can also affect the ability of some statins to lower LDL.[39]

LIPC. This gene codes for hepatic lipase (HL), an enzyme the liver produces that plays a role in lipoprotein metabolism. In people with a gene form that produces an enzyme with high activity, it breaks down HDL rapidly. Conversely, if you carry an alternative form of the gene for a less active enzyme, your HDL cholesterol level is higher.

LPL. This gene codes for an enzyme that breaks down the triglycerides (a type of fat consisting of three building blocks called **fatty acids**) that are carried in LDL particles. Once broken down, the resulting fatty acids can be used for energy. Turns out that the heart especially likes these fatty acids, preferring them to glucose. So, those of us with an enzyme that doesn't work as well have lower fatty acid levels, and consequently the heart has to work a bit harder, which may predispose one to heart disease.[40]

Prothrombin (aka Thrombin). This gene determines a protein of the same name that is involved in clotting blood. The most common, and certainly most problematic, variant of this gene is called Prothrombin G20210A. This risk allele increases the risk of blood clots. The most serious such clots are deep vein thrombosis and pulmonary embolisms.

Whew! What does that mean? When a blood clot breaks free from a vein and travels in the blood, this is called a venous (i.e., in the vein) thrombosis (fancy way to say clot). Veins return blood to the right side of the heart, so if a clot formed in a vein breaks off, that's where it goes. From here, the blood flows to the lung. So, if the clot continues on to the lungs, it is called a pulmonary embolism, meaning a clot that has gotten stuck. This type of embolism can be serious: they are thought to cause 15 percent of sudden deaths in the United States.

People with one copy of the risk allele have an increased risk for developing blood clots, from 1 in 1,000 (for people without this gene form), to 2.5 in 1,000. If you have two copies the risk can rise to 20 in 1,000. By comparison, most people never develop a blood clot in their lives.

A related gene, which is necessary for prothrombin to activate a clot, is called Factor V. It, too, has a well-known risk allele for thrombosis. Having one copy of the mutant form increases one's risk by about four times. Men were at slightly higher risk (five times), as were women taking oral contraceptives (six times).

Angiotensin-Converting Enzyme (ACE). This gene codes for an enzyme that indirectly affects blood pressure. The variant of the gene that produces more of the enzyme elevates BP slightly. Interestingly, the effect on BP is worse when people with this gene eat a diet high in saturated fat.

Many drugs for controlling BP act by blocking this enzyme. The most common variant of this gene has been shown (in a relatively small study) to influence how rapidly people carrying that form will respond to the BP-lowering effects of some drugs.

FTO. This gene contains the instructions to make the "fat mass and obesity-associated" protein. This is one of those enzymes that interacts with your DNA to turn on a lot of genes. Many of these are involved in your brain's decisions about eating. The gene has a number of variant forms, some of which have been shown to increase obesity and type 2 diabetes; thus they might predispose one to CVD.

CONCLUSION

Cardiovascular disease has been the number one cause of death in the United States for almost a century. With new drugs and interventional treatments, CVD is beginning to yield that position to cancer. For many of us, it is possible to forestall those extreme approaches by lifestyle and supplement approaches. I provide more detail on these in the final two chapters.

ACRONYMS

AICLI: Angitis-induced critical limb ischemia
ATP: Adenosine triphosphate (the energy molecule)
BP: Blood pressure
CV: Cardiovascular
CVD: Cardiovascular diseases
ED: Endothelial dysfunction
EDD: Endothelium-dependent dilation
LDL: Low-density lipoprotein
MI: Myocardial infarction
NO: Nitric oxide
PEF: Preserved ejection fraction
ROS: Reactive oxygen species

8

The Brain and Cognitive Decline

One scientific mystery has yet to be solved: the mystery of the human brain and how it gives rise to thoughts and feelings, hopes and desires, love and the experience of beauty, not to mention dance, visual art, literature, and music. —Paul Churchland

OVERVIEW

Of course, there is no organ called cognition, but this may be the brain function most of us are concerned with as we age. The brain holds our self-hood, and that may be the aspect of aging whose loss we fear most. In this chapter, I will explore brain anatomy and function to give you a basis for understanding cognition and the potential loss of cognitive abilities. Next, I will look at "normal" age-related changes in the brain, certain pathologies that can affect our cognitive abilities, and, of course, what to do to keep these losses to a minimum.

Wikipedia defines cognition as "a faculty for the human-like processing of information, applying knowledge and changing preferences." Pretty broad, but essential to the human experience. Our cognitive processes can be both conscious and unconscious, and include such abstract concepts as mind, reasoning, perception, intelligence, learning, and memory.

These processes arise in complex interactions among cells in the brain in ways that are not well understood. Many breakthroughs in this area have come about as a result of an imaging system called magnetic resonance imaging (MRI), which I introduced in chapter 5. Its use has been expanded to assess the activity of different brain regions. This methodology is called functional magnetic resonance imaging (fMRI).[1]

Using fMRI, scientists can ask experimental subjects to perform different tasks while their brain is being imaged in the MRI machine. The machine detects increased blood flow. As the blood flow is a measure of cell activity, an increase to a specific brain region implicates it in the task being performed. Commonly examined tasks include problem solving, musical performance, reading, and writing. Results from fMRI can lead one into the trap of saying such and such a brain region is responsible for X (fill in your favorite process). In reality, many brain areas cooperate to do X, but certain areas may be critical to the task or to coordinate its completion.

Having just said that one brain region is not responsible for a given task, I have to contradict myself. It really depends on the task. Let me give you two examples. First, starting in the 1950s, neurosurgeons discovered they could reduce or even cure the seizures from some types of epilepsy by cutting the band of nerves that connects the two halves of the brain. This connection is called the **corpus collosum**. During the surgery, patients were awake. This sounds horrifying until you realize that the brain itself has no pain sensors. The scalp is easily anesthetized with local anesthetic. Many of the surgical patients consented to take part in experiments in which the surgeon touched various brain regions with a small instrument carrying a slight electrical charge. The neurosurgeons found that a given region could reliably elicit a specific response: depression, the scent of a rose, the visual image of a cat, and so forth.

Second, many somewhat bizarre neurological conditions are caused by pathology (e.g., tumor) or trauma to a specific brain region. The archetypical disorder is the "visual agnosia" (**agnosia** just means the inability to take in and translate sensory information) that Oliver Sacks described in *The Man Who Mistook His Wife for a Hat*.[2] In this case, a type of Alzheimer's disease caused the degeneration of a brain region that integrates visual information, resulting in a scrambled collage of his seen world. Bottom line: big, complicated tasks require putting together inputs from many brain regions, each of which has its own specific job to do.

I'll start by introducing you to the structural organization of the brain to highlight a few important areas. Then I'll give you a short tour of the cell types and how they work to produce the activity that defines our nervous system. Then we'll get into the good stuff: what happens to the cells and functions as we age and results from new research on how to slow or prevent cognitive decline.

WHAT IS THE BRAIN, AND HOW DOES IT PRODUCE OUR COGNITIVE ABILITY?

Anatomy. Broadly speaking, our brains can be subdivided into three regions: **forebrain**, **midbrain**, and **hindbrain**. The hindbrain consists of the brain stem and cerebellum. These develop very early during the development of the embryo and eventually give rise to highly specialized regions. For example, the forebrain will develop into the outer layer of **cerebral cortex**, which is involved in our conscious processes of perception, learning, and voluntary movement. The cortex is the brain region that distinguishes us—by its extensive size— from other mammals. Its highly convoluted folds are distinct to humans, providing a huge amount of surface area where very specialized cells reside.

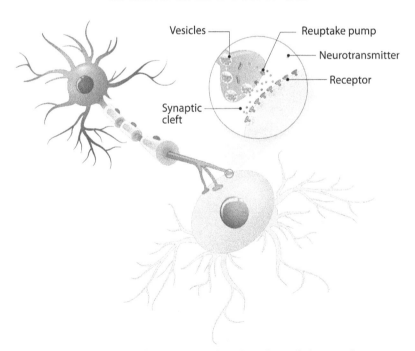

Figure 8.1. Two connected neurons. The inset box shows their synaptic connection. © iStock / ttsz.

The forebrain also includes deeper regions involved in processing sensory information and regulating physiologically important behaviors such as hunger, thirst, fight or flight, and sex. We share lower brain levels, such as the cerebellum and brain stem, with other vertebrates. These regions control movement and balance (cerebellum) and automatic physiological functions such as breathing, heart activity, and digestion (medulla).

Neurons and the "Wired" Brain. The brain, like other organs, is assembled from a variety of different types of cells. The cellular workhorse of the brain is called the **neuron**. The special thing about these cells is that they can talk to each other. Without going into all the chemical details of how they do this, it's a little like an electric current moving down one wire and then transmitting a signal to a second, adjacent wire. What is important is the complexity of the messages that can be assembled from the huge number of interacting neurons in the brain.

You can see two of these neurons in figure 8.1. Notice that each one has many branches pointing away from the central round cell body. These are extensions of the cell membrane, called **dendrites**, that connect to other neurons. A single neuron can have hundreds or thousands of dendrites. All of them can receive signals, called **impulses**, into this cell. All of these inputs are collated in the cell body and a decision is made, depending on how many and what types of inputs come in, if an output signal should be sent. If yes, then the long sausage-like tube down to the second cell, called an **axon**, is activated, and the impulse reaches its end. The junction between the two cells is shown in the inset. Note that the two cells don't actually touch. This

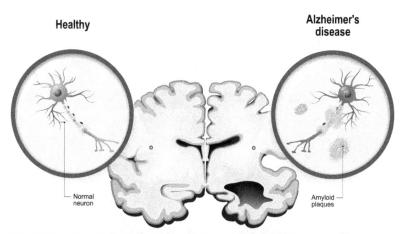

Figure 8.2.   Healthy and Alzheimer's disease brains showing a healthy neuron and neuron with amyloid plaques. © iStock / ttsz.

junction is called the **synapse**. Here the electrical signal releases the little dots of **neurotransmitter (NT)**, a chemical that crosses the microscopic gap of the synapse to pass into the second cell.

When the NT contacts the second neuron, a new electrical signal is generated, which will then produce the output of this cell. The brain has dozens of different NTs. Often any single neuron can produce more than one. The signals elicited by different neurotransmitters can cancel each other out, which is one way that neurons "decide" to transmit their secondary signal. For example, let's say there are inputs from two dendrites on a single neuron. One releases an activating NT at its synapse, while the second releases an inhibitory NT. As a result, that neuron doesn't send a signal down the chain.

Let's consider the implications of the interactions of neurons. An isolated neuron "decides" to transmit a signal to downstream cells. Each subsequent synapse can trigger the same output from yet another cell in a chain. Given that the human brain has perhaps ninety billion neurons (although this estimate is a moving target, ranging from fifty to one hundred billion), and each can develop thousands of synapses with other cells, a staggering amount of cross talk can go on.

Some signals will involve input from the body, perhaps on temperature, blood pressure, blood chemistry, and so on. These signals will be received in "lower" brain regions such as the brain stem or cerebellum. A receiving neuron can connect to response cells that will signal back to the body part. Let's say the incoming signal indicates skin temperature. That same receiving cell could also transit the message on, perhaps to a sensory center in the cortex, which would make you aware of the temperature. This reception of this signal in the cortex might then trigger an impulse to a motor center lower in the brain that would tell you to move away from the fireplace. For you to consider the aesthetics of fire or the environmental implications of burning wood, the signal would travel through different pathways or networks of neurons.

Many of these paths are simple **signal transduction** loops. This just means that a signal of one type (e.g., heat) is converted by a sensory neuron in the skin to an electrical signal (aka impulse) in the axon. That message then travels to a relay cell in the spinal cord, where it crosses its first synapse. The axon of the neuron in the spinal cord would then synapse with multiple cells in the brain, eliciting responses that will travel back down the spinal cord to places in the body that should respond (e.g., blood vessel dilation, sweating, etc.).

For the purpose of our discussion here, on cognitive processes, we are interested in what happens mainly in the cortex. Based on experiments done with fMRI, we know that most of the regions associated with our cognitive abilities are in the cortex—that wrinkled cover over much of the surface of the brain.

Abilities for language, music, and art arise here. Some memory functions are also found here. These abilities depend on the smooth flow of information (signals, impulses) among the neurons in these areas.

Take music, for example. In order to play a piece of music, you depend on visual input from the score, if you use one, or neuronal input from your memory of the melody. This information is further broken down. Some signals carry the sound of the notes, others arise from activity in neurons holding memory of the note patterns and how they are played, and still other signals travel to the areas of the cortex controlling voluntary movement. These latter signals are then passed on to lower brain regions communicating with the spinal cord for sending signals along motor neurons to contract or relax the muscles that manipulate the instrument.

Memory. Learning is the main activity of our brains. Whether we learn consciously, aware of storing facts and experiences; or emotional and physiological responses, which are stored unconsciously, our brains are engaged in learning. Learning involves what neuroscientists call **encoding**, or what you and I might call committing something to memory.

For example, when you perceive an object, neurons in different brain areas process information about shape, color, smell, sound, and so forth. Your brain then makes connections among these neurons. Afterward, when you recall the object, you activate those connections. But—and this is a big but—when your cortex activates that network, the neuronal connections are changed. In other words, memories are never purely preserved and recalled. Now, we have a lot of different types of memory (short term, long term, episodic, working, to name a few), and they all withstand the aging process differently.[3] Regardless, all types share the reliance on networks among neurons. Any process that damages neurons and the connections between them will also affect memory. We'll see how aging can influence these damaging processes.

Neurons and the "Hormonal" Brain. In the "wired" brain (i.e., those networks connected through synapses), information is communicated rapidly. Consider this speed when you are slicing vegetables, and the knife blade touches your finger. The tactile signal races along a sensory neuron to its first synapse in the spinal cord, where it is processed, then a motor signal returns to the hand and you pull back, often before you slice your finger.

Our brains also create long-lasting states such as attentiveness, sleep, anxiety, and pleasure. These states are created by neurons that send their axons through larger brain regions, where they release their neurotransmitters (NT) diffusely, thus affecting many synapses simultaneously. A single such neuron can modulate the activity of thousands of other neurons as if it were a vast broadcast network. How? The single neuron releases its NT into the space between cells, where the NT can diffuse into all the synapses in a large network containing thousands of cells.

Neuroscientists call this large-scale NT release and its effects **neuromodulation**. The effect of neuromodulation is to modify the signal received at the synapses of the wired brain, much as a volume control on a phone modifies the loudness of a signal but not its content. Neuromodulation takes longer to establish and lasts longer than a synaptic signal.

Neurons that produce the NTs used by the "hormonal" brain are found in small, distinct regions of the brain stem and midbrain. Specific clusters of cells are responsible for releasing individual neurotransmitters. The axons of these cells travel into large areas of the forebrain and midbrain to deliver their NT modulatory signal. For example, the neurons that release **dopamine** (a specific NT associated with rewards or pleasurable feelings and muscle control) in this way are found in three clusters in the midbrain. As a consequence, the connections among these regions are known as the **reward pathway**. When your brain rewards itself for certain behaviors, this neuromodulatory system is activated. Many drugs of abuse also activate this pathway. Its activation then rewards drug-taking behavior, contributing to addiction. It can also produce delirium and hallucinations if it is overactive.

One of the dopamine-producing clusters is located in an area called the **substantia nigra** (this means black structure in Latin, because early microscopists described its dark color). This region sends its dopamine to brain regions controlling movement. This cell cluster is damaged in **Parkinson's disease**, explaining the tremor and control issues associated with the disease.

Glia. More than 90 percent of the cells of the central nervous system (brain plus spinal cord) are not neurons. The **glia** make up most of these cells. Originally thought of as connective tissue "glue" that held the helpless neurons in place, we now know that glia play many important roles in the function of our brains. A subset of these functions includes structural support (yes, glue), oxygen and food transport to neurons, immune function (protect against disease-causing organisms and toxins), and waste removal. Basically, neurons are so specialized to communicate their messages that they don't do a lot of other things very well and rely on the glia to do them.

WHAT HAPPENS AS WE AGE?

We have all noticed that age-related changes in cognition are extremely variable. One person can recite long poems from memory or solve difficult mathematical problems at ninety-five years of age, whereas another will develop dementia at age fifty. There are many reasons for this, including overall health, education, socioeconomic status, and genetics. In most healthy older people, cognitive abilities don't decline much. In fact, the wisdom of accrued experience increases, and we can continue to learn new skills throughout life.[4]

Age-related changes in the brain have been studied for more than two centuries, but we still can't say much about what constitutes "normal" change. Much of the uncertainty is due to the difficulty of examining a brain in a living person. Recent advances in technology, such as the MRI, are changing this. The most obvious change is in brain weight, which is pretty stable until about midlife, then begins to decline. Brain volume, which correlates well with weight, drops 0.1–0.2 percent a year from thirty to fifty years, then falls off the cliff to 0.3–0.5 percent a year after the age of seventy.[5]

What Do We Lose? Scientists used to think that we lost more and more neurons as we aged. More recent studies found that, in general, neuron loss with age is either undetectable or relatively mild. Once you pass eighty years, though, all bets are off. After eighty, neurons are lost due to the processes that sometimes result in Alzheimer's disease, which I discuss in more detail below. Neuron populations are also affected by cerebrovascular disease (i.e., damage to blood vessels, which I introduced in the previous chapter), which, of course, is also more common with age.

When neurons die, they are replaced with glial cells because, with some exceptions (read on to learn about these), we don't make new neurons as adults. Interestingly, the number of neurons in the brain stem remains fairly constant throughout life, perhaps because of the many regions in this part of the brain controlling vital physiological functions such as breathing and heart rate. The few places in the brain stem that do shrink with age are areas that, first, control the physiological response to stress and fear, and, second, produce dopamine, the so-called reward NT. A third region, the hippocampus, an important memory area in the middle of the brain, also shrinks with age.[6] We can, therefore, expect some changes in behaviors affected by these areas. In the hippocampus, for example, with age-related shrinkage, memory can be impaired.

So, if we don't lose that many neurons as we get older, why do our brains get smaller? Turns out that individual neurons shrink. Specifically, dendrites are lost.[7] Recall that **dendrites** are the branching portions of the neuron that "talk" to other neurons. In other words, most inputs to a neuron come through its dendrites. Remove this cross talk provided by dendrites, the neuron receives less information, and the system shrinks. Think about your cell phone connection: if some cell towers go offline, you can't make calls. Those same neuronal connections play a vital role in memory.

Dendrites are constantly being replaced throughout life. Of course, when they are lost, communication between neurons is reduced, but in general, this is not a contributing factor to cognitive decline. And if we stay healthy as we age (i.e., resist cardiovascular disease or metabolic disorders such as diabetes), neurotransmitter levels don't decrease much either.

That said, changes in NT levels can and do account for some changes in our brains with age. One of the best-known degenerative diseases of the nervous system is Parkinson's disease (**PD**). In PD, there is a decline in levels of dopamine, which controls the activity of some **motor neurons** (nerve cells that activate muscles). When dopamine drops while levels of **excitatory** neurotransmitters (that cause muscle activity) stay the same, small muscle contractions are not controlled. The characteristic PD tremor results.

Some sensory perceptions decline when neurons that detect this type of input die and are not replaced. What happens then? We don't hear, see, or smell as well as we once did. And as you lose some of this input, then the brain's output will be affected, too. This is why older people don't regulate temperature as well. Another function that is affected, as discussed in chapter 5, is the ability to control posture and balance. Yet another effect of aging is to reduce the speed of messages traveling through neurons. The result is slower reflexes. The good news is that we can learn to expect and compensate for this.

Unwelcome Gains. One thing we get more of with age is a yellowish-brown goo called **lipofuscin**. Lipofuscin accumulates in many organs as we age. Its origin is not well understood, but scientists think it is kind of a trash can for broken down cellular structures such as membranes and organelles. When these cellular components are damaged, say, by reactive oxygen (ROS), they are partially broken down and recycled. I talked about this process (autophagy) in chapter 3. **Autophagy**, like other processes, doesn't work as well as we age. The breakdown and recycling become less thorough, and the residual gunk is stuck together as lipofuscin. This may or may not be harmful in and of itself, but it does take up space in our cells, so other things that should be there get crowded out. The amount of lipofuscin varies a lot from one type of neuron to another, but it tends to accumulate more in large neurons in the cortex and in motor neurons.

Neurodegenerative Diseases May Be Due to Plaque and Tangles. Another type of stuff we get more of as we age is **plaques** and **tangles**. Plaques are globs of protein that accumulate between neurons in the brain, as shown in figure 8.2. So-called **amyloid plaques** are a characteristic hallmark of Alzheimer's disease (AD). Amyloid is a general term for protein fragments that the body produces normally. Beta amyloid, the type associated with AD, is a piece snipped from a specific protein found in the cell membrane of neurons. In a healthy brain, these protein fragments are broken down and eliminated. In AD, the fragments accumulate to form hard chunks called plaques. People with AD typically have a lot of these plaques, though people without the disease may have them, too. Many researchers think that large amounts of the plaque are toxic, thereby damaging neurons, but it's a hotly debated topic.

Plaque is formed when the starting protein is chopped up by enzymes to produce the fragments that clump together. The amyloid beta fragment is particularly toxic to synapses in neurons grown in the lab. Remember that the synapse is the place where neurons communicate, so damaging this contact can cause extensive disruption to the brain. This is one reason past therapies for AD targeting only specific synapses or NT types have failed. A promising new therapy involves targeting the enzyme that does the initial chopping. Called BACE inhibitors, these drugs are currently in clinical trials.[8]

Neurofibrillary tangles are globs of protein that accumulate inside neurons. In AD, the tangles consist primarily of a protein called **tau**. Normally, tau functions to move nutrients and other important substances from one part of the nerve cell to another. In AD, the tau protein has become abnormal and it eventually breaks down, causing the tangles to form. Of course, the normal function of tau is also lost, meaning that the neuron slowly starves. The end of the axon forming the synapse, which, of course, communicates with other neurons, is the first to go. As a result, affected neurons can't talk to other cells, and brain circuits start to break down.

Researchers have tried a lot of ways to clear out plaques and tangles in efforts to treat AD. None has worked. A recent finding in some AD patients that the plaques and tangles are due to **prion** activity provides hope for novel treatments.

Prion is not a word you come across routinely, and for a good reason. A prion is a protein or piece of a protein that has the wrong shape, called misfolded. This shape acts like an infection, by converting normal forms of the protein into the misfolded form, the prion. Then these newly created prions can do the same, and the process spreads. A prion is responsible for the brain-destroying disease known as mad cow disease. This prion cause of AD is most common in younger, early-onset patients, but less so in the elderly for reasons that are still not understood.[9]

It is probably no coincidence that the two most common neurodegenerative diseases of aging, AD and PD, are characterized by the loss of cells that take the biggest hits from aging. In the case of AD, these are **cortex** and **hippocampal** cells; in PD, **substantia nigra** neurons. The former cell types are critical in learning and memory whereas the latter impact movement.

Almost everyone experiences some declines in memory and motor performance with age. These functions depend on networks involving the neurons in the regions bolded in the preceding paragraph that are affected in AD and PD. But some memory or motor loss is normal with age and isn't a diagnosis of AD or PD. In other words, we will all experience age-related changes in our brains where the extreme end point is neurodegenerative disease—but most people don't live long enough to get there.

Unlike other chronic illnesses, AD is becoming more common in our aging population. Recent estimates suggest that AD has become the third leading cause of death in those over sixty-five in the United States after coronary disease and cancer. It's not surprising that many of us are concerned about it.

Problems Due to Changes in Blood Flow. The first—and possibly key event in the origin of many dementias—is impaired circulation to the brain. When you consider that neurons are large, metabolically active cells, the importance of good blood flow to the brain is obvious. The brain, which accounts for less than 5 percent of body weight (much less in some cases), uses almost 25 percent of the body's energy budget. Blood flow in the brain decreases when **nitric oxide (NO)** levels fall. Recall from chapter 7 the role of NO in the peripheral, or body, circulatory system, where it causes vessel dilation. A reduction in cerebral blood flow reduces the clearance of the plaque protein, beta amyloid, which then can build up to high levels in the brain of AD sufferers.[10]

The reduced blood flow is relatively easy to detect, and may be a good early diagnostic tool for AD. So what, you say; why bother with a diagnosis? For one thing, if you know you are at risk for developing AD, you can start implementing some of the lifestyle changes I describe later in the chapter. The culprit seems to be a type of blood cell called a white blood cell, which sticks to capillary walls, gumming up these little vessels. In mice that were genetically altered to have AD, treatment with an antibody that prevented the white blood cells from sticking to the capillaries restored blood flow. Like humans, these mice had lost memory, but this was restored by the antibody treatment, even in really old mice with advanced stages of Alzheimer's disease.[11]

In some cases, it may be beneficial to inhibit NO in the brain. Don't throw up your hands yet; read on. Researchers believe that when glia are activated and subsequently release inflammatory compounds, this process can contribute to the development of neurodegenerative diseases. If these glia can be inhibited, the degeneration of neurons might be blocked. **Securinine** is a natural product from a plant root used in the treatment of neurological conditions such as amyotrophic lateral sclerosis (ALS, aka Lou Gehrig's disease), poliomyelitis, and multiple sclerosis. A recent study from the Buck Institute for the Study of Aging found that securinine significantly suppressed nitric oxide (NO) production in a type of glia. They also found that an extract from cells grown in the lab, which had been treated with securinine, reduced the degeneration of neurons whose loss results in Parkinson's disease.[12] In addition, more iron accumulates in the brain as we age. Why? No one really knows. Iron is an essential component of many enzymes in the brain, but high concentrations of iron, a reactive substance, can contribute to oxidation damage. I'll have more to say about this shortly.

You may recall that I detailed some of the deleterious effects of **AGEs** (advanced glycation end products) in chapter 4. Guess what? These also build up in the brain, where they also cause problems because they gunk up the circulatory system.

WHY IS ALL OF THIS HAPPENING?

Energy Demands of Neurons. Neurons use a lot of energy. The brain, which is only about 5 percent of your body weight at most, can suck off more than 20 percent of your body's total energy supply. That happens for two reasons: first, neurons are really big relative to other cells. Simply transporting nutrients around these big cells takes a lot of energy. Second, neurons have to maintain a constant electrical charge in order to send their signals. It's like needing to have your phone constantly plugged in to work.

Getting energy from food means that your mitochondria have to be active. And you no doubt recall that the more the mitochondria are active, the greater the potential for ROS (reactive oxygen species, or free radical) production. In excess, ROS can damage proteins, membranes, DNA, and, of course, the mitochondria themselves. Damaged mitochondria are not only less efficient at generating energy, thus limiting the activity of the neurons, but are also more likely to produce even more ROS. If DNA in neurons is damaged, as autopsies have shown, important genes won't function, which will also adversely affect the neuron's activity.[13]

Low Oxygen Level. As you learned in the previous chapter, age is a risk factor for coronary disease (CVD). When the heart doesn't pump effectively, even for brief periods, oxygen levels in the blood fall. In addition to increasing the production of ROS by mitochondria, low oxygen levels in the brain cause an increased release of a neurotransmitter called NMDA. This NT, in turn, allows more calcium into neurons. Too much of anything can wreak havoc in cells, and excessive calcium in neurons is no exception; it can disable or kill the cell.[14]

Inflammation. Yes, even in the brain. I wrote a lot about the mechanism of inflammation in chapter 3 as this is a biggie in the aging process. One recently recognized aspect of inflammation is a specific set of symptoms that cytokines, those inflammatory compounds introduced in chapter 5, generate in the brain. These include fever and associated metabolic effects such as loss of appetite, as well as some behavioral changes, including fatigue, depression, and mild cognitive impairment. These behavioral effects are collectively called "sickness behavior." **Microglia**, the immune system of the brain, along with the brain's vascular system, initiate and sustain these behavioral changes.[15]

We are all familiar with this sickness behavior when we are fighting off a bug. The fatigue and depression can be adaptive, causing us to lie low, saving resources to the immune system for healing. This behavior can become entrenched, however, if the inflammation persists, and can even exacerbate neurological conditions. For instance, AD patients with high levels of inflammation experienced much greater cognitive declines following bacterial infections than did AD patients who were not sick and consequently had low inflammation.[16]

In mice, it's possible to remove the microglial cells. Why would you want to do this? Well, just as in other tissues, these cells can become senescent (another factor contributing to aging that was introduced in chapter 3) and start cranking out chemical cocktails that may contribute to inflammation. When researchers killed off the microglia in mice, the cells grew back in a few weeks, and the lab treated animals did better on a number of tests that measure cognitive function in mice. Of course, doing better on tests of spatial ability and displaying lower levels of anxiety may not measure up to our hopes of restored cognitive function. The treated animals still showed enhanced inflammation. What do these results mean? It could be that microglial replacement would be a step in restoring or protecting cognitive function. That's debatable. It does seem that the aged brain, aside from its microglia, may be doing something else that causes the inflammation. These are preliminary results and definitely need further study.

Role of mTOR. I introduced **mTOR** in chapter 3. It may not surprise you that, due to its central role in cellular metabolism, it can greatly affect brain function. Specifically, mTOR has been implicated in the development of Alzheimer's disease and other dementias. To understand how this can happen, we have to back up and look at the brain's circulatory system. Like other body organs, the brain relies on continuous blood flow pumped by the heart. This amounts to about 15 percent of total cardiac output in typical adults. The delicate tissue and metabolic demands of the brain require a tightly regulated blood pressure within the brain: too much pressure, and tissue is damaged; too little, and not enough oxygen is delivered, with subsequent problems.

Experiments, primarily with rodents, have shown that even a slight decrease below the optimal pressure can result in cognitive impairment, synaptic changes (not usually good ones), and beta amyloid fragments sticking together (a precursor to plaque).

What's important about mTOR is that it decreases the amount of nitric oxide (NO) in the brain. Recall that NO is important in the vascular system as it causes dilation of the endothelial layer in blood vessels, allowing for increased blood flow. Conversely, blocking mTOR with **rapamycin**, an mTOR blocker that I revisit in detail in chapter 10, reverses the effect. Lifestyle modifications, such as exercise and low-carb diets (especially the ketogenic diet; more on this in chapter 9), have also been shown to alter the activity of mTOR. A related factor is that decreased circulation in the brain reduces the natural clearance of waste products such as beta amyloid, which are typically removed by internal blood flow. Rapamycin also increases the rate of clearance of beta amyloid.[17]

WHAT TO DO?

Exercise. The beneficial effect of exercise on brain health should come as no surprise. Since the 1970s, researchers have found that older athletes have outperformed nonathletes on a variety of perceptual, cognitive, and motor tasks. Though, these are typically modest effects, they persist for decades after the initial assessment and continue going in the right direction. Amazingly, frontal cortex and hippocampus actually grow in size with regular aerobic exercise.

When scientists combined different studies (remember my caveat on this procedure), they were able to pinpoint very specific benefits resulting from exercise:[18]

- executive function (a higher-order mental process characterized by attentiveness, focus, and organization) increased more than other cognitive processes
- women got more benefit than men
- combining strength training and aerobic exercise produced more gains than aerobic training alone
- working out for longer than thirty minutes was more beneficial than shorter sessions

An added benefit to frequent aerobic exercise, at least in mice, is that it protects against damage to the retina that results in glaucoma.

A Deep Dive into Why Exercise Is So Good for Our Brains

What about exercise challenges for the brain? Here's where we have to take a trip down evolution lane. **Hominins** (the group that includes modern humans and our close extinct relatives) split from the group that includes our closest living relatives, chimpanzees and bonobos, some six million years ago. In that time, hominins evolved a number of anatomical and behavioral adaptations that distinguish us from other primates. Two of these evolutionary changes may have provided the link between exercise and brain function that is still important to modern humans.

First, our ancestors shifted from walking on all fours to walking upright. This so-called **bipedal posture** means that at times our bodies are precariously balanced over one foot rather than two or more limbs as in apes. Your brain has to integrate a lot of positional and sensory input data and then generate the appropriate muscle control output just for you to stay balanced. At the same time, our ancestors would have had to be watching for bumps in the trail, possible predators, and, of course, any food that might be lying around. Just because we are bipedal, our brains were more cognitively challenged than those of our four-legged ancestors.

Second, the hominin way of life involved more aerobic activity. By two million years ago, the environment of these ancestral hominins was cooling and drying; the plants they had eaten previously began to disappear. Hunting and gathering replaced the earlier subsistence vegetarian diet, for nearly two million years, until agriculture was developed about ten thousand years ago.

Hunter-gatherers have to travel longer distances than our more sedentary vegetarian primate cousins. This travel means more aerobic exercise in our evolutionary past.

If you are traveling farther, you have to store more location data in your brain so you can get home. This suggests a link between bigger travel distances and growth of the hippocampus, the region of the brain primarily involved in storing memory. In addition, hunter-gatherers have to process sensory information about food availability, another task that challenges the hippocampus. And, they have to make decisions and plan their routes— cognitive tasks supported by the hippocampus and the prefrontal cortex, as well as other brain regions. Hunter-gatherers also often forage in groups, in which case they may have conversations while their brains are maintaining their balance and keeping them spatially located in their environment. All of this multitasking is controlled, in part, by the prefrontal cortex, which also tends to diminish with age.

Modern humans don't have to travel long distances to get food unless we have a long drive to the grocery story. The brain atrophy and memory and cognitive declines that often occur during aging may be related to our new (in an evolutionary sense) sedentary habits. But just going for a couple runs a week may not be the best thing you can do to reverse these declines. If the link between exercise and brain growth evolved due to the challenges I described above, then our exercise regime should incorporate some cognitive activity. That could potentially increase the ability of exercise to boost our thought processes as we age and potentially alter the course of neurodegenerative diseases such as Alzheimer's.

The combination works in mice. When mice exercised in a cognitively enriched environment where they had access to a variety of sensory stimuli, the result was better than in a boring cage. There was an additive effect: exercise alone was good for the hippocampus, but combining physical activity with cognitive demands in a stimulating environment was even better, leading to even more new neurons. Using the brain during and after exercise seems to improve the survival of the new cells.

Extending this idea into people is just beginning in laboratory experiments, but no reason to wait. In fact, I suspect a lot of us already incorporate cognitive challenges into our workout routines. It's more interesting to walk or run trails than roads, and more fun to hike or bike with friends while you carry on a conversation. So, keep it up. You're reprising your ancient hunter-gatherer ancestors, who blessed us with these big brains.[19]

Diet.[20] Diet is emerging as an important protective factor for brain health. Many studies show a diet rich in fruits, vegetables, and nuts is protective of brain health as well as cardiovascular health. The protective role of fruits in particular may be due to their flavonoid compounds, which have the ability to inhibit inflammatory effects of the brain's microglia. Flavenoid is a catch-all term for compounds made by plants in our diets that have health benefits. These findings support diets such as the Mediterranean and DASH that are high in plant foods and monounsaturated oils. Recent studies have also shown a protective effect of the high-fat ketogenic diet on cognitive abilities. These findings are not necessarily at odds with one another: the Mediterranean and similar diets are high in carbs (though these are good carbs as opposed to highly processed ones) whereas ketogenic diets are low in carbs. First, individuals vary in their metabolism, so the diet that works for me may not work for you. Second, exercise and lifestyle (e.g., dietary restriction) can keep blood sugar low despite a diet containing relatively high levels of carbs. Although large clinical trials have not yet been done on the efficacy of such diets as protective against cognitive decline, Dr. Steven Masley has described a number of smaller trials he has conducted supporting a similar diet. As always, keep in mind my caveats about small sample size and uncontrolled studies that I spelled out in the first chapter.

Good Fats, Bad Fats. Numerous large studies of older adults (one combined analysis examined 23,688 adults over the age of sixty-five) highlight the protective effect of long-chain omega-3 fatty acids, typically found in cold-water fish such as salmon or tuna, to cognitive health.[21] The long-term Chicago Health and Aging Project found that higher total intake of omega-3 fats was significantly associated with a lower risk for AD. One of these fats, DHA, provided the strongest association; a second one, EPA, had no association; and a third, α-linolenic acid, was associated with lower risk only among persons with the APOE-ε4 allele, which is a known risk factor for AD.[22]

I don't make any dietary recommendation regarding cholesterol, as views seem to change yearly. However, cholesterol may be an important player in AD. For example, cholesterol is involved in both the generation and deposition of amyloid beta. The single most important genetic risk factor for AD is a gene known as APOE-ε4, which produces the main cholesterol transporter in the brain (more on this in the final section in this chapter, on the role of genes). Experiments in animals have shown that diets that produce high blood levels of cholesterol also increase amyloid beta deposits in the brain. Conversely, the animals whose diets contained mostly unsaturated fat were faster learners and had better memories.[23] I want to stress that this subject is really controversial, and opinions are changing rapidly at this time. Later in the chapter I will give you some resources that will update you on the current views.

Although the internet teems with claims for the role of various supplements in protecting against cognitive decline, clinical trials are lacking. An important exception is the B vitamin, **folate**. Folate is essential for brain development and function. Low folate status or high homocysteine levels (which accumulates if you are low in folate) are associated with cognitive dysfunction in aging. You may have come across references on the internet to homocysteine testing. This is a way to determine whether you are low in folate. You can refer to figure 3.1 if you want more detail as to how folate is involved in regulating homocysteine.

Another caveat is warranted here: if you've come across references to homocysteine, you've probably seen recommendations to have your MTHFR gene tested. (If not, don't worry about it.) But if you've been considering it, most of the stuff I've seen about the role of MTHFR is gross oversimplification. Many people claim that if you have certain forms of the gene (aka **SNPs**, or **variants**, also discussed in chapter 3), you will have problems with **methylation** (some call this, incorrectly, detoxification). MTHFR is one of many genes involved in this important process, which, among other things, repairs DNA damage and helps break down toxic and unnecessary substances in the body. Think of methylation, which simply means adding methyl (a carbon plus three hydrogens) to other molecules, as a relay race. The MTHFR is the fastest runner, so with some variants your team will be slower, but most forms still work. Evidence exists for supplementing with other B vitamins. (Folate, which is essentially the same as folic acid, is one of the many B vitamins.) In a two-year randomized, placebo-controlled trial, 168 elderly subjects with mild cognitive impairment were given daily doses of 800 µg of folic acid, 500 µg of vitamin B_{12}, and 20 mg of vitamin B_6. Both groups had experienced the shrinkage in brain regions typically caused by AD. Further, this atrophy correlated with cognitive decline. The good news is that the loss was smaller in the group taking the B vitamins. A greater benefit was seen in subjects who had higher homocysteine levels at the start of the study. Thus, lowering homocysteine may be one component in preventing cognitive decline and dementia.[24] Clearly, the role of B-vitamin supplementation should be studied in larger, longer-lasting trials.

Finally, and this may seem like beating a dead horse, **caloric restriction (CR)** can maintain brain function. CR can achieve this through several pathways, including increased repair and maintenance activity in neurons and enhanced production of protective proteins. In addition, simply avoiding the metabolic activity associated with excessive food intake can minimize many of the risk factors for cognitive decline such as high cholesterol and blood pressure.[25]

Brush Your Teeth. New studies are showing that the bacteria that cause gum disease can get into the brain, where they trigger damage to the proteins involved in AD. If you want more information: the bacteria produce compounds that chop up brain proteins, and voila! The fragments that are implicated in AD are produced. In mice, a drug that sops up the bacterial products reversed the production of amyloid (that chopped up brain protein found in the brains of people with AD). A preliminary clinical trial in people yielded similar results; larger trials are in the works.[26]

Other infections have also been implicated in the development of AD. These findings support a protective role of the precursor protein whose breakdown results in amyloid plaque. The integrative approach, described below, includes assessment of bacterial or viral infections and treatment as one aspect of AD treatment.

Integrative Approaches. Despite numerous efforts, drug treatments for AD have not panned out. In fact, of the thousands of drugs tested in this effort, less than 1 percent have been approved by the FDA. Three currently are marketed for early, moderate AD. These are all drugs, called **cholinesterase inhibitors**, that block the action of an enzyme that breaks down a neurotransmitter (NT) called **acetylcholine**.

No one understands why inhibiting the enzyme, which prolongs the action of the NT, works to reduce the symptoms of dementia. One hypothesis is that acetylcholine is an important NT in the communication pathways among brain regions involved in attention, memory, and cognitive activity. Inhibiting the breakdown of acetylcholine can improve memory, as well as helping people with AD or dementia from Parkinson's to remain independent and retain their personality. It seems to be more effective in people with a more aggressive form of dementia (e.g., those with younger onset ages, poor nutritional status, or experiencing symptoms such as delusions or hallucinations).

A fourth type of drug, memantine, approved for more severe AD, affects the activity of a different NT. Unfortunately, like the cholinesterase inhibitors, its beneficial effect is limited while its side effects can be severe. That said, some evidence shows that combining one of the cholinesterase inhibitors (called rivastigmine, brand name Exelon) with memantine can improve memory and mood in some people.[27] This conclusion is based on a meta-analysis of a small number of studies, each of which had relatively few subjects. (And you may recall my hesitancy, expressed in chapter 1, on meta-analyses.) The improvement the authors describe is small, but it is an average. Some currently unidentifiable subset of us may benefit significantly from such a treatment. But all of the drugs can have side effects, making this choice a serious one.

This lack of drug therapies has led some researchers to look for alternatives. Intensive study over the past few decades has uncovered many potential causal factors for AD. A group at the Buck Institute for the Study of Aging has worked on identifying and using these factors, which include blood sugar and hormone and stress levels to develop a personalized approach for the treatment of cognitive decline due to neurodegenerative disease such as Alzheimer's. This approach, which has shown some success in small trials, is similar in concept to individualized immune therapies for cancer in that each person is evaluated for a panel of **biomarkers**—measures that are easily collected such as cholesterol, homocysteine, blood sugar, and so forth—that can be combined to generate a personalized therapy program.[28]

A similar approach was pioneered by a large interdisciplinary group at Weill Cornell Medicine and New York-Presbyterian Hospital, focusing on prevention. They, and other researchers, identified a number of risk factors for AD. Some of these are modifiable by lifestyle changes, such as exercise, blood sugar level, and blood pressure. Others factors are not changeable, such as age (the biggest risk factor for AD) and genetics. By combining data on each individual patient for these risk factors, and cognitive assessments, it's possible to predict future risk and determine a personalized strategy to reduce it. Interestingly, the biggest effects on risk reduction came from exercise and diet.[29]

An exciting therapy currently in an early stage of clinical trials is a vaccine against the beta amyloid protein. Remember that this is the chopped-up piece of a normal protein found in the brains of people with AD. The vaccine was shown to be effective in animal studies. In an early trial in people with mild AD, the vaccine did not cause any side effects and did activate an immune response. Ongoing trials are underway to determine whether the vaccine can reduce symptoms.[30]

Supplements, Nutraceuticals, Other Drugs. In chapter 10, I survey many alternative chemical treatments purported to extend health span and improve quality of life. Hold on till then, or skip ahead, to learn about the ability of stimulants, such as Adderall, hormones, vitamins, and other compounds to improve cognitive ability. Spoiler alert: evidence is sparse for most of these things.

Early Life Experiences. Several studies have reported that more cognitive activity early in life (building reading and writing abilities) correlated with a lower rate of cognitive decline later in life.[31] This finding raises the speculation that we can build up a reservoir of cognitive ability early that can protect us later in life. The intriguing question is: How much earlier do we have to engage in this training?

Brain Training. What do crossword puzzles, KenKen, Sudoku, and Luminosity all have in common? Lots of press touting their ability to enhance your cognitive ability. We have no evidence that these brain-training activities do anything except teach you to improve crosswords, Sudoku, and so forth. In fact, by spending time on these activities, you do fewer of those that actually can improve your mental abilities such as exercise or socializing.[32]

Vision and Hearing Loss. As we know, both of these impairments become commonplace with age. Less well known is that they are also risk factors for cognitive decline. Loss of visual ability affects 37 million Americans older than fifty years and one in four after eighty years. Most cases of vision loss in older patients are due to four common problems. Because good evidence shows that vision loss is a risk factor for cognitive decline, I describe prevalent causes and some available treatments.[33]

Macular degeneration is caused by the deterioration of part of the retina, the back layer of the eye that records the images we see and sends them from the eye to the brain. The retina is like film in old-fashioned cameras; the optic nerve carries that image to the brain. Macular degeneration is the leading cause of vision loss in the United States.[34] Vitamin supplements can delay its progression, and recently a drug has been developed that can preserve vision in some types of the disease.

Glaucoma is caused by fluid buildup in the front part of the eye. The extra fluid increases pressure in your eye, which damages the optic nerve. Once damaged, the nerve cannot be restored, but some treatments can prevent further damage. Medicated eye drops can delay the progression of vision loss in patients with glaucoma. The drops can reduce the amount of fluid the eye makes. Alternatively, other types can improve the natural drainage system of the eye. Two types of laser procedure have also been developed to relieve the pressure caused by some forms of glaucoma.[35]

Diabetes. One of the many side effects of diabetes is damage to the eye. The high blood-sugar level characteristic of the disease can damage the retina. Diabetes is also a risk factor for glaucoma and cataracts, as well as a less common problem called diabetic macular edema. Good control of blood sugar slows the damage, but in older adults, if blood sugar drops too low, the consequences can be serious. There are several treatment options, although, again, the damage can't be reversed.[36]

Cataracts become increasingly common as we age. In the United States, more than half of people over the age of eighty have cataracts. This form of vision loss is due to changes in the lens. The lens of the eye is a clear area that focuses light on the retina. The proteins in the lens focus the images we see. As we age, the proteins stick together, clouding the lens and reducing the light that reaches the retina. The clouding may become severe enough to cause blurred vision. Corrective glasses may help during the early stages, but as the blurring increases, the only effective treatment is surgery. Cataract removal is one of the most common operations performed in the United States. It also is one of the safest and most effective types of surgery. In about 90 percent of cases, people who have cataract surgery have better vision afterward.[37]

Sleep. A lot of studies on older adults with sleep apnea or other breathing issues have shown that these people have more cognitive issues and dementias than non-affected adults. In larger study populations where researchers have looked specifically at sleep quality (e.g., insomnia) there is an association between limited sleep and poor cognitive function. An increasing number of studies are showing a protective role of sleep in neurodegenerative diseases as well as other conditions. Although experimental studies so far are in short supply, they do suggest that good sleep could improve cognitive functioning in the aged.[38]

Poor sleep and shorter sleep times decrease your insulin sensitivity because growth hormone and cortisol levels are higher in the night when you are awake. These hormones, in turn, decrease your brain's ability to use glucose effectively. Melatonin is increasingly being used to treat sleep disturbances in AD and may reduce the risks associated with poor sleep. I revisit this topic in chapter 9 on actions you can take to improve health span.

Manage CVD Risk Factors. Due to the association between poor circulation and neurodegenerative disease and dementias, this caveat is clearly important. These factors include blood pressure, smoking, and diabetes. *Medication Alert.* Some drugs can affect cognitive and emotional states. Opioids (pain-relieving narcotics), benzodiazepines (a type of sedative), and anticholinergics (these block the action of the NT acetylcholine) carry an especially high risk of cognitive impairment. This risk increases when combined with other medications, a common practice in the elderly population. Be aware of this possibility and investigate potential side effects of all new medicines. This includes so-called nutraceuticals and even supplements and over-the-counter drugs, which can interact with prescription medications. High alcohol intake is an often-overlooked risk factor for dementia and cognitive impairment among older adults.

What Not to Do. Smoking is a big one, mainly because of its link to coronary disease, and as discussed above, how that can affect brain health. Smoking also contributes to stroke risk, which has obvious, often life-changing effects on brain health. Some evidence suggests that smoking in and of itself can have detrimental effects on cognitive ability, but the data are far from clear. Similarly, although limited research suggests that marijuana may affect cognition, these studies are not compelling.

Stress is another risk factor for cognitive decline and memory loss. Some 112 subjects in the Boston Longitudinal Study were followed for more than ten years and assessed for both daily stress and memory. Self-reported daily stress levels and higher cortisol (a blood biomarker of stress) were associated with more memory problems.[39] The same relationship between stress and cognitive performance was seen in more than six thousand older adults followed for almost seven years in the Chicago Health and Aging Project.[40]

Another potential contraindication is elective surgery. Anyone who has had general anesthetic knows the confusion that follows. Most of us recover quickly. Persistent suggestions are that this recovery is delayed in the elderly and could be due to pre-surgical conditions. A plethora of recent, but small, studies suggest there is no risk from anesthetic. Of course, you know the problems associated with small studies. Keep watching for more results on this topic, especially if you are considering elective surgery.

Finally, if you or those close to you are depressed, this is a risk factor for cognitive decline. Although the mechanism by which depression could affect cognition is not understood, some possibilities are heightened stress hormones such as cortisone, inflammation, and even increased production of beta amyloid fragments.[41] Given that depression is increasingly prevalent with age, this is a risk factor that should be monitored.

WHAT ABOUT MY GENES?[42]

As is the case for cardiovascular disease, a growing number of genes are implicated in the function and health of our nervous systems and cognitive health. Thus, the list that follows is constantly changing. The SNPedia.com site is an excellent resource for searching for genes and their effects in many diseases. Remember, in order to apply much of this information to yourself or another individual, you need access to specific data on your genes, such as that supplied by a growing number of commercial operations. I discussed this in depth in chapter 3 in the section on genes.

Presenilin. The protein produced by this gene plays a part in producing the amyloid protein that accumulates in AD. Some variants of this gene are known to cause early-onset forms of AD, which run in families.

ApoE. This gene codes for the main actor in the brain that moves cholesterol around. You can think of this creature as the Amazon delivery truck. Because of the important role of cholesterol in cell membranes, changes in its delivery system could affect brain health. It has three common forms, or alleles. Having one or two copies of one of them (the ApoE4 allele) puts you at increased risk for late-onset Alzheimer's disease. A second form (the E2 allele) is somewhat protective, and the most common form (the E3 allele) appears neutral for an AD risk.

The ApoE4 allele is not a direct determinant of AD—at least a third of patients with Alzheimer's disease don't have one, and some people with two copies never develop the disease. Overall, people with two copies have about a fifteenfold higher risk of developing Alzheimer's than those with the E3 form. These numbers reiterate a critical, but often forgotten, caveat of genetics. Genes are like blueprints. The way the genes are "interpreted" by our cells can be influenced by many lifestyle factors. It's extremely rare that a genetic instruction is expressed identically in everyone with the same form.

Amyloid Precursor Protein (APP). The APP gene codes for amyloid precursor protein. Remember, this is a shorthand way of saying the instructions for building the protein are found in this gene. The APP protein occurs in cell membranes and as such could be implicated in the activity of neurons. Its function is not known, but it has been implicated as playing a role in synapse formation and possibly iron export. APP is the parent of beta amyloid, which, in turn, is the major player in the plaque found in the brains of Alzheimer's disease patients. About twenty mutations in the APP gene are believed to be associated with AD.

TREM2 (Triggering Receptor Expressed on Myeloid Cells). A rare mutation in this gene causes a significant risk of AD, probably because of its anti-inflammatory function. The normal protein is believed to prevent the buildup of plaque.

CR1 (clusterin). Several forms of this gene, also known as APOJ, which plays a role in cleaning out waste products from cells, have been identified. One allele has a slight protective effect, while another increases the risk for late-onset AD.

CCL11 (C-C Motif Chemokine 11 or Eotaxin-1). This gene codes for eotaxin-1, an inflammatory protein. Eotaxin is found in the fluid bathing the brain and spinal cord. It increases with age and may contribute to the drop in neuron number observed with age. Several small studies found that people with one form of this gene may be protected from AD.

CONCLUSION

Maintaining our cognitive health is a priority for all of us as we age. Research in this area is relatively recent, and results are constantly changing, making it difficult to come up with many absolute pronouncements. That said, there are a few incontrovertible suggestions. First, stay active as long as possible. Exercise is good for the body, which means it is good for the brain. Avoid stress as much as possible. Exercise also helps relieve stress; more on this in the final chapter. And finally, eat well, which, though controversial, seems to mean fewer carbs, especially processed carbs; more on this in the final chapter as well. Dr. Rhonda Patrick has an excellent website, which she updates frequently, posting new findings in this area.[43]

ACRONYMS

AD: Alzheimer's disease
AGEs: Advanced glycation end products
ALS: Amyotrophic lateral sclerosis, aka Lou Gehrig's disease
CR: Caloric restriction
CVD: Cardiovascular disease
DHA: A fatty acid important in building cell membranes
EPA: Another fatty acid important in building cell membranes
FDA: Food and Drug Administration
MRI: Magnetic resonance imaging
fMRI: Functional magnetic resonance imaging
MTHFR: A gene important in the production of homocysteine
mTOR: Target of rapamycin, a protein that controls cellular activity
NMDA: An activating neurotransmitter
NO: Nitrous oxide
NT: Neurotransmitter
PD: Parkinson's disease
ROS: Reactive oxygen species, aka free radicals

9

Interventions Part 1

Actions You Can Take

We don't know how soon we're going to defeat aging. We should be able to keep people truly in a youthful state of health, no matter how long they live and that means the risk of death will not rise. —Aubrey de Grey, aging researcher

OVERVIEW

Well, by now you may be feeling overwhelmed by everything that happens to your body's systems as you age. Although dying is inevitable, poor health, by and large, is not. Sure, a lot of genes put you at risk for some diseases, but beneficial genes also give you a better chance at good health. In both cases, your environment, which includes the food you eat, the amount you sleep, and your stress level, will have an impact on the effects of your genes. You can take a lot of actions to improve long-term outcomes. Some of these actions will affect your genes, but most have a more direct effect, acting on specific body systems. Some of these may extend your life span, but the most important effect, in my humble opinion, is the benefit they confer to your **health span**—the portion of one's life lived in good health.

I've introduced many of these actions throughout the book, but in this chapter, I put them together and review the evidence supporting them and the most effective forms you can practice. The lifestyle actions, which I call **behavioral interventions**, are probably the most effective current means for promoting health and slowing the detrimental effects of aging. In other words, you can take these actions without supplements or drugs. For some people, these are easy, and for others, for various reasons, they are difficult. For this latter group, drug developers are working to identify the cellular mechanisms that account for the health-promoting benefits of these behaviors in order to target them with drugs. I will discuss some of these strategies in the next chapter along with supplements and nutritional compounds (called "**nutraceuticals**") that show promise in retarding aging.

The two best-known such interventions are caloric, or more broadly, dietary restriction and exercise. They are relatively inexpensive and have proven to be extremely effective in affecting health span and, possibly, life span. However, as a glance around any developed society will tell you, these may be the most difficult ways for many of us to achieve those desired effects. Thus, the search for pharmaceutical or "nutraceutical" options for achieving the same ends.[1]

Caloric Restriction (CR)

CR reduces calorie intake without causing malnutrition or impacting intake of essential nutrients. Clearly, reduce is a relative term. The reduction can be defined relative to your own intake or to an average person of similar body type. Caloric restriction is the most studied and robust nonpharmacological intervention for extending health span and life span in a range of animal models. In these studies, the reduction is typically about 30 percent below what the animal would eat left to its own devices. In yeast, fruit flies, and nematode worms, CR extends life span by 200–300 percent, which translates to a life span 2–3 times normal. And the animals stay healthier for most of that time. CR in some rats and mice prolongs life span by 50 percent and prevents or delays the onset of many chronic diseases, such as obesity, type 2 diabetes, cancer, cardiac disease, neurodegenerative diseases, and some autoimmune diseases.

In general, CR extends life span more in smaller animals than in humans and other primates. This makes sense from an evolutionary perspective. Think about the proportion of a mouse's life span (probably no more than a year in the wild) that would be affected by a season of famine. Yes, a big percentage. Then recall that the main evolutionary impetus for life extension is to extend the time the animal has to reproduce, as I discussed in chapter 2. Thus, a mouse that starves for a bad summer would need to extend its life span by at least a few months, or 50 percent, in order to reproduce. For humans, one bad summer is not a big percentage of a thirty-year life span, which may have characterized our ancestors, so we can't expect to gain as much as a mouse, but we can gain in health span.

Two long-term studies in primates (monkeys), despite some design problems, illustrate benefits of CR. As in humans, our primate cousins develop the same set of age-related diseases such as diabetes, cardiovascular disease, sarcopenia, bone loss, altered immune function, and cognitive decline. In both studies, CR monkeys lived longer and healthier than their counterparts who ate as much as they wanted, despite both studies using what I consider to be pretty awful diets. Because these (and other primate studies) brought in animals of different ages and changed some of their methods midway, it's hard to say just how much longer the CR monkeys lived, but their improved health was striking. In both studies, decreasing calories also decreased age-related diseases, such as heart disease, by more than 50 percent.

So, what about CR in humans? Caloric reduction was probably the norm for much of human history, but because malnutrition typically accompanies periods of famine, it's hard to tease out the effect of eating fewer calories. In one famous example during World War II, residents of Oslo experienced a 20 percent CR without malnutrition (because the Norwegian government rationed food) for four years, from 1941 to 1945. During this time, mortality was 30 percent lower than prewar level in both sexes.[2]

A number of clinical trials in humans support the benefits of CR. Interestingly, subjects on CR did not have less energy available for physical activity. In other words, despite eating fewer calories, they could expend just as many calories in typical activities such as walking, sitting, sleeping, and so forth. One explanation for this counterintuitive result could be that sensitivity to **insulin**, the hormone that controls blood sugar and fat storage, improved with CR. This sensitivity is a measure of how well and rapidly you respond to carbohydrates. In other words, you get more bang for your buck from the calories you do take in. It's like having a more fuel-efficient car: you can drive further on less gas. Another factor has to do with mitochondrial activity, and I'll revisit this shortly.

Even in young people, 25 percent CR for six months resulted in a reduction of almost 30 percent in the ten-year risk for cardiovascular disease. In this study, the subjects were assessed for risk factors for CVD such as total and HDL cholesterol, blood pressure, and age. Measures of **oxidative stress**, which is a measure of damaged **mitochondria** (see chapter 3), declined with CR; and in muscles, the number of mitochondria increased by 35 percent. If that's not enough, numerous other markers for health improve with CR (as well as other forms of dietary restriction), including fat, both total and visceral, osteoporosis, brain health, arthritis, sarcopenia (remember muscle loss from chapter 5), diabetes, colon health, incidence of cancer, and inflammation.[3]

Dietary Restrictions

Despite the evidence supporting the health and longevity benefits of CR, how many of us embrace cutting our food intake by 30 percent below what would keep us at a "normal" weight? Right, not too many of us. And, my guess is that long term, CR probably isn't healthy, especially as we age, when we require more protein (which I discussed in chapter 5). In many individuals older than 75–80 years, it is difficult to maintain body weight, which would also argue against CR in that population. Fortunately for us slackers, we have other, less painful ways to mimic CR.

Intermittent fasting (IF) is one promising alternative. IF strategies include alternate day fasting (eating every other day), as well as interval approaches (e.g., the "5:2 diet"—normal food intake five days of the week combined with fasting or significant calorie reduction two days a week). But fasting for one or two days is still tough. And, although the weight loss that goes along with both CR and IF is good for many people, it could be problematic for normal-weight older adults due to age-related declines in muscle mass and bone density. A more feasible approach is **time-restricted feeding (TRF)**, or a specially formulated diet that "mimics" fasting (**fasting-mimicking diets [FMDs]**). Under TRF, normal calorie intake is confined to a 6–12-hour window, and you fast for the remainder of the day. An example of this time window, which is easiest for me, is to eat an early dinner, between 5 and 6 p.m., then skip breakfast and eat my first meal of the following day between noon and 1 p.m. Longer fasts are certainly more difficult, but many people regularly engage in them, either for health or spiritual reasons. One intriguing benefit of fasting from the animal literature is that both long fasts and FMDs promote the toxic effects of chemotherapy in cancer cells, while simultaneously enabling normal cells to resist the toxicity and regenerate more rapidly after treatment.[4]

After all that, I have to say that researchers have reached no agreement on how long to restrict your fasting period. There aren't any completed studies in humans to pin this down. At this point, the evidence for the beneficial effect of DR is strong. I play around with it a lot because I believe in it. You should certainly read some of the references in the notes if you want to pursue it and make up your own mind.

Macronutrient restriction. Now that you're convinced that CR is beneficial, I'll muddy the waters. When researchers limited only lipid calories in mice, without reducing their caloric intake, their life span showed no benefit. When protein was restricted, while allowing the animals to feast away, the life span increase was half of what was seen with pretty restrictive CR. What?

Recall the role of the **mTOR** system (which I introduced in chapter 3 and discuss in more detail below) on life span. Briefly, mTOR is like an orchestra conductor integrating many independent inputs that together produce the metabolic pathways that build us up. When protein is reduced, mTOR slows down. Less rampant growth, in turn, means that your cells have to be more efficient, cleaning up and recycling anything that's not essential. Interestingly, restricting just a single amino acid (methionine), out of the twenty that humans use to build proteins, has the same life extension effect. The slowdown wanes a bit less when plant proteins are substituted for animal sources, suggesting a protective role for plants.[5] However, as I discussed in detail in chapter 5, protein requirements increase with age, partially because aging digestive systems become less efficient at extracting the amino acid building blocks from our foods.

Another macronutrient whose restriction has been shown to be beneficial is carbohydrate. Yes, I know, for years we were told to eat a high-carb, low-fat diet, but, as you know by now, these dietary recommendations are based primarily on epidemiological studies. These studies have a number of problems, which I talked about in chapter 1. Many recent studies (and, yes, take these with a grain of salt, too) show that restricting carbohydrate in an otherwise unrestricted diet confers longevity and health benefits.[6] The advantage to looking at recent studies is that science learns from previous work by incorporating earlier findings into new predictions and tests. New findings include better understanding of how carbohydrates affect insulin and the variety of body systems that insulin controls. Remember that when you eat a carbohydrate meal, your pancreas releases insulin, which normally activates your body cells, especially muscle and liver, to grab the sugar in your blood (which results from rapid breakdown of carbs). Eat a diet high in carbs, though, especially the simple sugars found in processed foods, and the body is constantly releasing insulin. And, sugar in your blood that isn't pulled out by cells that need it is rapidly sent off to storage in fat cells.

All of the body systems I discussed in this book are affected in one way or another by insulin and, more important, by the development of resistance to insulin. You can think of insulin resistance as the little boy who cried wolf. Too much insulin, released too often, and our cells quit listening. What happens? Blood sugar levels rise. The most prevalent and damaging consequence is type 2 diabetes, but high blood sugar has various other nasty effects. You've already heard about some of these, like glycation of proteins (see chapter 4), inflammation (see chapter 3), and neuronal damage (see chapter 8). In addition, insulin also tells your fat cells to pull sugar out of the blood and store it as fat. It's not surprising that an increase in obesity has accompanied high-carb diets, and the prevalence of insulin as a treatment for type 2 diabetes.

A Deep Dive into How Energy Restrictions Work

Basically, reducing calorie intake, whether for your lifetime or a twelve-hour window, seems to have the same effects on your cells. Many of these effects are processes that I introduced in chapter 3. Let's revisit the appropriate cellular and molecular processes to answer this question of how CR/IF/TRF all work.

First, remember the vital role your **mitochondria** play in your life. Without these little guys in your cells, and most of your cells have hundreds of them, constantly cranking away, making the all-essential ATP, the energy currency of the body, you would be dead in minutes. Fewer calories mean less input into the bucket brigade for electrons in the mitochondrial membrane. But, of course, electrons can inadvertently spill out of their buckets, forming reactive oxygen species (**ROS**), aka **free radicals**. These free radicals can damage the DNA in the mitochondria, the DNA in the cell nucleus (your genes), and important proteins in your cells. This damage is called oxidation. Bottom line: less food energy coming in means fewer electrons going out to cause oxidation.

Unfortunately, the previous paragraph oversimplifies the situation. Researchers have noted that in animals undergoing CR, mitochondrial activity actually increases. And remember the human studies I mentioned earlier, where people on CR didn't have any problem generating energy for physical activity? This finding is easily explained by increased activity of these energy-generating organelles. But then we have to ask, what about an increase in ROS production that you would expect?

New findings show that increased ROS levels, from active mitochondria, turn on protective genes. These genes, like the first domino down, then turn on numerous adaptive responses, including defense mechanisms and improved stress resistance, which confers better health outcomes and extended longevity.

All along the mitochondrial membrane are stations where ATP is made, using the energy from food passed through the electron bucket brigade. Less food energy in means less ATP is made, which sounds bad. But when ATP supplies drop, a sensor mechanism is activated. This situation is a little like what happens when the temperature in your house drops below the set point in the thermostat. The furnace kicks on to bring the temperature back up.

The ATP sensor is triggered by something called AMP. This is such a clever mechanism that I have to describe it in a little detail. ATP is a molecule with three P-groups (phosphates for the interested). I can diagram it as A-P-P-P. When your cells use ATP in reactions that require energy (this is like you spending money on anything that requires a financial transaction), the last P-group is removed. The resulting molecule, called ADP (the D is for di-phosphate, meaning it has two of the Ps), looks like this: A-P-P. If a second P is lost, AMP (mono-phosphate: A-P) is formed. These are typically returned to the mitochondria, where the energy culled from the electron bucket brigade attaches a second or third P. Both ADP and AMP are signals to the cell that ATP supplies are running low, like an overdraft notice from the bank. ADP and AMP can both activate the actual signal molecule, which is another first domino in the chain of energy production.

The downstream events not only produce more ATP, but also set in motion a whole host of maintenance and repair processes that keep the cell lean and mean and also mitigate against many of the degenerative processes of aging.

Autophagy. **Autophagy** is one of these protective processes. Autophagy is the sum of all the house-cleaning processes in our cells. When proteins and other structures in cells are damaged, they get tagged with a sort of bar code that tells the cleaning system to get rid of them. The cleaning system consists of microscopic structures similar in size and shape to mitochondria that act like vacuum cleaners. The cleaning structures do one better than vacuum cleaners, because they spit out the building blocks of the stuff they broke down, which can then be reused. If autophagy doesn't happen, crud builds up in cells, eventually damaging them and initiating the formation of senescent cells (see chapter 3); these, of course, contribute to aging-related diseases.

Many of the behavioral interventions I present in this chapter such as CR, time-restricted feeding, and exercise, and life-extending compounds such as rapamycin and resveratrol that I discuss in the following chapter, exert at least part of their effect by activating autophagy.[7]

Mitophagy is a form of autophagy, which breaks down and recycles damaged mitochondria. But wait, you say; if we get rid of mitochondria, don't we run out of ATP? Well, cleverly the AMP signal also activates the process that causes healthy mitochondria to divide and produce more.

That's not all. The AMP signal also turns down mTOR. Recall that mTOR is the master switch that coordinates cellular building processes (these are collectively called **anabolism**, the part of metabolism that builds rather than breaks down). When food is plentiful, the volume control of mTOR is turned up, and resources are used to build new cellular components and new cells. Sometimes that's a good thing, but often, mTOR is turned up because we are taking in too many calories. Our thrifty bodies never waste resources, so we use them, maybe building bigger muscle cells, but also adding to fat cells. Conversely, if food energy is limited by CR/IF/TRF, then mTOR is turned down because resources are limited. If you're curious, I'll come back to mTOR in a few pages.

The Starvation Hormone

Another compound that seems to be important in mammals is called **FGF21**, nicknamed the starvation hormone. It's produced by the liver when

. FGF21 is then released into the blood, where it travels telling cells to mobilize and burn fatty acids for fuel. In mice that produce more of this hormone, even without food restriction, they live longer and are more insulin sensitive than their control counterparts. Recall that insulin is the pancreatic hormone that tells cells to pull sugar out of the blood after a meal. People, and mice, that are less sensitive (i.e., resistant) to this message from insulin are at risk for developing type 2 diabetes.

The mice making more FGF21 are also smaller, because they don't respond to growth hormone and insulin-like growth factor (IGF-1, introduced in chapter 3). This makes sense: if you are starving, you don't want to shunt your limited energy reserves into growth. Although we don't want to make people smaller, like these mice, there is interest in using FGF21 in treating some diseases.[8]

A Deep Dive into Why We Have These Complicated Responses to Eating

If the evolutionary explanations appeal to you, read this section. Our cells generate daily rhythms in cellular metabolism, repair, cell division, and growth. These up-and-down cycles are found in virtually all organisms, though their exact nature varies by species and depends on the life cycle of each species. Consider that most organisms have built in clocks, called **circadian clocks**, telling their cells where they are in a twenty-four-hour day. This information provides a survival advantage as behaviors and metabolism can be coordinated to specific times of day.

In most animal species, including our ancestors, feeding would only have occurred during a limited window during the day. By contrast, in modern life, we have more frequent meals and shorter fasting periods. This pattern will increase the metabolic activity that follows eating.

After we eat, insulin is released and mTOR activity soon follows, with the concomitant buildup of proteins and other cellular structures. On the other hand, a period of fasting activates the AMP system, which triggers repair and catabolic, or breakdown, processes. The AMP system also inhibits mTOR activity. This inhibition makes sense: you don't want to push on the gas pedal (mTOR, which I introduced in chapter 3 and returned to in the following chapter) when the braking AMP system is on.

Both eating and fasting send signals that affect the circadian clock by producing proteins that turn various genes off or on. This is a long-winded explanation for how our eating patterns can affect the circadian patterns in metabolism. Over billions of years of life, our many ancestors evolved these patterns to take advantage of availability of food and to time repair and maintenance to alternative periods.

If you are thinking that other things that disrupt a "normal" circadian pattern, such as night-shift work, will also affect your metabolic patterns, you are quite right. In fact, altered sleep patterns have been found to contribute to obesity, type 2 diabetes, and cardiovascular disease. Finally, and not surprisingly, age also affects our built-in rhythms. But whatever the source of the altered rhythms, restricting food to a window of twelve hours or less can restore a normal pattern to the metabolic components of repair and maintenance.[9]

Alcohol

Some studies suggest that moderate drinking may confer some health benefits, but these results are controversial. I discussed some of the problems of these studies in chapter 7. Red wine is often singled out for its antiaging benefits, though more research is needed into how that might work. I discuss one of the chemicals that may contribute to this, resveratrol, in the next chapter. The cardiac benefit may be offset by an increased risk for cancer, particularly breast cancer. And, particularly germane here, alcohol consumption can pack on the calories.

Exercise

If you haven't read enough yet about the benefits of exercise, I'll summarize. If there is one thing you can do to improve your health span and quality of life, it's probably moderate exercise.[10] At all ages, both aerobic and strength training confer rapid benefits to every physiological system. Improved functioning in the vascular system probably underlies many of these effects. As we age, it becomes increasingly important to maintain muscle mass, another benefit of exercise, as I discussed at great length in chapter 5.

Not only do our muscles move us around, a function we want to preserve as long as possible, but active muscle tissue releases a variety of compounds that offset inflammation, one of the prime contributors to age-related diseases. As you exercise, the contraction of a muscle actually damages some of its cells. As with any injury, acute **inflammation** results. This is a process that signals the immune system to send help. During its repair, the muscle cell then releases **anti-inflammatory** compounds. For this reason, avoid taking anti-inflammatory drugs, if possible, when you exercise. I described some of the novel ideas for extending muscle mass in later life, and avoiding sarcopenia, in chapter 5.

Both **aerobic** (e.g., brisk walking, running, cycling) and **resistance exercise** (e.g., weight training) have positive effects on your mitochondria. If you want to pick one to maintain and enhance your muscle mass as you age, recent research gives a slight edge to resistance training. This type of exercise increases both the function (measured by oxygen use) and protein synthesis (which allows more mitochondria to be produced) of these all-important structures. Keep in mind that aerobic exercise is beneficial for the cardiovascular system in ways that resistance training is not. And aerobic exercise will indirectly build muscle mass, thus producing some of the same good effects on mitochondria.

Regardless of the kind of exercise you do, it is a big component of your real, or biological age, as opposed to your chronological age, which is the number of years you've been alive. In a recent European study that examined more than 125,000 patients who took an exercise stress test, a common way to diagnose heart problems, the researchers found that performance on the test was the best predictor of survival over the next ten years. And this was after taking into account chronological age, sex, smoking, body mass index, coronary artery disease, and high blood pressure.[11]

If that's not enough, another study that analyzed surveys from more than 1.2 million Americans tells us that mental health improves significantly with exercise. (But remember from chapter 1 the accuracy issues with self-reporting.) The analysis compared people who exercised and those who did not on the basis of self-reported "bad days." Exercisers had fewer days of poor mental health in the month before the survey than non-exercisers. More good news: all kinds of exercise improved mental health. Although the researchers looked at a small number of sports, the biggest positive effect was seen with team sports, cycling, and gym workouts, lasting approximately forty-five minutes and occurring 3–5 times a week.[12]

Now, you're probably thinking, sure, exercise sounds like a fountain of youth. The reasonable question that follows is: How much and how often? Well, as in the case of restricted eating, there haven't been any big studies in humans to nail down an answer. A lot of studies, some of which I discussed in chapter 5, illustrate the beneficial action of various types of exercise in older adults.

A growing body of literature is also systematically looking at the best "dose" of exercise. For example, one study compared old (60–75 years) to young (20–35 years) adults, specifically looking at the amount of exercise required to maintain muscle after it developed. I have to tell you the details to clarify. Seventy adults, divided into two age groups, participated in a two-phase experiment. The first stage consisted of weight (i.e., resistance) training three times/week for sixteen weeks (phase 1). During phase 1, both young and old subjects gained strength and muscle mass. The young subjects started at a higher baseline, but both groups gained similar amounts. And we aren't just talking tape measure around the leg measurements; everyone had muscle biopsies as well as leg size and maximal weight lifted determined.

Phase 1 was followed by thirty-two weeks (phase 2) where everyone was randomly assigned to one of three groups: no exercise, one-third of the phase 1 level (i.e., one day per week of the same amount of weight and type of exercise attained in phase 1), or one-ninth of the phase 1 level (i.e., one day per week of the same amount of weight and type of exercise attained in phase 1 but only one repetition of each of three exercises versus three repetitions in group 2). Not too complicated, right?

Here's the kicker. In the young subjects, both one-third and one-ninth routines preserved muscle mass. However, despite a decline in muscle mass in both groups in the older people (less in group 2 than group 3), both of these retained some of the increase they had achieved during phase 1. And, importantly, neither group of the older subjects lost much strength. Let me summarize: you can reap large benefits from weight training of three exercises, three sets each, three times/week in four months. This benefit is maintained with a smaller investment in time over eight further months. The study ended after a year, so no telling what kind of decline, if any, occurred after that point. Bottom line: weight training at any age gives a big bang for the buck. One caveat: if you've never weight trained, work with a trainer or take a class with a certified professional to get started. It's easy to injure yourself if you do it wrong.[13]

Heat and Cold Exposure

If you're like me, you don't like temperature extremes. We heat and cool our homes for a reason. But scientists are beginning to find that in humans, short-term exposure to these extremes can promote healthy outcomes. This is an example of the concept of **hormesis** that I introduced in chapter 3. Hormesis is the idea that a little stress, such as cold or heat extreme, turns on defense mechanisms in our cells. These protective mechanisms then stay online, resulting in better health. Exposures to temperature extremes have long been noted in model organisms, such as nematode worms, fruit flies, and mice, as promoting increased longevity, as well as increased ability to withstand other stresses.

The effect of regular sauna was studied in a large Finnish cohort of middle-aged men, about half of whom used a sauna regularly. The men who used a sauna once a week were compared to more frequent users. The sauna fanatics had much-reduced risk of several types of heart disease as well as all-cause mortality (78 percent of the control group events for 2–3 saunas per week, and 39 percent of the controls for 4–7 per week). The 4–7 per week group showed a

66 percent lower risk of any form of dementia, and the risk of Alzheimer's disease was 65 percent lower than among those taking a sauna just once a week. The researchers found similar reductions in blood pressure, inflammation, stroke, and respiratory diseases.[14] Personally, I'd rather run ten miles than sit in a sauna for ten minutes, but given that exercise is not possible for everyone, regular saunas are nothing to sneeze at.

The beneficial effect of heat is probably mediated by a group of proteins called **heat shock proteins** (HSP). HSP were first found in flies and occur in virtually all living organisms, from bacteria to humans. They are also released by exposure to other stresses, including cold, UV light, wound and tissue healing. The HSP act by stabilizing proteins that may be disrupted by heat or other stressors, thus protecting the integrity of the cell. Because of this role, the HSP act in many important metabolic functions, including cardio protection, immune-system activity, and autophagy. In mice, the heat stress, and subsequent activation of HSP, following daily sauna-like exposure actually reversed mitochondrial and oxidation damage in muscles.[15]

Some evidence indicates that cold exposure, like sitting in an ice bath (which sounds worse than a sauna), can have beneficial effects. These include reducing inflammatory compounds and stress hormones, and changes in blood chemistry. These effects have been shown to improve the immune system's response to infection and inflammation.[16] But it also seems you can achieve the same results by meditating through control of the breath. Read on.

Intermittent Living?

By now you probably wonder which of these actions to take. Not surprisingly, some scientists are suggesting a combined approach. Let me remind you of our evolutionary background. Our ancestors were exposed to cold, heat, (relatively) short periods of low food intake (dare I say starvation?), and regular consumption of small amounts of "toxic" (e.g., spoiled) foods that triggered internal repair systems. Recall the concept of hormesis: a small amount of a bad thing will elicit a healthy response to overcome it. The few surviving populations of hunter-gatherers today eat a remarkably varied diet, determined by seasonal availability. Most of us would probably not choose to eat the same foods our ancestors were forced to eat: reptiles, bitter plants, insects, and so forth. Yet, that food diversity could also provide a source of both hormesis and nutrients.

Several small studies in Europe showed that combining some of the aforementioned stresses (cold, heat, fasting) produced improved measures on metabolic markers such as body weight, insulin, blood levels of glucose, and various lipids including cholesterols. The researchers called this approach **intermittent living**, as it mimics the lifestyle of ancestral humans. They think using this combination of several factors for several days each month could act as a sort of vaccine, to encourage our cells, which are essentially the same as those of our ancestors, to develop mechanisms protective against numerous modern lifestyle challenges.[17]

Reduce Your Chronic Stress Level

Our ancestors faced many environmental challenges of short duration. An acute, or short-term, stress response allowed them to funnel resources to the systems that needed them. Once the stress was over, so was the stress response. Modern lifestyles teem with long-term stresses, and many of us keep our stress response systems turned on for long periods, or for lots of short periods each day.

An important component of the stress response is the hormones that are released to get it going. These include adrenaline and cortisol. Cortisol, in particular, is released by emotional stresses. Some of its effects include breaking down muscle tissue (to generate energy for an anticipated emergency) and contributing to stomach ulcers (by increasing the formation of stomach acids). Maybe worst, high and sustained levels of cortisol reduce the ability of our brains to adapt and learn from new situations, and to store the memory of how to do that.

We can make numerous changes to our lifestyles—too numerous to describe here—that include mindfulness and meditation, yoga, and cognitive behavioral therapy, among others. I include several good reads in the notes to get you started.[18]

Get Your Eight Hours Sleep

A fitting conclusion to this section on behavioral modifications is about sleep. We know that our circadian clocks control many biological processes. It's not surprising that disrupting these rhythms contributes to age-related pathologies, including neurodegeneration, obesity, and type 2 diabetes. Getting a good night's sleep, which I know can be hard to do, contributes to optimal health of all body systems, from brain to skin. One startling natural experiment, which illustrates the immediate role sleep plays in cardiovascular health, is the observation that in the twenty-four hours following the spring time change to daylight saving time, when we lose only one hour of sleep, heart attacks increase by 20 percent. Much recent research highlights the importance of sleep for health span and suggests ways to improve sleep quality. I include a few of these reads in the notes.[19]

CONCLUSION

You can have a profound effect on your health span as well as your life span by making some changes to your lifestyle. These will be easy or hard, depending on your current behavior patterns. Don't try to make too many changes too fast. Do try to incorporate one that you think could work, then, monitor yourself for a few months to see if it has a positive effect. I describe self-experimentation in more detail in the next chapter. And, if behavioral changes seem too hard at this point, read on. In the final chapter I introduce some of the growing pharmacopeia available to stem the aging tide.

ACRONYMS

ATP: Adenosine triphosphate; the energy molecule of the cell
ADP, AMP: smaller pieces of ATP, with 2 and 1 P's respectively
CR: Caloric restriction
DR: Dietary restriction
FGF21: The starvation hormone
FMD: Fasting-mimicking diets
HSP: Heat shock proteins
IGF-1: Insulin-like growth factor
IF: Intermittent fasting
mTOR: Mammalian target of rapamycin
ROS: Reactive oxygen species
TRF: Time-restricted feeding

10

Interventions Part 2

Drugs and Supplements You Can Take

> I don't want to achieve immortality through my work; I want to achieve immortality through not dying. —Woody Allen

OVERVIEW

Maybe you would like to do something more than the lifestyle actions described in the previous chapter. Or maybe dietary restrictions or exercise are not for you, but you still want to work toward improving your health span. Then this chapter is for you.

Keep in mind that many of the compounds I discuss here have only preliminary data supporting them, but in my mind the data are really good. Some of these compounds may be hard to find, and you may have to play around with dosing and timing because human data are limited. A lot of people are doing just that and sharing their experiences in what are essentially experiments with really small sample sizes. And you know my thoughts on small sample size. That said, you are your own best control. Compare and contrast how you feel with and without the supplement. Become an experimental scientist.

I describe some compounds here, with good evidence for their effect, distributed by small biotech companies. Keep in mind that I am not endorsing the drug/supplement or the company. Also bear in mind that the scientists who did the research typically are on the board of the company making the drug. This situation is a definite conflict of interest.

In the first section, I introduce drugs that have been found to have a positive effect on longevity and health span. Some scientists and physicians who specialize in aging are recommending and prescribing these drugs. Although many of these people advertise themselves as specializing in antiaging therapies, at most, they have access to the same information you are reading here. At worst, they are relying on the trove of misinformation that populates the internet. Remember my caveats in chapter 1 about sorting the wheat from the chaff.

In the second section, I discuss "**biologicals**," compounds made by living cells. For the most part, these are obtained by purification from cells grown in labs, rather than made from scratch. They include hormones, enzyme-activating substances, and therapeutic compounds that can destroy senescent cells.

In the third section, I introduce supplements and so-called natural compounds with evidence for promoting health span. These include vitamins and other supplements as well as compounds found in foods. They have become known as "**nutraceuticals**." As always, I discuss the ways in which these chemicals work to affect your health or life span.

Next, I discuss genes with known effects on life span and health span. More specifically, I provide a tutorial on how these genes can work. When you understand the many ways that genes interact, you can understand how different forms of the same gene can either protect you or put you at risk. I also introduce biomarkers, measurable markers of gene activity or of the effect of the interventions you read about in these final chapters.

Finally, I introduce the idea of self-experimentation. As many of the compounds described in this chapter are not widely commercialized, you will have to find them for yourself rather than getting a prescription from your doctor. Most have had no large clinical trials, so they have no established doses or dosing schedules. However, protocols exist, which I point you to, for addressing these issues on your own. The field of antiaging compounds is in its infancy. Our choices are to wait years or possibly decades for the pharmaceutical companies to pursue this path or do our own investigation.

CHEMICAL INTERVENTIONS: SMALL MOLECULES

So-called **small molecules** are what we typically think of as drugs: things such as aspirin, ibuprofen, and other pills we use routinely. These compounds are more readily synthesized by chemists than the larger molecules made in our bodies. Some of these drugs have been around for a while, so a lot of safety data are available. For a smaller subset, a lot of data exist based on correlations between the use of the drug and a certain outcome, such as extended life span.

The use of drugs in the context of extending health span and life span is a lot more speculative than the behavioral strategies described previously. I limit the list of drugs and supplements to those with strong experimental evidence; however, most of them lack large and long-term clinical trials on humans. That said, for me to include them here, the animal data and preliminary human trial evidence are pretty good. All of these drugs are in the process of further investigation. In my mind, this caveat means that if you want to take any of these, you should do a little research on your own. In that spirit, I provide starter citations in the notes and revisit my suggestion for finding more recent studies in chapter 1.

Rapamycin. Although I just said that all of these compounds have good experimental evidence, I'm starting with one, rapamycin, that is falling out of favor due to some unpleasant side effects. (Some rapamycin look-alikes are in clinical trials treating cancer.) And technically, rapamycin isn't even a "small" molecule, although it is now synthesized by chemists.

The reason to start here is that rapamycin illustrates how a potential anti-aging drug can influence the cellular processes affected by both behavioral and chemical interventions. The life span extension from rapamycin that I introduced in chapter 3 was noted during early studies in mice, when it was being investigated as an immunosuppressive drug (i.e., one used to turn down the immune system of transplant patients to allow their bodies to accept a foreign organ). In addition to increasing their life span, rapamycin also significantly increased health span in mice. The drug also had positive effects on many of the age-related pathologies (in mice) discussed in earlier chapters, such as cardiovascular disease, muscle loss, osteoporosis, and Alzheimer's disease.

Rapamycin inhibits the cell's master key for regulating growth, called **mTOR**, which stands for mammalian target of rapamycin, which I also introduced in chapter 3. Individual cells in multicellular organisms, such as humans, have to integrate all kinds of information to make decisions as to what to do with themselves. We are all familiar with this kind of integration when we think about our budgets and what we can and cannot do with the amount of money available.

Our cells use information such as nutrient availability (which determines the ability of the cell to grow and divide), **growth factors** (proteins that tell a cell to grow and divide), and **cyotokines** (chemicals produced by the immune system that affect other cells) to make decisions about what to do. These chemical messages travel through the blood and communicate the needs of the whole body. mTOR integrates four major signals that tell the cell if conditions are a go for growth:

1. growth factors (e.g., insulin and IGF-1—remember these signals from chapter 3; more on these below),
2. how much food energy is available,
3. oxygen, and
4. **amino acid** (the building blocks of proteins) levels.

Then mTOR can turn on cell growth. Any of these signals can activate mTOR to set in motion **anabolic** (a jargon way of saying pro-growth) processes such as protein and lipid synthesis, and reproduction of mitochondria. Not surprisingly, mTOR signaling is messed up in diseases such as cancer and type 2 diabetes. It may be that a high protein intake, which has been associated with increased cancer risk, turns up the mTOR system, which could then result in excessive cellular growth and reproduction—the hallmark of cancer.

Here's an interesting experimental finding related to the activity of mTOR. Think of mTOR as a volume control knob. High nutrient levels and growth factors, which are protein signals made by the body, turn it up. Then, growth happens. In mice, when one growth factor is turned up by researchers, activating its gene in skin cells, they got wrinkles. Lots of wrinkles.[1] Makes sense: if the cells get bigger, they will crowd each other and start to stack up. Read on for ways to minimize this.

Conversely, when mTOR is turned down, **autophagy** (also introduced in chapter 3), which breaks down cellular components and recycles them to provide nutrients, is turned up. mTOR, which is a protein, is often found attached to the recycling center. This location is obviously a prime site for a nutrient sensor to live.

Both rapamycin and **DR (dietary restriction)** increase life span in mice. Both interventions have similar effects on of mTOR (inhibiting it) and autophagy (activating it). These interventions also reduce **cellular senescence**. But—and this is a big but—they have opposite effects on glucose and its metabolism. DR increases insulin sensitivity, whereas rapamycin causes insulin resistance. Resistance to insulin is a risk factor for type 2 diabetes and not a desirable outcome, as this results in sugar levels staying high in the blood. Treating mice with rapamycin results in longer and healthier life, but the same might not be true in humans.

A further difference is that DR, but not rapamycin, stimulates breakdown of fats. These findings highlight the complex nature of mTOR's regulatory function. My take is that mTOR evolved to integrate numerous signals that occur naturally in cells. In other words, mTOR was designed to interpret events such as exercise and periodic starvation (simulated by fasting or DR) that occur often in nature. And to extend this naturalistic view of the mTOR system, its default is to be on. When it senses that some critical nutrient (glucose, leucine—which is a marker for amino acid availability, oxygen, etc.) is low, then mTOR shuts down anabolic processes. Then the coin flips, and maintenance and repair activities come to the fore. However, rapamycin affects a subset of the mTOR system, whereas exercise and DR are more global controls. Hence, the differing effects on health span with rapamycin.

A final twist to the mTOR story is that it is regulated differently in different parts of the body. For example, a low-carb diet will turn down mTOR in the liver but turn it up in muscles. Both of these are desirable. At this point, no chemical intervention can produce this naturally occurring specificity.

Bottom line: although rapamycin has its clinical uses, initially as an immunosuppressant in transplant patients, more recently in cancer treatment, and currently being investigated in controlling Alzheimer's disease, its use as an antiaging drug in humans is equivocal. Ongoing research in mice suggests that it may be possible to use low dose or intermittent doses to extend life span without the negative side effects. Another possibility is using chemically modified versions of the drug that produce the desirable effects without the down sides. Whatever the outcome of these studies, the role of rapamycin in elucidating the intricacies of the previously unknown mTOR system was invaluable.[2]

Metformin.[3] Metformin is one of the earliest drugs approved to treat diabetes. In fact, goat's rue, the plant from which metformin was originally extracted, may have been used to treat diabetes as long ago as the Middle Ages.[4] It reduces blood sugar, and thus the level of insulin in the blood goes down. By reducing insulin, the drug also diminishes the development of insulin resistance that defines type 2 diabetes.

In diabetics, the immediate effect of this drug, and others like it, is to decrease blood sugar. It also has an important long-term effect, which is to reduce **glycated hemoglobin**. That's a mouthful, so everyone calls it **HbA$_{1c}$**. We don't have to worry about what the acronym stands for, but the idea is important. Hemoglobin, the protein that carries oxygen in your blood, can get gobbed up with sugar—as can many other things in your body that I've talked about in previous chapters (recall the AGEs from chapter 4). As blood sugar levels rise, so does the amount of HbA$_{1c}$.

Here's the clincher: you can take a finger poke or other blood test to get your instantaneous blood sugar reading. As you may know, this can vary wildly over the course of the day. What you would really like to have is a longer-term measure, kind of an average. Enter the HbA_{1c}. Red blood cells, which carry the hemoglobin around the body, have a life span of about three months. Measuring HbA_{1c} can give you the long-term, more useful assessment of your blood sugar. Higher levels of HbA_{1c} are a good indicator of risk for cardiovascular disease as well as problems in kidney, nerve, and retinal function associated with diabetes. Thus, the beneficial effect of metformin in reducing this marker.

In addition, metformin targets some of the mechanisms that underlie aging. Specifically, metformin diminishes **IGF-1** (part of the insulin system that regulates growth) and mTOR signals (thus reducing anabolic activity—i.e., growth of cells). The drug also slows movement of electrons through the mitochondria, thus reducing production of **reactive oxygen species (ROS)**. If that isn't enough, it also increases **AMP** signals. In case you don't remember this important signal from the previous chapter, AMP tells the cell to produce more ATP, to reduce anabolic (growth) activity, to stimulate DNA damage protection, and to promote **autophagy** and anti-inflammatory activity.

All of these effects have been documented in mice. At most doses, metformin treatment in rodents also extends life span and health span. Although the drug results in the preceding list of favorable actions on different cellular pathways, the way in which it produces these benefits is not understood.

Metformin's effects have been tabulated in a number of human trials involving diabetics. Not only did the drug treatment significantly reduce mortality from diabetes, but it also was associated with improvements in cardiovascular disease risk factors, atherosclerosis, cancer development, and cognitive function. The caveat? All of these findings are observational. In other words, the benefits were noted in patients given the drug because of their diabetes. But the implications are striking, and rodent studies support these findings. A big longitudinal study on the effects of metformin in otherwise healthy older adults is now in progress.

That said, many middle-aged and older people are not waiting for these results and are starting to take metformin prophylactically to prevent diabetes and cardiovascular diseases in their future. One recent small study showed that metformin might reduce the beneficial effect of aerobic exercise. The study group of fifty people all participated in moderate aerobic activity for forty-five minutes three times a week. Half then received metformin. (Before I go further, keep in mind the small number of participants; additional larger studies to confirm this finding are in progress.) Aerobic exercise, as you know by now, has beneficial effects in many body systems and has consistently reduced risk for type 2 diabetes. In some, but not all, of the group receiving metformin, several of the beneficial effects of exercise were reduced. This result appears to be due to differences in the mitochondria of the people getting metformin.

You may recall that taking antioxidants, which reduce ROS, is not always a good thing, as our bodies use the production of ROS as a signal to turn on our own internal antioxidants. You may also recall from my introduction of mitochondria in chapter 3 that mitochondria age at different rates. Put together these two pieces of the puzzle, and we can conclude that a drug such as metformin, which relies on the activity of the mitochondria, will be affected by individual differences in the level of activity and efficiency of one's mitochondria. Bottom line? I'd say the jury is still out on metformin, but, like other drugs, it certainly has off-label effects.

A Deep Dive into Nonsteroidal Anti-inflammatory Drugs (NSAIDS)

To understand the antiaging effects of NSAIDs, which include aspirin and ibuprofen, you have to know a little more about **inflammation**. Remember that inflammation is a normal response to injury or infection. These situations cause "acute inflammation," which increases blood flow, triggers the activation of the immune system, cleans up dead or dying cells and other debris, and initiates healing. All good. This acute response is then shut down. But for various, many poorly understood reasons, such as oxidation damage, the immune response that produces inflammation can become stuck in the on position as we get older. Then, the hallmarks of constant inflammation, increased blood flow and immune cell activity, can cause their own damage. This chronic inflammation, cleverly dubbed **inflammaging** in the geroscience community, causes many age-related problems.

One way to turn down chronic inflammation is through judicious use of NSAIDS. These drugs inhibit the synthesis of **prostaglandins**. These are signals made by the body that, among other things, cause blood vessels to dilate. As you no doubt know by now, this dilation increases blood flow to the area. What's relevant to the story here is that prostaglandins initiate and maintain acute inflammation. NSAIDS block the activity of two enzymes, **COX-1** and **COX-2** for those who like jargon, that control the manufacture of prostaglandins. COX-2 is particularly important in producing prostaglandins that activate the inflammatory process. Both forms of COX are found at higher levels in Alzheimer's patients, perhaps explaining some of the benefits of anti-inflammatory agents in slowing this disease.

At this point you're starting to get why it may be good to take NSAIDS prophylactically. Hold on. They can have some less desirable side effects, too. One type of prostaglandin, made by COX-1, protects the lining of the stomach and intestine. Most NSAIDs (called nonselective), which act against both forms of the COX enzymes, can cause gastrointestinal (GI) problems because they block this enzyme. That's why low-dose aspirin, such as baby aspirin, has been recommended as a nonselective preventive of inflammation that can contribute to heart disease.

Some selective NSAIDS target only COX-2. Sounds like these are the perfect solution to the GI problem caused by the nonselective NSAIDS. But, of course, nothing in biology is so simple. It turns out that in some blood vessel cells, COX-2 blocks some anticlotting mechanisms. This means that you risk getting blood clots if you take too much of the selective drugs.

Side Trip: Enzyme and Signal Specificity

I know I've alluded to this point on numerous occasions, but it's worth a paragraph of its own. It's a bit mind-boggling, but many of the important regulatory compounds our bodies make can come in a bunch of flavors. It's a little like going to a fancy ice cream shop: You don't just get vanilla or chocolate. Usually, you have dozens of choices. Enzymes, and other proteins, are similar, but you don't get just one flavor. You are born with a whole "family" of related proteins. To make things even more interesting, other people may have a different set of these flavors. And, finally, each individual flavor can have different effects in different tissues. That would be like vanilla being a condiment in cooking but a lubricant in your car. This complexity is one reason it's difficult to design and prescribe a single drug, such as a COX-2 inhibitor, for a condition that may be due to the effect(s) of some of the different forms of the proteins in different places. Going back to the vanilla example, in reality, it's useful in the kitchen but not in the car. In the body, the same molecule can be inflammatory in some contexts and anti-inflammatory in others.

A Deep Dive into Turning Off Inflammation[5]

Normally, acute inflammation is turned off, and the affected tissue returns to a healthy state. **Resolution**, or termination as it's sometimes called, is an active process that relies on "**mediators**" built from the (omega-3) **essential fatty acids** EPA and DHA. This is an important point, because pro-resolution and anti-inflammation are not the same. Some NSAIDS can actually block the resolution process, but in healthy people low-dose aspirin can facilitate it. Obesity reduces levels of the resolving compounds, but supplementation with DHA/EPA or omega-3 oils reverses that effect. Just like essential amino acids, essential fatty acids, can't be made by your body and must be taken in from foods such as nuts, seeds, and fatty fish. The omega-3 variety refers to the chemical structure; in the United States another type of fatty acid, the omega-6 is more commonly consumed as a component of oils such as corn, safflower, and soy. Some practitioners are starting to recommend that older individuals supplement with specialized pro-resolving mediators (SPMs), mixtures of the omega-3 oils that turn off the inflammatory response. The immune system has another tool in its tool kit for resolving inflammation. This is a type of cell called an **eosinophil**. These cells are mostly called on to protect us against parasites. A special group of them in belly fat keeps the immune system in check. As we age, the number of these anti-inflammatory cells drops off, allowing the cells that promote inflammation to gain the upper hand. Voila, inflammaging. In experiments in mice, this inflammation was reversed by injecting eosinphils from young mice into old mice. In the treated mice, local and whole-body inflammation was reversed. The results were quite amazing: the old mice appeared rejuvenated. Their physical strength and endurance increased, as did the responses of their immune systems to challenges. We may be getting injections of young immune cells in the future.

Back to NSAIDS. NSAIDs reduce blood flow everywhere, not just where we have inflammation. When blood flow to the kidneys slows, they work more slowly. And when your kidneys slow down, fluids can accumulate in your body, raising your blood pressure. So, if blood pressure is an issue for you, you probably don't want to take NSAIDS regularly. High blood pressure also contributes to risk for stroke, explaining why long-term NSAID use increases this possibility. A slightly increased risk of heart attack is associated with use of NSAIDs, though not with baby aspirin.

Interestingly, ibuprofen inhibits the ability of cells to bring in an essential amino acid, tryptophan. As you may recall, the aspect of our metabolism that builds large molecules, such as proteins, is called anabolism. Many anabolic reactions involve the mTOR system discussed above. It seems that ibuprofen blocks one part of this system. So, this drug can have age-blocking effects independent of its anti-inflammatory properties. Indeed, in the big three invertebrate model organisms—yeast, nematodes, and fruit flies—ibuprofen extends life span.

One final thing that some nonselective NSAIDS such as aspirin and ibuprofen can do is activate the energy sensing AMP system (described in the previous chapter). Because AMP builds up when ATP (the energy supply of the cell) is low, it, like a gas gauge, tells the cell that fuel is low and to conserve. And, of course, this conservation strategy, which is also induced by caloric/dietary restrictions, produces many favorable outcomes for our cells and ourselves.[6]

Side Trip: Mitochondrial Antioxidants[7]

I know the whole issue of **antioxidants** is confusing. Should you, or shouldn't you? Well, as in so many cases, the answer is, it depends. As I discussed in chapter 3, when I first introduced the bombshell of oxidation damage and free radicals (aka reactive oxygen species [ROS]), it may be counterproductive to take a broad-spectrum antioxidant, such as vitamin C or vitamin E. This kind of supplement can send your body the message that it has plenty of antioxidant, so your body doesn't have to make its own. Then, if the situation arises where you need more, or if the supplemental stuff isn't available, then you end up with oxidation damage because your own supply had gotten cut off.

On the other hand, if you could put an antioxidant right where ROS are being produced and have the ability to cause the most damage, in the mitochondria, this could potentially be a good thing. Scientists have been looking for just this kind of targeted antioxidant and have come up with a few candidates. The best tested of these is called Mito-Q. It's made by chemically modifying the naturally occurring antioxidant Coenzyme Q10, aka CoQ10, to target it specifically to mitochondria. You may be familiar with CoQ10, as it's often recommended for people with heart disease. A small clinical trial in older people gave them Mito-Q for six weeks. After six weeks on the supplement, several markers of blood vessel health (that I talked about in chapter 7) looked twenty years younger.

Other drugs in development selectively target the mitochondria to protect them against oxidation damage, but none have undergone much testing at this time.

Cross-Link Breakers.[8] Way back in chapter 4, I introduced the idea that sugars circulating in the blood can attach to proteins, causing them to stick together. This so-called glycation, as occurs in hemoglobin described above, or cross-linking, causes all kinds of problems because then the proteins don't do their jobs like they should. This process is worse in diabetics because of the increased amount of sugar in their blood. Glycation also increases in the bones with age, because bone remodeling, which removes cross links, slows down as we get older. I described this process in chapter 6. In the skin, glycation can cause wrinkling and sagging because the collagen protein that support the skin gets clumped up. In other systems, such as the vascular or nervous system, the damage caused by these cross-linked proteins can be life threatening. A lot of things can prevent the formation of the cross-links. Reducing sugar intake (e.g., with a low carb diet) will do so, but a lot of drugs and nutraceuticals can minimize the glycation process, too. These include a lot of compounds with unpronounceable names but also some of the B vitamins; we'll come back to these later in the chapter.[9]

Some compounds can break these cross-linked proteins, aka **AGEs (advanced glycation end products** for the curious). Compounds that can remove these are called AGE-breakers. In rodents, several have been shown to break cross-links that had formed in blood vessels, and even reverse damage that had been done. One small study of human cells showed that bone loss due to cross-linkage was reversed by one of these compounds. Unfortunately, studies in real people didn't have the same result, probably because we have different types of AGEs than mice. One human AGE, glucosepane, makes up the majority found in our tissues. Although this is a promising target, the one clinical trial to target it so far had no success removing it. This is an ongoing, and promising, area of research.

CHEMICAL INTERVENTIONS: BIOLOGICALS/LARGE MOLECULES

Chemists aren't very good at making large molecules because the processes they use to build them tend to stop working well after just a small piece has been put together. Imagine making a ten-foot-high tower from Legos. It's a lot easier to make a ten-inch tower and quite difficult to get the ten-foot version to stand up. In the past few decades, however, biochemists have perfected their ability to extract compounds made by cells, or tricking other cells into making them. These compounds can be carbohydrates, proteins, nucleic acids (e.g., DNA), hormones, or even living cells. These so-called **biopharmaceuticals** or **biologics** include vaccines, blood components, gene therapies, immune system proteins, and cell therapies.

Hormone Replacement Therapy (HRT). Hormones are important in every body system. I introduced their effects in earlier chapters on skin, muscle, and bone. Evidence is increasing that for both sexes HRT can affect both health span and longevity.

As you know by now, we can all expect some chronic, low-grade inflammation or inflammaging as we age. This ultimately damages every body system, including the stem cells that could repair the damage. Inflammaging is more pronounced in men than women and may explain why men have a shorter life expectancy than women. And we can't forget the vital role that muscles play in keeping us healthy and active as well as influencing some of the many actions of insulin in our metabolisms. Anything that contributes to muscle decline, such as lower hormone levels, will impact our health. All of these points argue for HRT, but as I discussed in previous chapters, some problems are associated with this therapy.

A new approach to HRT follows from the fact that estrogen is found in both men and women. Estrogen, as you may recall from chapter 6, has a number of protective effects, primarily thought to be due to its anti-inflammatory and antioxidant nature. HRT in postmenopausal women, though not without some controversy, is not considered unethical. However, giving estrogen to men, which can have "feminizing" effects, is not generally acceptable.

It turns out that the body has several forms of estrogen. One of these, called **alpha estradiol**, has the same protective effects as the more active form (called beta estradiol, for the interested) but without its feminizing action. In a recent study in middle-aged and old male mice, alpha estradiol reversed the inflammation and metabolic disturbances that went along with aging. The HRT did this by reducing body mass and fat, apparently by creating an internal milieu like that of CR. Another benefit of the HRT-mediated fat loss was to improve liver function. I suspect this effect, if it replicates in humans, would have a positive effect on insulin resistance and type 2 diabetes. Of course, these findings are very preliminary, but nonetheless, promising.[10]

A Deep Dive into NAD+ Stimulants[11]

NAD^+ is a complicated story, but a growing body of evidence from the past five years confirms it as a major player in aging. Early human trials suggested that supplementation may be beneficial in reducing some age-related declines, and a lot of current research is looking at the best way to increase levels in the body.

You may recall from chapter 3 that NAD^+ is a signal. It tells the mitochondria to activate their few genes, which then decreases ROS production. It also turns on genes in the nucleus of the cell that control antistress and antioxidant activities. NAD^+ declines with age in all organisms that have been investigated. Conversely, restoring NAD^+ in these animals reverses some aspects of aging. NAD^+ is increased by actions that increase life span and health span, such as dietary restriction and exercise, and decreased with aging or actions that decrease life span and health span, such as a high-fat diet. These observations support the conclusion that decreased NAD^+ levels contribute to the aging process. Further, NAD^+ supplementation can protect against some deleterious effects that accompany aging.

Side Trip: Signaling in the Body

I've talked a lot about signals in our cells and bodies, and maybe you wonder just what these are. Let's start with a traffic analogy. We are all familiar with the many traffic signals we use on a regular basis. Stop lights, stop signs, yield signs, speed limits; I don't need to go on. Our bodies make a multitude of signals with equivalent function: conveying a message about what should be done at a specific point in space and time. Whereas traffic signals are usually visual, our signals are chemical. An important difference is that the same chemical signal may have different meanings in different neighborhoods. Imagine if a stop sign meant go on another street. Our bodies are amazingly sophisticated, however, and deal with this apparent ambiguity by having different readers for the same signal in different regions. This would be equivalent to your eyes seeing go on one street and stop on another for the same sign. Fortunately for us, chemical signals are read by interpreters known as receptors, which can produce different actions even when reading the same signal. Imagine your eyesight changing when you went from one intersection to another; you would actually get a different message as to how to proceed from the same (e.g., stop) sign.

Back to NAD⁺: its best-known function is to carry electrons from food molecules in the cell to the mitochondria. The 1929 Nobel Prize in Chemistry was awarded to Sir Arthur Harden and Hans von Euler-Chelpin for figuring out the structure and function of this important molecule.

Recently, it was discovered that NAD⁺ can talk to the mitochondria and the nucleus, telling them to turn certain genes off and on. This function makes sense in that the affected genes are often related to mitochondrial activity, so the NAD⁺ acts a bit like a gas gauge, telling the cell what the mitochondria are doing. Subsequently, another function was discovered, where NAD⁺ acts in concert with some important enzymes. These enzymes, which I describe below, simply don't work without NAD⁺.

One final point about NAD⁺: Its levels fluctuate with our circadian rhythms (i.e., our innate biological clocks). This means that NAD⁺ levels can vary in different cells and even different parts of one cell, as we have different regional "clocks." As I discussed in the section on sleep in the previous chapter, one common complaint of older people is a worsening sleep cycle. One potential effect from sleep disruption is lowered NAD⁺. I haven't seen any studies yet to look at an effect of NAD⁺ supplementation on improving sleep. A related point is that in order for dietary restriction to exert its protective effects in animal studies, the animals' circadian clocks must be working. This finding highlights the beneficial role of these internal cycles in aging.

Sounds good, right? OK, let me explain a little more about NAD⁺ and what it does so you can decide if these supplements might be for you. First, I have to start by telling you about the group of enzymes I mentioned above, called **sirtuins, SIRT** for short. Sirtuins, like mTOR, have their fingers in all kinds of pies in the cell. A short list includes stress resistance, inflammation, cell death, cancer, gene regulation, and metabolism. Increased SIRT levels in the brain are protective against many neurodegenerative diseases.

When plentiful, sirtuins regulate our cellular metabolism. Essentially, they are recognizing when our bodies are experiencing stress and coordinating protective responses, typically by modifying epigenetic tags. These, you may recall from chapter 3, are tags added to our genes to turn them on, off, up, or down. One example of this effect of SIRT is the benefit from calorie restriction. It's also been found that SIRTs reduce inflammation, reduce cell death, and increase the number and vitality of our mitochondria, the energy factories of our cells. So, it's not too surprising that when SIRTs are turned down, some pathological effects of aging emerge. In a comparison study of a bunch of rodent species, the ones that naturally live longer all had more active forms of the SIRT enzymes. Finally, and not surprisingly, SIRT and mTOR have opposite effects in cells. If you recall that mTOR promotes growth and thus some of the pathologies that hasten aging such as cancer and cardiovascular disease, then the antiaging effects of SIRT make sense.[12]

But sirtuins don't do all this on their own. They depend on the molecule I introduced a few paragraphs ago, NAD+, to exert their positive effects. In other words, when sirtuins are high, then NAD+ is high, and health and longevity benefits follow. Some specifics?

Let's start with mice. Increasing SIRT protects their stem cells from becoming senescent by protecting telomeres and DNA. Telomeres were introduced in chapter 3; these are the ends of chromosomes that, when lost, result in DNA damage and the subsequent chaos in cellular activity. Senescent stem cells just don't work, and the tissues where they are found lose their ability to regenerate. CR, fasting, and exercise are all ways to increase NAD+ and thus the protective activity of SIRTs in mice and other animals.

One sirtuin activator that you may have heard of is resveratrol. **Resveratrol** was first purified from the grapes that make red wine and was suggested as one reason for the remarkable cardiac health of the French despite their high-fat diets. Resveratrol, which is made by plants, acts to protect them from fungal infection. This is reminiscent of the rapamycin story: rapamycin is made by bacteria to protect them from fungi. Rapamycin blocks the activity of TOR, and resveratrol (and similar compounds), in turn, affects some equally important protective cellular process.

Early studies showed that resveratrol increased the life spans of yeast, worms, fruit flies, fish, and mice. However, more extensive studies have shown that resveratrol does not extend life span in healthy mice but does lessen many age-related changes, as well as early mortality in obese animals. One especially encouraging result in mice is the finding that supplementation with resveratrol slowed damage to and loss of **NMJs** (these **neuromuscular junctions** are the places where the nerve controlling your muscle connects to the muscle; when the NMJ is damaged, the muscle stops working). Resveratrol also made the NMJs in old mice look more like those from young mice, in effect reversing aging. One final caveat: in these mice, CR (caloric restriction) produced the best results, with NMJs virtually identical between old mice (granted, they had lived virtually their entire lives on CR) and young mice.[13]

At this time, there are only a few small studies with resveratrol in humans. These do show some effect of the supplement in increasing antioxidant levels, improving insulin sensitivity, and increasing **NO** production (which protects blood vessels, as discussed in chapter 5). In these studies, people took huge amounts, much more than you get from a glass or two of red wine. Bottom line: the data are just not in, but resveratrol supplements seem pretty safe. Keep in mind, though, that the amounts you have to take are high, 1–2 grams/day, because our bodies are not very good at either getting it from the gut or getting it into cells.[14]

NAD+ Supplementation. Restoring NAD+ levels in aging mice to those of young animals actually reversed mitochondrial dysfunction, which I discussed, perhaps in too much detail, in chapter 3. Briefly, mitochondrial dysfunction shows up as a decline in ATP (the energy currency of our cells) production and an increase in ROS (free radical) production and DNA damage.

These results make it sound like increasing either SIRTs or NAD+ levels can have antiaging benefits. True, but you can't simply pop an NAD+ pill, as it won't get into your cells. You have to supplement with the building blocks for NAD+. Two commercially available supplements are precursors to NAD+. One of these is called NMN, and the second, cheaper one is called NR. If you want to know what the acronyms stand for, check out my notes and the table at the end of the chapter.

In figure 10.1, I illustrate the relationships among sirtuins, NAD+, and its precursors. NR is used to build NMN, which then is used to build NAD+. NAD+ is constantly being used up for the reactions that are activated by the sirtuins. Both NR and NMN supplements increase NAD+ levels. NMN is more stable, but it can't get into our cells directly. NR can get across the cell

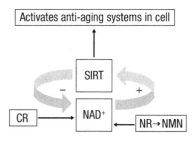

Figure 10.1. NAD+activates sirtuins. NAD+ is used up in the process. CR and supplementation replenish NAD+, aging and high-fat diets deplete it. Beth Bennett.

membrane. A modified form of NR called NRH has been shown in test tubes and mice to increase NAD$^+$ levels more than any other form, but it is not commercially available.

Both NR and NMN supplements in mice increased NAD$^+$ levels and SIRT activity. NMN specifically improved cardiovascular markers in aged mice, despite it not being able to cross the cell membrane. The way in which NMN can promote NAD$^+$ production is not clear and hotly debated. We see lots of suggestive tidbits from the animal work for pursuing this avenue, and several of these researchers publicly admit to taking either NMN or NR daily. Let's turn to the human work.[15]

NAD$^+$ levels have been determined in people in a few different ways. In one study, tissue was collected from adult and infant surgical patients of various ages. Another study looked at three groups of about ten people each, 20–40 years, 40–60 years, and 60+. Across all studies, the older the person, the lower their NAD$^+$ levels (and SIRT). Interestingly, this correlation was stronger in males than females. In a small trial done in my hometown of Boulder, Colorado, supplementation with NR stimulated NAD$^+$ production in thirty healthy middle-aged and older (50–79 years) adults of both sexes. It showed suggestive decreases in both blood pressure and arterial stiffness with NR, but these findings should be replicated in a larger trial. A clinical trial in ten men showed that NMN is safe, but no long-term efficacy studies have been reported yet. In case you need more evidence that the SIRT system is central to the role of energy processing in aging, consider this: **FGF21**, the starvation hormone I introduced earlier, is another example of a hormone activated by SIRT.

In a clinical trial of 120 healthy adults (60–80 years), using a combination of NR and a form of resveratrol that is more active in the body (this is a commercially available product described in the notes), supplementation increased NAD$^+$. People taking the recommended dose saw NAD$^+$ levels increase by an average of 40 percent over baseline after thirty days, a number that was sustained at sixty days. Those taking twice the recommended dose saw their NAD+ levels increase by 90 percent over baseline after thirty days and 55 percent at sixty days. And those taking the placebo had no NAD+ increase at all. No serious adverse events were reported in the study. Before you rush out to buy this supplement, recall my warnings in chapter 1 about clinical trials, especially those done by organizations that can benefit from positive results. To be fair, this study was conducted by an independent group, though it was designed by the company that makes the product.[16] This is a rapidly evolving field of study, so expect more changes weekly.

Senotherapeutics and Senolytics. Of course, you remember **senescent cells**, which I introduced you to in chapter 3 and have referred to ever since. These unpleasant little critters increasingly populate our aging bodies but have lost the ability to divide and make more cells. They can't divide, in part because their telomeres, the ends of the chromosomes, are too short. Nonetheless, they can still produce chemical signals that are released into their surroundings and, unfortunately for us, can cause neighboring cells to become senescent. And these senescent cells aren't harmless. They also release compounds that cause inflammation and damage mitochondria in neighboring cells. **Senolytics** are drugs that target and kill these little monsters, whereas **senotherapies** are treatments that reduce their effects. At this point, we don't have much data on the latter, but a lot of mouse studies show that the targeted destruction of senescent cells extends life and, even better, has a rejuvenating effect. The converse experiment has been done also—namely, injecting senescent cells into mice. The injected mice got old much faster than the untreated siblings.

Here's how the targeting works: molecules on the outsides of cells help the cells interact with their surroundings. Each type of cell has different surface molecules, which can serve as markers, or ID tags for that cell type. Think of these surface markers as unique street address numbers on houses (e.g., liver cells have a different group of surface molecules than blood cells). In the case of senescent cells, they have their own unique surface molecules, making them an attractive target for this removal therapy. Oncologists, physicians who treat cancer, already use this approach with new drugs that target cancer cells, either killing them directly or telling the immune system to do the job.

Our immune systems naturally use this type of strategy by making **antibodies**. These are proteins, kind of like heat-seeking missiles, that can find a specific senescent cell marker, latch onto the cell, and kill it. When old mice were treated with an antibody targeting senescent cells, twice a week for three weeks, they had a big drop in senescent cells, but even better, their muscle mass jumped up. Treated mice didn't experience any adverse effects from the treatment, and they retained the bigger muscles, typical of young mice, in the nine-week follow-up. That's a long time for old mice.[17]

In a similar way, senolytics can selectively destroy senescent cells without causing any great harm to normal cells. Some senolytics target key proteins inside the senescent cells. Although these treatments are supposed to be specific to the senescent cells, they can always cause collateral damage because their administration is systemic. In other words, if the targets occur on other types of cells, they, too, would be destroyed. To avoid this issue, a new strategy uses nanocapsules, tiny little beads (1/10,000,000 of a meter in diameter) that carry the drug into cells. They are released only in senescent cells because their coating is dissolved by a process that is found exclusively in these cells.[18]

Another approach injects an inactive "suicide gene." Although this may sound scary, all of our cells carry these, and I've discussed their action in previous chapters (**apoptosis**). In a lot of situations in the body, when it needs to get rid of cells, these genes are like remotely activated bombs. In this type of senolytic, the gene is only turned on when the drug gets inside a senescent cell. Poof, and the cell is history. Good results in mice.[19]

The senolytic agents furthest along in their development are just starting clinical trials in people. This drug is like a Trojan horse; it gets inside the cell, then messes with some of the "traffic signals" in the senescent cells that control their activity. When these signals are turned off, the suicide genes in the senescent cells are activated. There are currently two trials for this therapy, the first for osteoarthritis, the second for some of the age-related eye diseases I described in chapter 8.[20] As usual, keep in mind that when the company developing the drug or treatment is doing the clinical trials, the potential for bias is always there.

A final strategy, still in its infancy, relies on boosting the immune system, which normally clears senescent cells, but as we have seen, its efficacy declines with age. In fact, some of this decline is due to the increased demand that clearing these cells places on the system. So, improving overall immune system activity and improving its specific anti-senescent cell functions are components of this strategy. As you now know, based on the preceding description of how antibodies work, the immune system targets cells by looking at what is on the outside. This method is conceptually similar to some of the new anticancer therapies that involve genetic engineering of your own immune cells to boost their ability to recognize the cells we want to eliminate.[21]

And, don't forget, one senolytic has been developed not as a drug but as a cosmetic cream, targeting senescent cells in the skin. The product has been approved by the FDA and is in large-scale clinical trials in people. I described this approach in detail in chapter 4.

Blood Transfusions. For more than a decade, scientists have been joining the circulatory systems of old and young mice in a science fiction-y technique called **parabiosis**. They found that when old mice get blood from young mice, they look and act younger. Subsequently, the method was refined to use only the filtered plasma, which gave the same remarkable results. The age reversal was especially notable in expanding the ability of old mice to learn and recall new information. Heating the plasma removed the effect, suggesting that proteins, which are disabled by high heat, are the causal factors.[22]

A number of clinical trials are underway to investigate the possibility of treating diseases such as Alzheimer's and a type of cerebral palsy using this method. Not surprisingly, a clinic in California is selling this technique to people, in a poorly designed (in my opinion) clinical trial, at a cost to participants of thousands of dollars.[23] The trials in humans hope to replicate the animal findings, but, unfortunately, in many such extrapolations, it has become clear that we are not big rats.

CHEMICAL INTERVENTIONS: NUTRACEUTICALS AND SUPPLEMENTS

For various reasons, such as financial, educational, or cultural, many of us don't or can't use the behavioral interventions described in the previous chapter. These people need alternatives that can contribute to healthy aging. Many of us would prefer more "natural" treatments, such as **nutraceuticals**—individual food ingredients with properties that may benefit one's health. But keep in mind that the active agents in these natural substances can have unwanted off-target effects, just as synthetic drugs do.

Nutraceuticals. These substances include dietary supplements such as vitamins and so-called functional foods. The latter are foods that have been modified to have an effect beyond the simple nutrients they contain. Some examples of nutraceuticals are antioxidant vitamins (e.g., vitamins C and E, which are plentiful in most high-fruit/vegetable diets) and omega-3 polyunsaturated fatty acids (anti-inflammatory compounds abundant in Mediterranean and other diets using olive oil). Earlier in this chapter, I mentioned some issues with broad spectrum antioxidants, but what about the omega-3 oils? Diets emphasizing this "healthy" fat are typically healthier than the average American diet. Dietary studies are a mess! That's probably not surprising when you think about how they are conducted. Either people are asked about what they have eaten over many years (I couldn't answer that very accurately), or they are assigned to a specific diet with little oversight (I probably wouldn't follow it very closely).

Let's start with the simpler example of vitamins. Folate, a B vitamin, and vitamin D, have shown promise in studies looking at specific diseases, such as cardiovascular disease. The results in healthy adults have not been so clear-cut. Vitamin K deficiency may be a risk factor for age-related diseases such as osteoporosis, osteoarthritis, dementia, and arteriosclerosis. See chapter 6, where I talked about the benefits of this supplement in osteoporosis sufferers. Its role in other diseases is less clear, and because the evidence comes from epidemiological studies, is less compelling.[24]

There is some evidence for vitamin D's protective role in the bones (which I reviewed in chapter 6). However, the human studies are sometimes contradictory. I talked about some of the reasons for this in chapter 1, so you should take study results with a few grains of salt, especially small trials, or studies based on associations and not on experimentation. I say all of this to preface some potentially positive results about vitamin D in the context of Alzheimer's disease (AD). Vitamin D deficiency is a risk factor for AD. When supplements were given to rats with an AD-like condition, some factors that promoted neuron death were reduced. But, with no data from humans, it's probably too early to recommend this.[25]

Some other promising candidates are compounds found in coffee (called terpenes and polyphenols) and green tea (a polyphenol called **chlorogenic acid [CGA]**), as well as some found in soy and cocoa. **Polyphenols** are a type of plant compound, and the name just refers to their structure, which we don't have to worry about here. Many of them have been tested in lab animals and in test tubes and shown a variety of beneficial effects, which include protection from oxidation damage and reversal of protein glycation (our AGEs: advanced glycation end products). CGA extends life span and protects neurons in nematode worms at a relatively high dose (equivalent to a few quarts of coffee or tea a day, which is unrealistic for me but maybe not for some), but has not been tested in mammals.[26] Another compound in green tea may stimulate NAD⁺ production, providing some evidence for many of the health claims made for this beverage. A wide variety of fruits and vegetables also contain chemicals that are protective in lab tests (i.e., not yet in people). These include apples, garlic, onions, broccoli (and related vegetables, known as crucifers), tomatoes, and peppers.

One such nutraceutical, made from unripe avocados, contains an unusual sugar (called mannoheptulose if you're curious) that blocks the breakdown of glucose. Studies in mice and dogs showed that the avocado extract improved insulin sensitivity and increased life span.[27] There is a lot of interest in compounds like this (and rapamycin and metformin, discussed earlier, which have similar actions) for treating cancer, because many tumors use glucose as their major energy source.[28]

One problem with nutraceuticals such as omega-3s and antioxidants such as vitamins C and E is that they are broad spectrum. In other words, they don't "target" any specific cellular activity or structure. Consequently, interest is growing in more targeted compounds for treating specific causes of aging and energizing the cells' abilities to protect themselves (such as autophagy or mitochondrial repair).

Let's delve a little deeper into a couple of these nutraceuticals that have been tested in specific body systems. One is **nitrite** (and a related compound, nitrate), found in high concentrations in green leafy vegetables and beets. You may recall the role of **nitric oxide (NO)** in vascular flexibility from chapter 7. If you don't, in brief, it stimulates the muscle layer in your arteries to relax, so it keeps the vessels supple and resistant to the process that initiates **atherosclerosis** (hardening of the artery). If you eat foods high in nitrite/nitrate, or the NO precursor citrulline, you have the building blocks for NO, which, in turn can prevent and minimize damage from oxidation and inflammation. These diets have been shown in mice and older adults to reverse arterial damage. Nitrite specifically improved muscle and cognitive functions in small studies of older adults, although the results for citrulline are mixed. Larger clinical trials to confirm and extend these results are underway.[29]

But wait, you say, aren't nitrates bad? Aren't they linked to cancer? Actually, no. The reason this possible link was publicized years ago is that nitrite and its cousin nitrate are added to processed meats such as bacon, ham, sausages, and hot dogs. These nitrogen compounds preserve the meat and affect its color, keeping meats red or pink. Without the added nitrates/nitrites, meats will rapidly turn brown. If you're interested in why this happens, recall that nitrite is converted in the body into the beneficial signal NO. NO in meats reacts with oxygen, which on its own, is a browning agent. Think about how sliced apples turn brown if left exposed to air.

As you know, our bodies use nitrite to produce NO. Plants do this, too. In fact, plants are the biggest source of nitrate/nitrite in our diets. And, of course, diets containing plenty of plants appear to be protective against cancer. So, probably something else in processed meats may increase one's risk of cancer. I did speculate a bit on this in chapter 5.

Another nutraceutical that affects NO is curcumin. **Curcumin** is a chemical found in the spice turmeric. It activates the same pathway targeted by some active compounds in broccoli and the other crucifers (cauliflower, kale, Brussels sprouts). Taking oral supplements of curcumin improved vascular health and reduced inflammation in both mice and older adults (men and postmenopausal women, 45–74 years).[30]

Curcumin also has been shown to reduce plaque development in mouse brains, suggesting that it may be protective against Alzheimer's disease (AD). Again, we don't have much human data, but one study found that 90 mg, taken twice a day, produced memory and attention benefits in non-demented adults over sixty years of age. But another small study showed that curcumin didn't help people already diagnosed with AD.[31] Yet another reminder of the problems of small sample sizes.

Many other nutraceuticals (e.g., polyunsaturated fats and berberine) are touted to have antiaging properties, but evidence is slowly emerging for them. For example, berberine (BBR), a natural alkaloid found in the herb Chinese golden thread, has a long history of medicinal use in traditional Chinese medicine. Recent work in human cells and mice showed that BBR can reverse cellular senescence. It may achieve this by inhibiting mTOR, much like rapamycin does.[32]

SIRTs (which I introduced above for their overall protective effects in aging) also play a role in vascular health. SIRT activates the enzyme that produces NO in the blood vessel walls (refer back to chapter 7 for more details). This means more SIRT, which we get from restricting food intake in all the delightful ways described in the previous chapter, is good for blood vessel health.[33]

Curcumin, and a compound in broccoli (**sulfurophane**; it's especially concentrated in sprouted broccoli seeds), activate anti-inflammatory and antioxidant mechanisms in our cells. If you're curious, this pathway is named after the protein that controls it, Nrf2 (pronounced nerf 2).

Finally, a few nutraceuticals seem to activate autophagy. Remember that autophagy (described in some detail in chapter 3) is the cellular vacuum cleaner that not only cleans out old stuff, but actually recycles it into new, useful structures. One of these is **trehalose**, a sugar found in mushrooms and honey. In mice, trehalose boosted autophagy and reversed oxidation damage. Another natural compound that stimulates autophagy is **spermidine**. This funny-sounding stuff is found in grapefruit and fermented soy products. Mice that were given spermidine also were able to repair damaged arteries. One study of trehalose in middle-aged and older adults showed improvement in arterial function. Clearly, more study of these nutraceuticals is warranted.[34]

You can find additional study results online for some of the compounds discussed here. The National Institute for Aging (NIA) is testing a large number of possible antiaging drugs and other compounds in its Interventional Testing Program. Its website lists the experiments and, when available, the results.[35] The Geroprotectors.org database includes more than 250 life-extension experiments in eleven model organisms (including mice and worms). The data are based on more than two hundred chemicals promoting longevity, including compounds approved for human use. This database integrates information about life span-increasing experiments and related compounds, suppression of aging mechanisms, activation of longevity mechanisms, and age-related diseases obtained from research papers and databases. Personally, I found the search engine here inefficient, and the list of compounds was not up to date. That said, if you are looking for information on a chemical in the database, the information is very complete. The Found My Fitness website follows quite a few nutraceuticals and their effects on health span and longevity. I reference several of these in the notes to this chapter. Finally, I maintain and update a list of websites with similar information on my website.

WHAT ABOUT MY GENES?

In previous chapters I've discussed the admittedly limited information available on risk and protection alleles. Here, I want to present a series of caveats about the pseudoscience that is rampant now, especially on the internet, making claims regarding the role of your genes in health and disease.

In figure 3.1, I introduced the idea of biochemical pathways by illustrating how homocysteine (bear with me; soon you'll know what this is) is produced and participates in various activities in our cells. I want to go into some detail about this story, because it relates to many of the misinterpretations and misapplications of genetics.

Let's start with **homocysteine**. It's an amino acid (AA) but not one the body uses to make our proteins. The diagram shows you that it is produced from one of the protein-building AAs (**methionine**) and can, in turn, be converted to another of those AAs used to build our cells' proteins (cysteine). Some medical practitioners recommend testing for homocysteine, because high levels have sometimes been associated with an increased risk of cardiovascular and Alzheimer's diseases. However, this association is still controversial.

You can also see from the diagram that many B vitamins are important in the reactions that remove homocysteine. These vitamins can be obtained from a diet high in fruits and leafy vegetables, as well as from supplements. Imagine removing the parts of this interconnected path that rely on the B vitamins. Much of the output would simply not occur. Imagine these parts of the path as a road map. Take out connecting roads, and it would be difficult, if not impossible, to get from point A to point B.

Where the story gets derailed in the telling by internet health gurus is in the top portion of the diagram. One role of methionine, outside of its protein-building function, is to give away its "methyl" group. **Methyl** is a simple little compound that has a variety of important functions in our cells. When it's added to another compound, in a process called **methylation**, it's a bit like the charge that's added to your purchases when you use a credit card. You aren't aware of the charge, but it's ubiquitous and allows the purchase to go through. Methylation, too, is an important and ubiquitous process in the body that facilitates other actions.

When methionine donates its methyl group for a cellular reaction, the leftover piece is homocysteine. Then, either folic acid or vitamin B6 can give their methyl group to homocysteine to regenerate methionine. Keep in mind that you also get methionine from protein that you eat, so this regeneration process isn't the only source for all of your methyl donations. I want to emphasize here that the pathway is not the only source of methylation, as suggested by many on the internet.

If you are low in the critical B vitamins, or if you have a form of the enzyme that is not very good at providing the methyl to donate to the homocysteine, then homocysteine levels can rise. This may or may not be a risk factor for heart disease, but high homocysteine definitely inhibits some methylation reactions. Imagine having a block on your credit card: you can't make any more purchases until it's removed. Too much homocysteine acts in a similar way by blocking those critical reactions.

If you have a family history of heart disease or Alzheimer's disease, and unlimited resources, you may want to get tested for your homocysteine level. Alternatively, you can have your genome tested (e.g., by one of the genome-testing services such as 23andMe) to identify the forms of the enzymes you have in this and other pathways. A big caveat here is that it's not easy to interpret the results of these screens yourself.

Back to some genetic basics. Remember that enzymes are proteins. Many genes are instructions for making proteins. Drilling down, a gene is a long sequence of DNA. DNA, in turn, is a really long string of the four letters of the DNA alphabet. In our human chromosomes, the string can be millions of letters in length. These letters can be arranged differently in a given gene to produce different **alleles**, or forms, of the same gene. Each allele can then produce a different form of the same protein. Sometimes one such is better than the common allele, sometimes worse.

If you have your DNA tested, say by 23andMe or Ancestry.com, they identify those changes in the DNA of most of your twenty-thousand-some genes. Ignoring some complicating factors, what this process does is essentially like distinguishing between alternate spellings of the same name (same gene): Alicia, Elicia, Elissa, Alissa, and so forth. For some of these genes we know that one spelling (i.e., allele) works better than another. For other genes, we know that one spelling predicts trouble for you.

Going back to the homocysteine story, what you don't see in the diagram is that the process that makes the compound that actually donates the methyl (the one on the lower left in the box) takes about a half dozen steps. Each of these steps has its own enzyme to make it happen. The last enzyme, called MTHFR, is the slowest, so it's the most important one in getting rid of homocysteine in this way. Think about your commute to work, for example. Maybe you have to go through six stoplights, and at the last one, you have to turn left on an arrow. This particular arrow stays on for a short time some days, so only a few cars get through, like a slow enzyme. On other days, the arrow can stay on for longer, and more cars get through; this would be like a more-efficient form of MTHFR. But you don't have to take that particular path to get to work. Several alternative routes are a little longer in mileage but don't involve a left turn. So, depending on how backed up traffic is on a given day, you can take another path. Your cells can do the same thing.

This was a long-winded way of illustrating that although you may have an MTHFR allele that is suboptimal, your cells can sneak around it. However, the functional medicine community has seized on MTHFR as a huge problem and recommends genetic testing for it (there are three common alleles) as a risk factor for almost every imaginable disease. This mischaracterization is based on extreme oversimplification and misunderstanding of the complex chemistry that goes on in our cells.[36]

Many other genes have similar stories. In other words, there is no simple explanation for how one gene will affect your health. Deciphering the story is complicated and time-consuming. If you really want to know, you will have to invest time and energy into understanding some biochemistry and working with a genetic counselor.

Biomarkers. Before wrapping up this chapter, I want to introduce you to the idea of **biomarkers**. This may seem an obscure and irrelevant topic, but I think I can convince you of its significance.

What is this thing I'm calling a biomarker? Wikipedia defines it as "a measurable indicator of the severity or presence of some disease state . . . More generally, an indicator of a particular disease state or some other physiological state." What Wiki doesn't come out and say directly is that these are really useful because it's not always easy to gauge the disease or underlying state. Take coronary disease, for instance. We're all familiar with stories of people, usually men, in their forties, who seem healthy but drop dead of a heart attack. With a good biomarker of this disease, these people could be identified and treated much earlier. Convinced now?

Let's extend this idea to aging. Yes, I know, it's pretty easy to identify older people. My wrinkles are a dead giveaway. But seriously, if you want to use some of the interventions described herein, and to be able to assess their effects, you need good biomarkers. Another "wrinkle" here is that they will greatly accelerate the pace of development in aging research. If geroscientists had an assessment of biological age (i.e., a biomarker) that could be measured immediately before and after a treatment, that would greatly facilitate experimentation and validation in aging research, making it faster and cheaper.

Right now, we lack affordable and reliable biomarkers of aging. The only widely accepted approach for identifying such a beast is to carry out life-span studies. Mouse life-span studies are not cheap, and their relevance to human outcomes is not clear-cut. Primate studies are even more costly and really long-term. I've already discussed the limitations of these in an earlier chapter. I used a systems approach in the chapter structure of this book. Now, you can appreciate that some biomarkers may be system-specific. For example, there is fluorescence screening for glycation compounds in the skin (AGEs, chapter 4). It is possible, though still controversial and definitely not cheap, to measure plaque formation in the brain to test for Alzheimer's (chapter 8). An aging biomarker, on the other hand, would indicate the amount of accumulated damage in a person. This measurement could then be used to assess specific systems. Maybe you have a lot of health-conferring genes. Your biological age, at a chronological age of seventy, could be a lot younger, meaning you wouldn't need a lot of expensive testing or treatments. Or vice versa.

One such measure is a kind of **cytokine** (remember, these are compounds released by a cell that can affect other cells, for good or ill). One particular cytokine, called **MCP1**, recruits immune system cells that attack invading pathogens.

MCP1, which has been studied primarily in mice, is a good candidate for an aging biomarker for several reasons. First, its levels increase with age. Second, in mice that mimic **progeria** (diseases that accelerate aging), MCP1 levels are even higher than in normal aged mice. In these mouse models, treatments that slowed aging also lowered MCP1. Finally, in older people with certain types of heart disease, MCP1 levels were higher in those who were sicker. These results support this compound as a potential marker of biological age. Even better, the finding that MCP changes with interventions highlights its utility as an index to testing efficacy of new therapies.[37]

Remember oxidative stress? This condition occurs when the amount of reactive oxygen species, coming mostly from our mitochondria during aerobic metabolism, overwhelm our innate abilities to neutralize them (known as antioxidant mechanisms). Not surprisingly, intense physical exercise, which activates our mitochondria, increases oxidative stress. Other conditions that have a similar effect include high levels of stress hormones and long periods of being in a cold environment.

We know that too much **oxidative stress** can be damaging, so biomarkers for this stress could be useful indicators of damage. But we also know that a little stress can be a good thing (**hormesis**). A study in birds looking at the effect of "intermittent living" stresses on markers of oxidative damage provides an example of using biomarkers to assess aging. I include this story here because this group of researchers used four easily measured assays of oxidative stress and came to interesting conclusions about the role of hormetic stress (specifically intermittent food restriction) and life span.

Let's look at each of the markers the researchers used. They chose markers based on the fact that ROS damage both DNA and proteins. The first is produced when DNA is damaged. (If you're curious, it's called 8-OHdG, and is found in the plasma, kind of like blood stains on pavement can indicate an injury occurred there.) When proteins are damaged, the second marker, a compound found in red blood cells, called PC, is produced. The other two markers they looked at are antioxidants. Both of these are found in blood plasma. The first is a general defensive mechanism, relying on vitamins C, E, and others that simply grab ROS, much like a magnet picks up metal. This marker is called **OXY**. The fourth marker is another antioxidant found in plasma, a protein that specifically targets ROS. It's called **SOD**.

Now that you know what the biomarkers are for oxidative stress, what did the study find in birds and, more important, how can those findings be extrapolated to humans? Not surprisingly, as the birds got older, levels of the two damage markers increased. You would expect this, if, as we suppose, oxidative stress occurs throughout life and contributes to age-related damage. The availability of food (hormetic stress) also affected the markers of stress. In food-restricted birds, DNA damage was higher but did not increase mortality, whereas in control birds fed freely, higher levels of DNA damage did increase their chance of dying younger. In both groups of birds, more protein damage meant increased death rates.

The situation was more complicated with the antioxidant defenses. Levels of the enzyme SOD increased with age in the control birds but not in food-restricted ones, whereas the opposite was true for OXY. Here's the weird thing. You would think that SOD going up would be good (i.e., more protection). But the higher it was, the more likely the birds were to die. Maybe it went up because the bird was trying to reduce an already high level of damage.

The study had a lot of hand waving to try to explain the results, but we can skip that and go directly to what's more interesting to me—how to use these markers for humans. A few small studies in people show the same general trend: confusing. We shouldn't be surprised by this. In uncontrolled studies of humans, especially small studies, we expect a lot of variation. My point is that if we had markers that can clearly correlate with mortality, they would be useful in a lot of different aging studies. I'm hopeful we will be seeing more biomarkers identified in the coming years and that their use will grow. In the meantime, don't be convinced by ads for reliable biomarkers.[38]

Then there is the so-called epigenetic clock. This biomarker measures specific changes to DNA. These added pieces are **epigenetic**, meaning on top of the DNA, because they are made of another compound that the cell adds to the DNA. Think of them as Post-it notes stuck onto your genes. It was developed by Dr. Steve Horvath, using publicly available data from more than eight thousand samples from fifty-one healthy tissues and cell types. Horvath's approach was to look at the same (350) DNA regions in all the samples. He found consistent changes in the epigenetic markers with age. By comparing samples across ages from newborn to elderly, he calibrated the clock.

Then he used the known age of the sample, combined with the amount of change in that DNA, to predict biological age. Remember that people age at different rates. This variability is the basis for the notion of biological age. Your chronological age is the number of years since your birth. Your biological age is harder to define but basically measures how healthy and functional you are.

More recently, the clock has been expanded to many more regions in the DNA used to examine a host of age-related factors, including all-cause mortality, cancers, physical functioning, alcohol dependence, Alzheimer's disease, and even skin aging as described in chapter 4. Each of these is related to biological age. In other words, someone with an age-related disease would have a biological age, determined by the clock, that was greater than their chronological age. Changes in the clock (i.e., one's biological age) are partly genetic—think of the families that tend to be long-lived—and partly environmental (more on this in the next section on telomeres). Other types of clocks based on genetic information are also being developed. If you're curious about your biological age, this could be useful, but be forewarned, it's not cheap, and its applicability to health span has not been conclusively demonstrated, although a recent modification of the clock seems to predict one's remaining time to live.[39] Not sure I want to know.

One intriguing spin-off from the epigenetic clock is the possibility of turning the clock backward. It sounds like science fiction, but theoretically it would be possible to change those Post-it notes on the DNA to encode a younger you. Something like this has been seen in people getting bone marrow transplants from younger donors. The epigenetic marks of the recipients changed to match those from the donors. A small clinical trial to reverse aging, by a combination of treatments that restored immune system activity in people who had lost theirs, appears successful. But note that these people had a serious disease that damaged or destroyed their immune systems.[40]

Another measurement sometimes used as a marker of age is telomere length. Telomeres were introduced in chapter 3 (if you need a refresher). These definitely shrink with age, so measuring them can provide an index.

Further, shorter telomeres are a risk factor for some diseases such as Alzheimer's and coronary disease. Their drawback as a biomarker is that they respond to environmental changes. In other words, you can change their length by your behaviors and exposures to various environmental attributes such as pollution. On the other hand, you may be able to increase their length by implementing a healthy lifestyle, including a plant-based diet, moderate exercise, and stress reduction.[41]

All of these biomarkers are a little like the old story of the blind men and the elephant. One felt the trunk and told the others the elephant was like a rope. Another felt the tusks and told the others an elephant was like a sword. Yet another felt the leg and told the others an elephant was like a tree trunk. You get the idea: looking at a single biomarker can give you some information but not necessarily the whole picture.

CONCLUSION

You can take a lot of drugs or supplements to affect your health span and, possibly, your life span. These range from commonplace drugs such as aspirin, to prescription drugs such as metformin that have been repurposed, to speculative compounds such as the NAD^+ boosters. None of these have been rigorously tested in large clinical trials. That said, many of them have strong suggestive evidence. And don't forget, some tried-and-true methods we know will increase your health span and maybe your life span. But they aren't necessarily easy.

I'm talking about exercise and dietary changes. Compounding the problem, we have no formula for how to implement any of these compounds or even the lifestyle changes. And, of course, because we are all different, each person will have to come up with a unique recipe. This is the allure of "personalized medicine." Getting that individualized information from our doctors and health-care providers is in the future. Right now, we can experiment on ourselves. Try tweaking your diet or exercise regime in some of the ways described, for a few weeks, and see how you feel.

Side Trip into Self-Experimentation[42]

If you want to experiment on yourself, plenty of self-help books describe specific regimens with detailed formulas. Here's an example. Start by plugging into a search engine a term for the variable you want to experiment on, such as high-intensity strength training, intermittent fasting, or the supplement of interest, and go through the results. Warning: in either case, check the background of the author or the site to make sure it's not just a sales pitch for a product or a service. Remember my caveats in chapter 1 about websites. But don't trust opinions you might read online; go to the primary sources. This means read the scientific papers reporting human data: the observed results, side effects, and dosages. I provide a lot of these, and you can easily find others by searching PubMed, the NIH-curated database of scientific papers. Recall my suggestion from chapter 1; to find more recent publications, use the reference I give in the note and enter it into the search field in Google Scholar (https://scholar.google.com), which will search forward from its publication date.

Then you have to assess your results. For some of us, this is as simple as measuring your resting pulse, blood pressure, weight, or BMI (which I think is fairly meaningless). Many technological gadgets will track other markers such as activity level and sleep. If you want to dig deeper, you can get tests of blood chemistry and other physiological parameters. These would probably best be determined by discussing your goals with a physician or other clinician versed in health span or longevity issues. In any case, whether or not you choose to use the steps outlined by a dedicated self-experimenter, I suggest reading the post he created.[43] The material is detailed and includes a general overview with a specific formula for mitochondrial antioxidants. Even approximate costs are included. Spoiler alert: it's not cheap, but neither is a thorough workup at the Mayo Clinic. Whatever you do, inform yourself as much as possible. Good luck!

ACRONYMS

AD: Alzheimer's disease

AGEs: Advanced glycation end products

AMP: Adenosine monophosphate, a signal derived from ATP (the triphosphate or 3P form, the vital energy storage compound used by cells)

BBR: Berberine, the active compound in a Chinese herbal medicine

CGA: Chlorogenic acid, a compound found in green tea

COX-1/2: Cyclooxygenase-1 and 2, the enzymes that produce prostaglandins

CR/DR: Caloric/dietary restriction

EPA, DHA: Two essential fatty acids used to produce the compounds that turn off the immune response (eicosapentaenoic acid and docosahexaenoic acid)

HbA$_{1c}$: Hemoglobin type A1C (i.e., glycated hemoglobin)

HRT: Hormone replacement therapy

IGF-1: Insulin-like growth factor 1

MCP1: Monocyte chemoattractant protein 1, a protein that activates immune system cells to attack invading pathogens

mTOR: Mechanistic target of rapamycin

NAD$^+$: Nicotinamide adenine dinucleotide, a signal found in every cell involved in many metabolic processes

NMJs: Neuromuscular junctions, the places where the nerve controlling your muscle connects to the muscle

NMN/NR: Nicotinamide mononucleotide/nicotinamide riboside; both are building blocks of NAD$^+$

NO: nitric oxide, a gaseous signal molecule

Nrf2: Nuclear factor erythroid 2-related factor 2, a protein that activates production of antioxidant proteins

NSAIDS: Nonsteroidal anti-inflammatory drugs

ROS: Reactive oxygen species

SIRT: Sirtuins, a group of enzymes involved in stress resistance

SOD/OXY: Superoxide dismutase and glutathioine, naturally produced antioxidants

SPMs: Specialized pro-resolving mediators

Notes

CHAPTER 1. WHAT IS AGING, AND WHY DO WE GET OLD?

1. World Health Organization, "Ageing and Health," Fact Sheets. Last modified February 5, 2018. https://www.who.int/news-room/fact-sheets/detail/ageing-and -health.

2. A huge class of books describes spiritual, psychological, and mental growth that occur with age. This is decidedly not one. I will not attempt to list any, but they can be found by searching a variety of bibliophilic websites. For a great read on what wisdom is, including its neurological basis, see Elkhonen Goldberg, *The Wisdom Paradox: How Your Mind Can Grow Stronger as Your Brain Grows Older* (London: Free Press, 2005); also, an excellent volume on neurological aspects of aging, including the benefits to our processing systems provided by age: Daniel Levitin, *Successful Aging: A Neuroscientist Explores the Power and Potential of Our Lives* (New York: Dutton, 2020).

3. World Health Organization, "International Statistical Classification of Diseases and Related Health Problems (ICD)," Classification of Diseases. Last modified November 20, 2020. https://www.who.int/classifications/icd/en/.

4. For a good synopsis on the Framingham Heart Study, see M. W. Higgins, "The Framingham Heart Study: Review of Epidemiological Design and Data, Limitations and Prospects," *Progress in Clinical and Biological Research* 147, no. 1 (1984): 51–64. PMID: 6739495.

5. You can read about the breakfast cereal study and its problems in S. Stanley Young and Alan Karr, "Deming, Data and Observational Studies. A Process Out of Control and Needing Fixing," *Significance* 8 (2011): 116–20. The Bradford Hill criteria are described by Wikipedia, "Bradford Hill Criteria." Last modified December 9, 2020. https:// en.wikipedia.org/wiki/Bradford_Hill_criteria. For a deep dive into the shortcomings of

many types of studies, see Peter Attia, "Studying Studies: Part II—Observational Epidemiology," Topics, January 15, 2018, https://peterattiamd.com/ns002.

6. As a research scientist, I studied genetic mechanisms contributing to alcoholism and other types of substance abuse. My life was made easier by my study subjects: rodents, not humans. I sympathize with those who have ethical concerns about using animals for research, but some experimental research is impossible to conduct outside of living organisms. If I could have done my experiments in test tubes, I would have. That said, most scientists doing animal research, including me, try really hard to provide the best living conditions for our animals. There are three main reasons to do so. First, it is the right thing to do, to care for other sentient beings. Second, if my animals were suffering or deprived in important ways, the data I obtained from them would be suspect. Third, the grant agencies, usually the federal government, impose strict rules protecting the welfare of experimental animals. In fact, laboratory animals live in, and are treated, much more humanely than most animals raised for food.

7. R. A. Davidson, "Source of Funding and Outcome of Clinical Trials," *Journal of General Internal Medicine* 1, no. 3 (1986): 155–58. doi: 10.1007/BF02602327. PMID: 3772583.

8. A lot of publications are on the WHI site. For a summary of the conclusions, see J. E. Rossouw, J. E. Manson, A. M. Kaunitz, and G. L. Anderson, "Lessons Learned from the Women's Health Initiative Trials of Menopausal Hormone Therapy," *Obstetrics and Gynecology* 121, no. 1 (2013): 172–76. doi: 10.1097/aog.0b013e31827a08c8. PMID: 23262943. The WHI draws plenty of criticism as well. For an excellent discussion of these critiques, as well as additional information on hormone therapy, see Avrum Bluming and Carol Tavris, *Estrogen Matters: Why Taking Hormones in Menopause Can Improve Women's Well-Being and Lengthen Their Lives—Without Raising the Risk of Breast Cancer* (New York: Little Brown Spark, 2018). If reading an entire book on this issue is daunting, a very condensed version is on my website (Beth Bennett, "What Exactly Is Osteoporosis?" Blog post. February 28, 2019. Topic Affecting All Women--The Role of Hormone Replacement Therapy through Menopause and beyond--The Compelling Case for Long-Term HRT and Dispelling the myth that it Causes Breast Cancer http://senesc-sense.com/what-exactly-is-osteoporosis/ or Peter Attia, "Controversial topic affecting all women—the role of hormone replacement therapy through menopause and beyond—the compelling case for long-term HRT and dispelling the myth that it causes breast cancer." Podcasts. February 25, 2019. https://peterattiamd.com/caroltavris-avrumbluming/.

9. WebMD, "Curcumin May Prevent Clogged Arteries," Heart Disease. Last modified July 20, 2009. https://www.webmd.com/heart-disease/news/20090720/curcumin-may-prevent-clogged-arteries.

CHAPTER 2. THE WHY OF AGING, OR EVOLUTIONARY EXPLANATIONS FOR WHY WE GROW OLD

1. Leonard Hayflick, "Biological Aging Is No Longer an Unsolved Problem," *Annals of the New York Academy of Sciences* 100, no. 4 (2007): 1–13. doi: 10.1196/annals.1395.001. PMID: 17460161.

2. A good overview can be found in the editorial by Felipe Sierra, "Moving Geroscience into Uncharted Waters," *Journals of Gerontology. Series A, Biological Sciences and Medical Sciences* 71, no. 11 (2016): 1385–87. doi: 10.1093/gerona/glw087. PMID: 27535965. This was a special issue on the future of aging research. The interested (and ambitious) reader can peruse the tables of contents of some excellent scientific publications such as *Aging, BMC Geriatrics, Aging Cell, Journal of Aging and Health, Journal of Nutrition, Health and Aging,* and *Experimental Aging Research.*

3. An editorial perspective by John C. Newman, Sofiya Milman, Shahrukh K. Hashmi, Steve N. Austad, James L. Kirkland, Jeffrey B. Halter, and Nir Barzilai, "Strategies and Challenges in Clinical Trials Targeting Human Aging," *Journals of Gerontology. Series A, Biological Sciences and Medical Sciences* 71, no. 11 (2016): 1424–34. doi: 10.1093/gerona/glw149. PMID: 27535968, gives a good overview. For a good discussion of health span, and a related concept, compression of morbidity, see Douglas R. Seals, Jamie N. Justice, and Thomas J. LaRocca, "Physiological Geroscience: Targeting Function to Increase Healthspan and Achieve Optimal Longevity," *Journal of Physiology* 594, no. 8 (2016): 2001–24. doi: 10.1113/jphysiol.2014.282665. PMID: 25639909. Seals joins forces with Simon Melov to expand further into what they call "translational geroscience," in which basic research findings on aging are translated into biomedical applications to extend health span, or what they term optimal longevity. Douglas R. Seals and Simon Melov, "Translational Geroscience: Emphasizing Function to Achieve Optimal Longevity," *Aging* 6, no. 9 (2014): 718–30. doi: 10.18632/aging.100694. PMID: 25324468.

4. Demographers struggle with the statistics of aging to address issues such as identifying the causes of death in different age groups. Some good sources in that field can be found in Kenneth W. Wachter and Caleb E. Finch, eds., *Between Zeus and the Salmon* (Washington, DC: National Academy Press, 1997). A good review of the genetics of aging in people is presented by Andrzej Bartke and Nana Quainoo, "Impact of Growth Hormone-Related Mutations on Mammalian Aging," *Frontiers in Genetics* 9 (2018): 586. doi: 10.3389/fgene.2018.00586.

5. Dan Buettner, *The Blue Zones: 9 Lessons for Living Longer,* 2nd ed. (Washington, DC: National Geographic Partners, 2012).

6. Life expectancy is a statistic calculated by examining the mortality or death rates in specific populations. For example, white Americans born in 2010 are expected to live until age 78.9, but black Americans only until age 75.1. Within a race, females tend to live longer; thus, the average figure is skewed upward because of women's increased life spans. According to the latest estimates, life expectancy at birth is still in the low- to mid-40s in some African countries but is almost universally above 50 years elsewhere; in Japan and a few other countries, the mean length of life is now around 84 years. For more statistics, see National Vital Statistics Reports on the Centers for Disease Control (CDC), posted April 19, 2006, www.cdc.gov/nchs/data/nvsr/nvsr54/nvsr54_14.pdf.

7. For a technical, in-depth discussion of the evolutionary theories, see Wachter and Finch, *Zeus and the Salmon.* For an entertaining, if somewhat biased discussion, read Joshua Mittledorf and Dorian Sagan, *Cracking the Aging Code: The New Science of Growing Old—And What It Means for Staying Young* (New York: Macmillan, 2016). For great historical perspective on the theories and scientists studying aging, read Bill Gifford, *Spring Chicken: Stay Young Forever (or Die Trying)* (Waterville, MA: Thorndike Press, 2015).

8. As discussed on the National Cancer Institute (NCI) website, https://www.cancer.gov/about-cancer/causes-prevention/risk/age, posted April 29, 2015.

9. John Wilmoth, "In Search of Limits," in *Between Zeus and the Salmon*, edited by Kenneth Wachter and Caleb Finch, 38–64 (Washington, DC: National Academy Press, 1997) discusses evidence suggesting that early levels of human life expectancy were around twenty-five years. At the beginning of the twentieth century, many poorer countries still had life expectancies in this range, although by 1900 the mean life span in the most advantaged countries had already risen to around fifty years. Dr. Charles Raison has developed a persuasive twist on this idea that connects defense against pathogens to major depression. Read his review: Charles L. Raison and Andrew H. Miller, "Pathogen-Host Defense in the Evolution of Depression: Insights into Epidemiology, Genetics, Bioregional Differences and Female Preponderance," *Neuropsychopharmacology: Official Publication of the American College of Neuropsychopharmacology* 42, no. 1 (2017): 5–27. doi: 10.1038/npp.2016.194 or listen to an interview with him (https://www.foundmyfitness.com/episodes/charles-raison).

10. Nick Lane has written extensively on this and other topics concerning mitochondria and cellular biochemistry. A good introduction for the interested reader is *Life Ascending: The Ten Great Inventions of Evolution* (New York: Norton, 2009).

11. For a current review of caloric restriction in humans, see the review by Most et al., "Calorie Restriction in Humans: An Update," *Ageing Research Reviews* 39 (2017): 36–45. Also see the website of the Caloric Restriction Society, www.crsociety.org/. For information on the CALERIE study, see James Rochon, Connie W. Bales, Eric Ravussin, Leanne M. Redman, et al., "CALERIE Study Group. Design and Conduct of the CALERIE Study: Comprehensive Assessment of the Long-term Effects of Reducing Intake of Energy," *Journals of Gerontology. Series A, Biological Sciences and Medical Sciences* 66, no. 1 (2011): 97–108. doi: 10.1093/gerona/glq168. Epub 2010 Oct 5. PMID: 20923909.

12. Doug Seals has published on this and related issues affecting health span. See, for example, Christopher R. Martens and Douglas R. Seals, "Practical Alternatives to Chronic Caloric Restriction for Optimizing Vascular Function with Ageing," *Journal of Physiology* 594, no. 24 (2016): 7177–95. doi: 10.1113/JP272348. Epub 2016 Nov. 29. PMID: 27641062.

13. Valter Longo, *The Longevity Diet* (New York: Avery Books, 2016).

14. Nick Lane has covered this and other topics associated with evolution. See especially *Power, Sex and Suicide* (Oxford: Oxford University Press, 2005). Also see Andre Klarsfeld and Frederic Revah, *The Biology of Death* (Ithaca, NY: Cornell University Press, 2004).

CHAPTER 3. THE HOW OF AGING

1. To read brief interviews with a dozen leading researchers on the basic mechanisms, see Linda Partridge, Toren Finkel, Amita Sehgal, Pankaj Kapahi, et al., "Focus on Aging," *Cell Metabolism* 23 (2016): 951–56, 2016. An excellent video, produced by

the National Geographic Channel, titled *The Age of Aging*, is part of a program called Breakthrough.

2. If you're interested in seeing how this actually works, this YouTube video, https:// www.youtube.com/watch?v=q8mJZOuaMLY, is pretty accessible.

3. To read about the U.S. project, see https://www.reuters.com/article/us-usa -obama-precisionmedicine-idUSKBN0L313R20150130; you can learn about the European Union effort at https://www.ictandhealth.com/news/next-country-joins-the -1-million-genomes-initiative/, the Chinese project at https://futurism.com/discovery -make-invisibility-cloak, and 23andMe at https://www.23andme.com.

4. Elizabeth Blackburn and Elissa Epel, *The Telomere Effect* (New York: Grand Central Press, 2016).

5. https://www.zymoresearch.com/pages/dnage.

6. The first of many early life separation experiments was reported by Ian C. G. Weaver, Nadia Cervoni, Frances A. Champagne, Ana C D'Alessio, et al., "Epigenetic Programming by Maternal Behavior," *Nature Neuroscience* 7, no. 8 (2004): 847–54. doi: 10.1038/nn1276. PMID: 15220929. For a less technical exploration of epigenetics in this context as well as the clock, see https://www.whatisepigenetics.com/cuddling-can -leave-positive-epigenetic-traces-babys-dna/; the clock was developed by Steve Horvath, "DNA Methylation Age of Human Tissues and Cell Types," *Genome Biology* 14, no. 10 (2013): R115–35. doi: 10.1186/gb-2013-14-10-r115. PMID: 24138928. Alejandro Ocampo, Pradeep Reddy, Paloma Martinez-Redondo, Aida Platera Luenga, et al. (about twenty other researchers) describe a risky way to reverse the aging in mice, "In Vivo Amelioration of Age-Associated Hallmarks by Partial Reprogramming," *Cell* 167, no. 7 (2016): 1719–33. doi: 10.1016/j.cell.2016.11.052.

7. A. J. Hulbert, "Metabolism and Longevity: Is There a Role for Membrane Fatty Acids?," *Integrative and Comparative Biology* 50, no. 5 (2010): 808–17. doi: 10.1093/ icb/icq007. PMID: 21558243.

8. Lee Know has written a well-researched and accessible book on this subject, *The Future of Mitochondria in Medicine: The Key to Understanding Disease, Chronic Illness, Aging, and Life Itself* (White River Junction, VT: Chelsea Green Press, 2018). For a comprehensive deep dive into mitochondria, including their evolutionary origin and all kinds of implications for health, disease, and philosophy, see Nick Lane, *Power, Sex, Suicide: Mitochondria and the Meaning of Life* (Oxford: Oxford University Press, 2005). And if you really want to delve deeply, see Douglas C. Wallace's review, "A Mitochondrial Paradigm of Metabolic and Degenerative Diseases, Aging, and Cancer: A Dawn for Evolutionary Medicine," *Annual Review of Genetics* 39 (2005): 359–410. doi: 10.1146/annurev.genet.39.110304.095751.

9. Nathan Basisty, Dao-Fu Dai, Ami Gagnidze, Lemuel Gitari, et al., "Mitochondrial-Targeted Catalase Is Good for the Old Mouse Proteome, But Not for the Young: 'Reverse' Antagonistic Pleiotropy?," *Aging Cell* 15, no. 4 (2016): 634–45. https://doi .org/10.1111/acel.12472. For a thorough but technical overview of this and many of the other mechanisms in this chapter, see Ines Figueira, Adelaide Fernandes, Aleksandra Mladenovic Djordjevic, Andre Lopez-Contreras, et al., "Interventions for Age-Related

Diseases: Shifting the Paradigm," *Mechanisms of Ageing and Development* 160 (2016): 69–92. doi: 10.1016/j.mad.2016.09.009. PMID: 27693441.

10. A lot has been written lately on the so-called NAD⁺ world, as this is a recent and popular topic of research in the aging field. The Firewall on Aging website, http://www.anti-agingfirewalls.com/, has a number of more or less comprehensible blog posts and links. For a thorough but dense mechanistic explanation of how NAD⁺ impacts our mitochondria as we age, see A. P. Gomes, Nathan L. Price, Alvin J. Ling, Javin J. Moslehi, et al., "Declining NAD(+) Induces a Pseudohypoxic State Disrupting Nuclear-Mitochondrial Communication during Aging," *Cell* 155, no. 7 (2013): 1624–38. doi: 10.1016/j.cell.2013.11.037. PMID: 24360282.

11. Wallace, "Mitochondrial Paradigm"; and see Matthew Walker, *Why We Sleep: Unlocking the Power of Sleep and Dreams* (New York: Scribner, 2017), for much more on the role of sleep in regulating these pathways.

12. Andrzej Bartke and Westbrook Reyhan, "Metabolic Characteristics of Long-Lived Mice," *Frontiers in Genetics* 3 (2012): 288. doi: 10.3389/fgene.2012.00288. And for a thorough but technical dive into the effects of TOR, see Mikhail V. Blagosklonny, "Aging and Immortality: Quasi-Programmed Senescence and Its Pharmacologic Inhibition," *Cell Cycle* 5, no. 18 (2006): 2087–2102. doi: 10.4161/cc.5.18.3288. PMID: 17012837.

13. Know, *The Future of Mitochondria in Medicine*.

14. Judith Campisi has written widely on the phenomenon of chronic inflammation and its role in age-related disease. See, for example, C. Franceschi and J. Campisi, "Chronic Inflammation (Inflammaging) and Its Potential Contribution to Age-Associated Diseases," *Journals of Gerontology. Series A, Biological Sciences and Medical Sciences* 69, suppl. 1 (2014): S4–9. doi: 10.1093/gerona/glu057. PMID: 24833586. Also, Hae Young Chung, Mateo Cesari, Stephen Anton, Emmaneuelle Marzetti, et al., "Molecular Inflammation: Underpinnings of Aging and Age-Related Diseases," *Ageing Research Reviews* 8, no. 1 (2009): 18–30. doi: 10.1016/j.arr.2008.07.002. PMID: 18692159. Anne M. Minihane, Sophie Vinoy, Wendy R. Russell, Athanasia Baka, et al., "Low-Grade Inflammation, Diet Composition and Health: Current Research Evidence and Its Translation," *British Journal of Nutrition* 114, no. 7 (2015): 999–1012. doi: 10.1017/S0007114515002093. PMID: 26228057 provide an excellent review of the roles of diet on inflammation.

15. For summaries of these preliminary findings in mice, see the *Science Daily* article on the hypothalamic hormone, www.sciencedaily.com/releases/2013/05/130501131845.htm; and for a thorough description of the blood exchange process known as parabiosis, read the *Nature* summary, www.nature.com/news/ageing-research-blood-to-blood-1.16762.

16. For a comprehensive review of senescent cells and their role in aging, see Christopher D. Wiley and Judith Campisi, "From Ancient Pathways to Aging Cells-Connecting Metabolism and Cellular Senescence," *Cell Metabolism* 23, no. 6 (2016): 1013–21. https://doi.org/10.1016/j.cmet.2016.05.010. Sue Armstrong's *Borrowed Time: The Science of How and Why We Age* (London: Bloomsbury Sigma, 2019) features an interesting interview with Judith Campisi, who is credited with discovering these cells. This goes into more detail on the potential benefits of senescent cells in some

contexts. You can find an interesting non-technical interview with Angelika Amon, who wrote the cell size hypothesis on the MIT Spectrum, http://spectrum.mit.edu/fall-2019/taking-aim-at-cell-dysfunction/; for a quick read with plenty of links, see the Fight Aging site at www.fightaging.org/archives/2014/07/aiming-to-remove-the-senescent-cell-contribution-to-aging-and-age-related-disease/.

17. A thorough, but technical review by James L. Kirkland and Tamara Tchkonia, "Cellular Senescence: A Translational Perspective," *EBioMedicine* 21 (2017): 21–28. doi: 10.1016/j.ebiom.2017.04.013. PMID: 28416161; and a current list of candidate drugs at the Fight Aging site, www.fightaging.org/archives/2017/03/the-current-state-of-senolytic-drug-candidates/.

18. A great review by Vikramit Lahiri and Daniel J. Konski was published in the March 2018 issue of *The Scientist* ("Eat Yourself to Live: Autophagy's Role in Health and Disease") but it is a little heavy on jargon. For an excellent lecture, complete with labeled diagrams and on-screen definitions of jargon terms, see Rhonda Patrick's excellent site, which I will refer to again in this book: https://www.foundmyfitness.com/episodes/guido-kroemer.

CHAPTER 4. SKIN

1. In skin, cholesterol sulfate—produced, of course, from cholesterol—is located predominantly in the epidermis, where it functions as an important regulatory molecule. Here, the basement layer cells (see figure 4.1) begin the process of differentiation and migrate into the outer layer of living epidermal cells, where the amount of cholesterol sulfate reaches a maximum. It is then broken down in the dead outer layer of skin, creating what is called "the epidermal cholesterol sulfate cycle." The cholesterol sulfate in the skin is critical for holding the layers of skin together in a way that allows them to slide across one another. This smooth movement of one layer relative to another gives skin much of its elasticity. So, as cholesterol sulfate goes down, so does the elasticity of your skin.

2. Paraskevi Gkogkolou and Markus Böhm, "Advanced Glycation End Products: Key Players in Skin Aging?," *Dermato-Endocrinology* 4, no. 3 (2012): 259–70. doi: 10.4161/derm.22028. PMID: 23467327.

3. An excellent description of the decline in the vascular system with age can be found in Douglas R. Seals, "Edward F. Adolph Distinguished Lecture: The Remarkable Anti-Aging Effects of Aerobic Exercise on Systemic Arteries," *Journal of Applied Physiology* 117, no. 5 (2014): 425–39. doi: 10.1152/japplphysiol.00362.2014. PMID: 24855137.

4. Douglas R. Seals, "Edward F. Adolph Distinguished Lecture: The Remarkable Anti-Aging Effects of Aerobic Exercise on Systemic Arteries," *Journal of Applied Physiology* 117, no. 5 (2014): 425–39.

5. For more on the androgen paradox, a good review is provided by Shigeki Inui and Satoshi Itami, "Androgen Actions on the Human Hair Follicle: Perspectives," *Experimental Dermatology* 22, no. 3 (2013): 168–71. doi: 10.1111/exd.12024. PMID: 23016593.

6. To learn more about hair stem cells as a potential treatment for hair loss, a readable, nontechnical summary is given in "New Way to Activate Stem Cells to Make Hair Grow," *ScienceDaily*, August 14, 2017, www.sciencedaily.com/re leases/2017/08/170814134816.htm.

7. More on palmitoyl and other peptides in Roanne R. Jones, Valeria Castelletto, Che J. Connon, and Ian W. Hamley, "Collagen Stimulating Effect of Peptide Amphiphile C_{16}–KTTKS on Human Fibroblasts," *Molecular Pharmaceutics* 10, no. 3 (2013): 1063–69. doi: 10.1021/mp300549d. PMID: 23320752; the clinical trial was reported by L. R. Robinson, N. C. Fitzgerald, D. G. Doughty, N. C. Dawes, C. A. Berge, and D. L. Bissett, "Topical Palmitoyl Pentapeptide Provides Improvement in Photoaged Human Skin," *International Journal of Cosmetic Science* 27, no. 3 (2005): 155–60. doi: 10.1111/j.1467-2494.2005.00261.x. PMID: 18492182.

8. More on NO treatments in James Q. Del Rosso and Leon H. Kurcik, "Spotlight on the Use of Nitric Oxide in Dermatology: What Is It? What Does It Do? Can It Become an Important Addition to the Therapeutic Armamentarium for Skin Disease?," *Journal of Drugs in Dermatology* 16, no. 1 (2017): s4–10 PMID: 28095537.

9. To find out more about the hair transplant experiments, the original paper is Mingqing Lei, Linus J. Schumacher, Yung-Chin Lai, Weng Tao Juan, et al., "Self-Organization Process in Newborn Skin Organoid Formation Inspires Strategy to Restore Hair Regeneration of Adult Cells," *Proceedings of the National Academy of Sciences U.S.A.* 114, no. 34 (2017): E7101–10. doi: 10.1073/pnas.1700475114. PMID: 28798065. A brief, less technical summary is available in the USC press release, (https://stemcell.keck. usc.edu/usc-stem-cell-scientists-obtain-how-to-guide-for-producing-hair-follicles/).

10. The company is OneSkin (https://www.oneskin.co/blogs/reference-lab/oneskin-launches-molclock-the-first-skin-specific-molecular-clock-to-determine-the-biological-age-of-human-skin); the scientists who started the company have only published one paper on their process, namely, the use of the epigenetic clock to determine the biological age of skin samples: Mariana Boroni, Alessandra Zonari, Carolina Reis de Oliveira, Kallie Alkatib, Edgar Andres Ochoa Cruz, Lear E. Brace, and Juliana Lott de Carvalho, "Highly Accurate Skin-Specific Methylome Analysis Algorithm as a Platform to Screen and Validate Therapeutics for Healthy Aging," *Clinical Epigenetics* 12 (2020): article no. 105. doi.org/10.1186/s13148-020-00899-1. The company website does say that clinical trials in humans are in process.

11. The study identifying the role of the *IRF4* gene was done by Christian Praetorius, Christine Grill, Simon N. Stacey, Alexander M. Metcalf, et al., "A Polymorphism in IRF4 Affects Human Pigmentation through a Tyrosinase-Dependent MITF/ TFAP2A Pathway," *Cell* 155, no. 5 (2013): 1022–33. doi: 10.1016/j.cell.2013.10.022. PMID: 24267888; the SNPedia site gives an exhaustive review of other studies linking this gene to various cancers: https://www.snpedia.com/index.php/Rs12203592. This is a good site to search for information on specific genes, as is the NCBI site (https:// www.ncbi.nlm.nih.gov/gene).

12. If you really want to go down the rabbit hole, see the review by Sylvie Ricard-Blum, "The Collagen Family," *Cold Spring Harbor Perspectives in Biology* 3, no. 1 (2011): a004978. doi: 10.1101/cshperspect.a004978.

CHAPTER 5. MUSCLES

1. Jonathan R. Ruiz, Xuemei Sui, Felipe Lobelo, James R. Morrow, et al., "Association Between Muscular Strength and Mortality in Men: Prospective Cohort Study," *British Medical Journal* 337, no. 7661 (2008): a439. doi: 10.1136/bmj.a439. PMID: 18595904. This, like many other studies in the past, was done on male, typically white, subjects. Only recently have federally funded studies begun to require sex and gender balance in the design.

2. Marjolein Visser and Tamara B. Harris, "Body Composition and Aging," in *The Epidemiology of Aging*, edited by A. B. Newman and J. A. Cauley, 275–92 (New York: Springer Science, 2012).

3. Lots of great articles describe the causes of sarcopenia. An excellent recent summary of the many interacting causes can be found in the September 2018 issue of *The Scientist* by Gillian Butler-Browne, Vincent Mouly, Anne Bigot, and Capucine Trollet, "How Muscles Age and How Exercise Can Slow It." Also in September 2018, the *New York Times* published several pieces by Jane Brody on sarcopenia, its causes and preventions (https://www.nytimes.com/2018/09/03/well/live/preventing-muscle-loss-among-the-elderly.html). A thorough and readable summary of all of the processes affecting muscles as we age is given by Robin A. McGregor, David Cameron-Smith, and Sally D. Poppitt, "A Review of Muscle Quality, Composition and Metabolism during Ageing as Determinants of Muscle Function and Mobility in Later Life," *Longevity & Healthspan* 3, no. 1 (2014): 9–17. https://doi.org/10.1186/2046-2395-3-9. For a beautiful illustration of the replacement of muscle by fat, see https://www.routledge.com/Sarcopenia-Molecular-Cellular-and-Nutritional-Aspects-Applications/Meynial-Denis/p/book/9781498765138.

4. Lots of good information on this topic is in Alistair Farley, Charles Hendry, and Ella McLafferty, eds., *The Physiological Effects of Ageing* (Oxford: Wiley-Blackwell, 2011).

5. A multitude of books exist on exercise physiology, which is the basis of this section. One such is by Scott K. Powers and Edward T. Howley, *Exercise Physiology: Theory and Application to Fitness and Performance*, 9th ed. (New York: McGraw-Hill, 2015). A very readable, less technical choice is Doug McGuff and John Little, *Body by Science* (New York: McGraw-Hill, 2009).

6. Ronenn Roubenoff, "Sarcopenia: Effects on Body Composition and Function," *Journals of Gerontology. Series A, Biological Sciences and Medical Sciences* 58, no. 11 (2003): 1012–17. doi: 10.1093/gerona/58.11.m1012. PMID: 14630883.

7. For more detail on the role of the neuromuscular junction in sarcopenia, see Mikael Edström, Altun Erik, Esbjorn Bergman, Hans Johnson, et al., "Factors Contributing to Neuromuscular Impairment and Sarcopenia during Aging," *Physiology and Behavior* 92, nos. 1–2 (2007): 129–35. doi: 10.1016/j.physbeh.2007.05.040. PMID: 17585972. Also, Ruth J. Chai, Jana Vukovic, Sarah Dunlop, Miranda D. Grounds, and Thea Shavlakadze, "Striking Denervation of Neuromuscular Junctions without Lumbar Motoneuron Loss in Geriatric Mouse Muscle," *PLoS One* 6, no. 12 (2011): e28090. doi: 10.1371/journal.pone.0028090. PMID: 22164231.

8. To immerse yourself in the NMJ and its role in sarcopenia, start with P. Aagaard, C. Suetta, P. Caserotti, S. P. Magnusson, and M. Kjaer, "Role of the Nervous System in Sarcopenia and Muscle Atrophy with Aging: Strength Training as a Countermeasure," *Scandinavian Journal of Medicine and Science in Sports* 20, no. 1 (2010): 49–64. doi: 10.1111/j.1600-0838.2009.01084.x. PMID: 20487503. Also see Geoffrey A. Power, Brian H. Dalton, and Charles L. Rice, "Human Neuromuscular Structure and Function in Old Age: A Brief Review," *Journal of Sport and Health Science* 2, no. 4 (2011): 215–26, https://doi.org/10.1016/j.jshs.2013.07.001; and Marta Gonzalez-Freire, Rafael de Cabo, Stephanie A. Studenski, and Luigi Ferrucci, "The Neuromuscular Junction: Aging at the Crossroad between Nerves and Muscle," *Frontiers in Aging Neuroscience* 6 (2014): 208, https://doi.org/10.3389/fnagi.2014.00208. PMID: 25157231.

9. Marco A. Minetto, Ales Holobar, Alberto Botter, and Dario Farina, "Origin and Development of Muscle Cramps," *Exercise and Sport Sciences Review* 41, no. 1 (2013): 3–10. doi: 10.1097/JES.0b013e3182724817. PMID: 23038243; for the distinction between cramps and spasms, see http://www.emedicinehealth.com/slideshow_pic tures_muscle_cramps_and_muscle_spasms/article_em.htm.

10. On the role of inflammation in aging, and specifically in muscle loss, these articles will get you started: Hae Young Chung, Mateo Cesari, Stephen Anton, Emmaneuelle Marzetti, et al., "Molecular Inflammation: Underpinnings of Aging and Age-Related Diseases," *Ageing Research Reviews* 8, no. 1 (2009): 18–30. doi: 10.1016/j. arr.2008.07.002; Anne M. Minihane, Sophie Vinoy, Wendy R. Russell, Athanasia Baka, et al., "Low-Grade Inflammation, Diet Composition and Health: Current Research Evidence and Its Translation," *British Journal of Nutrition* 114, no. 7 (2015): 999–1012. doi: 10.1017/S0007114515002093; Christopher Nelke, Ranier Dziewas, Jens Minnerup, Sven G. Meuth, and Tobias Ruck, "Skeletal Muscle as Potential Central Link between Sarcopenia and Immune Senescence," *EBioMedicine* 49 (2019): 381–88. doi: 10.1016/j.ebiom.2019.10.034. PMID: 31662290; PMCID: PMC6945275, https://www.ebiomedicine.com/article/S2352-3964(19)30704-2/fulltext; and the classic, original work by Claudio Franceschi and Judith Campisi, "Chronic Inflammation (Inflammaging) and Its Potential Contribution to Age-Associated Diseases," *Journals of Gerontology. Series A, Biological Sciences and Medical Sciences* 69, suppl. 1 (2014): S4–9. doi: 10.1093/gerona/glu057.

11. Li Li Ji, Chounghung Kang, and Yang Zhang, "Exercise-Induced Hormesis and Skeletal Muscle Health," *Free Radical Biology and Medicine* 98 (2016): 113–22. doi: 10.1016/j.freeradbiomed.2016.02.025. PMID: 26916558; also, Jonathan M. Peake, James F. Markworth, Kazunori Nosaka, Truls Raastad, et al., "Modulating Exercise-Induced Hormesis: Does Equal More?," *Journal of Applied Physiology* 119, no. 3 (2015): 172–89. doi: 10.1152/japplphysiol.01055.2014. PMID: 25977451. Li Li Ji wrote a more technical review: "Redox Signaling in Skeletal Muscle: Role of Aging and Exercise," *Advances in Physiology Education* 39 (2015): 352–59. doi: 10.1152/ advan.00106.2014. PMID: 26628659.

12. Giovanni Vitale, Matteo Cesari, and Daniella Mari, "Aging of the Endocrine System and Its Potential Impact on Sarcopenia," *European Journal of Internal Medicine* 35 (2016): 10–15. doi: 10.1016/j.ejim.2016.07.017. PMID: 27484963.

13. To see pictures and read more about this, see Belgian Blue (https://en.wikipedia.org/wiki/Belgian_Blue) and Piedmontese (https://en.wikipedia.org/wiki/Piedmontese_cattle).

14. A. Besse-Patin, E. Montastier, C. Vinel, I. Castan-Laurell, et al., "Effect of Endurance Training on Skeletal Muscle Myokine Expression in Obese Men: Identification of Apelin as a Novel Myokine," *International Journal of Obesity (London)* 38, no. 5 (2014): 707–13. doi: 10.1038/ijo.2013.158. PMID: 23979219.

15. The effect of muscle on blood sugar and other aspects of metabolism is thoroughly discussed by Robin A. McGregor, David Cameron-Smith, and Sally D. Poppitt, "It Is Not Just Muscle Mass: A Review of Muscle Quality, Composition and Metabolism during Ageing as Determinants of Muscle Function and Mobility in Later Life," *Longevity & Healthspan* 3, no. 9 (2014): 2046–2395. doi: 10.1186/-3-9. PMID: 25520782.

16. A lot has been written about the role of the mitochondria and aging muscles and muscle loss. Keep in mind that some is contradictory as the field is evolving rapidly. Some of the better articles (some quite technical) are Chounghun Kang and Li Li Ji, "Role of PGC-1α in Muscle Function and Aging," *Journal of Sport Health Science* 2, no. 2 (2013): 81–86, /doi.org/10.1016/j.jshs.2013.03.005; R. T. Hepple, "Impact of Aging on Mitochondrial Function in Cardiac and Skeletal Muscle," *Free Radical Biology and Medicine* 98 (2016): 177–86. doi: 10.1016/j.freeradbiomed.2016.03.017. PMID: 27033952; Gregory D. Cartee, Russell T. Hepple, Marcus M. Bamman, and Juleen R. Zierath, "Exercise Promotes Healthy Aging of Skeletal Muscle," *Cell Metabolism* 23, no. 6 (2016): 1034–47. doi: 10.1016/j.cmet.2016.05.007. PMID: 27304505. Finally, although L. Know talks briefly about aging, his excellent and readable 2018 book on the mitochondria is a perpetually good source on the topic: *The Future of Mitochondria in Medicine: The Key to Understanding Disease, Chronic Illness, Aging, and Life Itself.*

17. You can read these studies if so inclined: Adam R. Konopka, Miranda K. Suer, Christopher A. Wolff, and Matthew P. Harber, "Markers of Human Skeletal Muscle Mitochondrial Biogenesis and Quality Control: Effects of Age and Aerobic Exercise Training," *Journals of Gerontology. Series A, Biological Sciences and Medical Sciences* 69, no. 4 (2014): 371–78. doi: 10.1093/gerona/glt107. PMID: 23873965; Gilles Gouspillou, Nicolas Sgarioto, Sofia Kapchinsky, Fennigje Purves-Smith, et al., "Increased Sensitivity to Mitochondrial Permeability Transition and Myonuclear Translocation of Endonuclease G in Atrophied Muscle of Physically Active Older Humans," *FASEB Journal* 28, no. 4 (2014): 1621–33. doi: 10.1096/fj.13-242750. PMID: 24371120.

18. For an extensive summary of the process, see Silvia Carnio, Francesca LoVerso, Martin A. Baraibar, Emaneula Longa, et al., "Autophagy Impairment in Muscle Induces Neuromuscular Junction Degeneration and Precocious Aging," *Cell Reports* 8, no. 5 (2014): 1509–21. doi: 10.1016/j.celrep.2014.07.061. PMID: 25176656; and the ultimate review of the NMJ and its role in muscle aging by E. Edstrom et al., "Factors Contributing to Neuromuscular Impairment and Sarcopenia during Aging."

19. Haley J. Denison, Cyrus Cooper, Alvin A. Sayer, and Sian M. Robinson, "Prevention and Optimal Management of Sarcopenia: A Review of Combined Exercise and Nutrition Interventions to Improve Muscle Outcomes in Older People," *Clinical Interventions in Aging* 10 (2015): 859–69. doi: 10.2147/CIA.S55842. PMID: 25999704.

20. Caterina Tezze, Vanina Romanello, Maria A. Desbats, Gian P. Fadini, et al., "Age-Associated Loss of OPA1 in Muscle Impacts Muscle Mass, Metabolic Homeostasis, Systemic Inflammation, and Epithelial Senescence," *Cell Metabolism* 25, no. 6 (2017): 1374–89. e6. doi: 10.1016/j.cmet.2017.04.021. PMID: 28552492.

21. All of the articles I extolled in note 3 discuss the benefits of strength or resistance training. If you want more detail on the cellular mechanisms that account for these benefits, see P. J. Atherton, J. Babraj, K. Smith, J. Singh, M. J. Rennie, and H. Wackerhage, "Selective Activation of AMPK-PGC-1alpha or PKB-TSC2-mTOR Signaling Can Explain Specific Adaptive Responses to Endurance or Resistance Training-Like Electrical Muscle Stimulation," *FASEB Journal* 19, no. 7 (2005): 786–88. doi: 10.1096/fj.04-2179fje. PMID: 15716393.

22. The articles I cited above by Li Li Ji et al. in note 11 detail the PGC results. Gene expression studies, which list specific genes active in the systems studied (e.g., human or rodent muscle cells) are proliferating. I'm not sure how much information we get from them because we don't know all the genes involved and how they interact; a few that focus on muscle are Aretem Zykovich, Alan Hubbard, James M. Flynn, Mark Tarnopolsky, et al., "Genome-Wide DNA Methylation Changes with Age in Disease-Free Human Skeletal Muscle," *Aging Cell* 13, no. 2 (2014): 360–66. doi: 10.1111/acel.12180. PMID: 24304487; PMCID; and Simon Melov, Mark A. Tarnopolsky, Kenneth Beckma, Kristin Felkey, and Alan Hubbard, "Resistance Exercise Reverses Aging in Human Skeletal Muscle," *PloS One* 2, no. 5 (2007): e465. https://doi.org/10.1371/journal.pone.0000465.

23. Denison et al., "Prevention and Optimal Management of Sarcopenia" give an overview of studies of exercise; motor unit loss is reviewed by Power et al., "Human Neuromuscular Structure and Function in Old Age."

24. These results are from Konopka et al., "Markers of Human Skeletal Muscle Mitochondrial Biogenesis and Quality Control."

25. For an interesting and important commentary on the effects of too much exercise, see Christopher C. Case, John Mandrola, and Lennard Zinn, *The Haywire Heart: How Too Much Exercise Can Kill You, and What You Can Do to Protect Your Heart* (Boulder, CO: Velo Press, 2017). Too much means that prolonged production of ROS and inflammatory cytokines can activate catabolic pathways, impede protein synthesis, and overwhelm endogenous defense mechanisms, causing adverse effects. For a discussion on the downside of too much exercise on the cardiovascular system, see James H. O'Keefe, Evan L. O'Keefe, and Carl J. Lavie, "The Goldilocks Zone for Exercise: Not Too Little, Not Too Much," *Missouri Medicine* 115, no. 2 (2018): 98–105. PMID: 30228692. For effects on the NMJ, see Gregorio Valdez, Juan C. Tapia, Hiyuno Kang, Gregory D. Clemenson, et al., "Attenuation of Age-Related Changes in Mouse Neuromuscular Synapses by Caloric Restriction and Exercise," *Proceedings of the National Academy of Sciences of the United States of America* 107, no. 33 (2010): 14863–68. https://doi.org/10.1073/pnas.1002220107; additional NMJ effects were described by Aagaard et al., "Role of the Nervous System in Sarcopenia and Muscle Atrophy with Aging." Finally, for easy-to-read articles on exercise (as well as a variety of other topics

related to the science of aging), the National Institute of Aging maintains an excellent website, https://www.nia.nih.gov/health/exercise-physical-activity.

26. Jonathon M. Peake, James F. Markworth, Kazunori Nosaka, Truls Raastad, Glen D. Wadley, and Vernon G. Coffey, "Modulating Exercise-Induced Hormesis: Does Less Equal More?," *Journal of Applied Physiology* 119, no. 3 (2015): 172–89. doi: 10.1152/japplphysiol.01055.2014. PMID: 25977451.

27. Peake et al., "Modulating Exercise-induced Hormesis: Does Equal More?"

28. Ji et al. (2015, 2016), cited in note 1.

29. EMS is described in more detail by Atherton et al., "Selective Activation."

30. Yuki Tamura, Yataka Matsunaga, Yu Kitaoka, and Hideo Hatta, "Effects of Heat Stress Treatment on Age-Dependent Unfolded Protein Response in Different Types of Skeletal Muscle," *Journals of Gerontology. Series A, Biological Sciences and Medical Sciences* 72, no. 3 (2017): 299–308. doi: 10.1093/gerona/glw063. PMID: 27071782.

31. For a readable review of protein sources and breakdown, though a bit dated, see M. J. Rennie, A. Selby, P. Atherton, K. Smith, V. Kumar, E. L. Glover, and S. M. Philips, "Facts, Noise and Wishful Thinking: Muscle Protein Turnover in Aging and Human Disuse Atrophy," *Scandinavian Journal of Medicine and Science in Sports* 20, no. 1 (2010): 5–9. doi: 10.1111/j.1600-0838.2009.00967.x. PMID: 19558380. Another good review is Siân Robinson, Cyrus Cooper, and Avan Aihie Sayer, "Nutrition and Sarcopenia: A Review of the Evidence and Implications for Preventive Strategies," *Journal of Aging Research*, article ID 510801 (2012). doi.org/10.1155/2012/510801; the experiments showing that exercise before eating protein enhances your ability to take in amino acids are described by Nicholas A. Burd, Stefan H. Gorissen, and Luc J. van Loon, "Anabolic Resistance of Muscle Protein Synthesis with Aging," *Exercise and Sport Sciences Review* 41, no. 3 (2013): 169–73. doi: 10.1097/JES.0b013e318292f3d5. PMID: 23558692. For a comprehensive review of the mTOR signaling system and how protein intake interacts with it, specifically in aging muscle, see George A. Soultoukis and Linda Partridge, "Dietary Protein, Metabolism, and Aging," *Annual Review of Biochemistry* 85 (2016): 5–34. doi: 10.1146/annurev-biochem-060815-014422. PMID: 27145842. Finally, the role of inactivity, coupled with nutrition, in muscle loss is described by F. W. Booth and K. A. Zwetsloot, "Basic Concepts about Genes, Inactivity and Aging," *Scandinavian Journal of Medicine and Science in Sports* 20, no. 1 (2010): 1–4. doi: 10.1111/j.1600-0838.2009.00972.x. PMID: 19602189.

32. Morgan. E. Levine, Jorge A. Suarez, Sebasttian Brandhorst, Priya Balasubramanian, Chia-Weh Cheng, Federica Madia, Luigi Fontana, Mario Mirisola, Jaime Guevara-Aguirre, . . . and Valter Longo, "Low Protein Intake Is Associated with a Major Reduction in IGF-1, Cancer, and Overall Mortality in the 65 and Younger But Not Older Population," *Cell Metabolism* 19, no. 3 (2014): 407–17. https://doi.org/10.1016/j.cmet.2014.02.006.

33. Oliver Perkin, Polly McGuigan, Dylan Thompson, and Keith Stokes, "A Reduced Activity Model: A Relevant Tool for the Study of Ageing Muscle," *Biogerontology* 17, no. 3 (2016): 435–47. https://doi.org/10.1007/s10522-015-9613-9. If you are dubious of these numbers, and I know most people cling to the idea that you have

to eat a lot of protein to build and maintain muscle, check out Peter Attia's blog at eatingacademy.com to see that you don't need a lot of protein to do so (but note that I'm not endorsing his particular diet).

34. B. Ramamurthy and L. Larsson, "Detection of an Aging-Related Increase in Advanced Glycation End Products in Fast- and Slow-Twitch Skeletal Muscles in the Rat," *Biogerontology* 14, no. 3 (2013): 293–301. doi: 10.1007/s10522-013-9430-y. PMID: 23681254.

35. For a review of evidence showing that some actions, such as CR, may result in life span extension by activating mitochondria that then form reactive oxygen species, in turn activating cellular antioxidant defenses, see M. Ristow and S. Schmeisser, "Extending Life Span by Increasing Oxidative Stress," *Free Radical Biology and Medicine* 51, no. 2 (2011): 327–36. doi: 10.1016/j.freeradbiomed.2011.05.010. PMID: 21619928.

36. Russell T. Hepple, David J. Baker, Jan J. Kaczor, and Daniel J. Krause, "Long-Term Caloric Restriction Abrogates the Age-Related Decline in Skeletal Muscle Aerobic Function," *FASEB Journal* 19, no. 10 (2005): 1320–22. doi: 10.1096/fj.04-3535fje. PMID: 15955841.

37. Caloric restriction, especially combined with exercise, reversed sarcopenia in rats: Stephanie E. Wohlgemuth, Arnold Y. Seo, Emmanuelle Marzetti, Hazel A. Lees, and Christian Leeuwenburgh, "Skeletal Muscle Autophagy and Apoptosis during Aging: Effects of Calorie Restriction and Life-Long Exercise," *Experimental Gerontolology* 45, no. 2 (2010): 138–48. doi: 10.1016/j.exger.2009.11.002. PMID: 19903516. In humans, calorie restriction without malnutrition inhibited inflammation and increased autophagy to protect muscles: Ling Yang, Danilo Licastro, Edda Cava, Nicola Veronese, Francesca Spelta, Wanda Rizza, Beatrice Bertozzi, Dennis T. Villareal, Gokhan S. Hotamisligil, and Luigi Fontana, "Long-Term Calorie Restriction Enhances Cellular Quality-Control Processes in Human Skeletal Muscle," *Cell Reports* 14, no. 3 (2016): 422–28. doi: 10.1016/j.celrep.2015.12.042. PMID: 26774472.

38. Ann-Sophie Arnold, Anna Egger, and Christof Handschin, "PGC-1α and Myokines in the Aging Muscle—a Mini-Review," *Gerontology* 57, no. 1 (2011): 37–43. doi: 10.1159/000281883. PMID: 20134150.

39. Valdez et al., "Attenuation of Age-Related Changes in Mouse Neuromuscular Synapses by Caloric Restriction and Exercise."

40. Vitale, Cesari, and Mari, "Aging of the Endocrine System and its Potential Impact on Sarcopenia"; Annabella La Colla, Lucia Pronsato, Lorena Milanesi, and Andrea Vasconsuelo, "17β-Estradiol and Testosterone in Sarcopenia: Role of Satellite Cells," *Ageing Research Reviews* 24, pt. B (2015): 166–77. doi: 10.1016/j.arr.2015.07.011. PMID: 26247846; Astrid M. Horstman, E. Lichar Dillon, Randall J. Urban, and Melissa Sheffield-Moore, "The Role of Androgens and Estrogens on Healthy Aging and Longevity," *Journals of Gerontology. Series A, Biological Sciences and Medical Sciences* 67, no. 11 (2012): 1140–52. doi: 10.1093/gerona/gls068. PMID: 22451474; John E. Morley, "Pharmacologic Options for the Treatment of Sarcopenia," *Calcified Tissue International* 98, no. 4 (2016): 319–33. doi: 10.1007/s00223-015-0022-5. PMID: 26100650.

41. Richard V. Clark, Ann C. Walker, Susan Andrews, Phillip Turnbull, et al., "Safety, Pharmacokinetics and Pharmacological Effects of the Selective Androgen Receptor Modulator, GSK2881078, in Healthy Men and Postmenopausal Women," *British Journal of Clinical Pharmacology* 83, no. 10 (2017): 2179–94. doi: 10.1111/bcp.13316. PMID: 28449232.

42. The MYOAGE project, conducted in the European Union to explore the basis of skeletal muscle aging, is introduced by Gillian Butler-Browne, Jamie McPhee, Vincent Mouly, and Anton Ottavi, "Understanding and Combating Age-Related Muscle Weakness: MYOAGE Challenge," *Biogerontology* 14, no. 3 (2013): 229–30, https://doi.org/10.1007/s10522-013-9438-3. You can read about IGF specifically in Laura Bucci, Stell L. Yani, Christina Fabbri, Astrid Y. Bijlsma, et al., "Circulating Levels of Adipokines and IGF-1 Are Associated with Skeletal Muscle Strength of Young and Old Healthy Subjects," *Biogerontology* 14, no. 3 (2013): 261–72. doi: 10.1007/s10522-013-9428-5. PMID: 23666343.

43. Clark et al., "Safety, Pharmacokinetics and Pharmacological Effects of the Selective Androgen Receptor Modulator."

44. LaColla et al., "17β-Estradiol and Testosterone in Sarcopenia."

45. Vitale et al., "Aging of the Endocrine System and Its Potential Impact on Sarcopenia."

46. Clark et al., "Safety, Pharmacokinetics and Pharmacological effects of the Selective Androgen Receptor Modulator."

47. LaColla et al., "17β-Estradiol and Testosterone in Sarcopenia."

48. Aagard et al., "Role of the Nervous System in Sarcopenia and Muscle Atrophy with Aging: Strength Training as a Countermeasure."

49. T. Brioche, R. A. Kireev, S. Cuesta, A. Gratas-Delamarche, J. A. Tresguerres, M. C. Gomez-Cabrera, and J. Viña, "Growth Hormone Replacement Therapy Prevents Sarcopenia by a Dual Mechanism: Improvement of Protein Balance and of Antioxidant Defenses," *Journals of Gerontology. Series A, Biological Sciences and Medical Sciences* 69, no. 10 (2014): 1186–98. doi: 10.1093/gerona/glt187. PMID: 24300031.

50. A good overview of creatine's actions and review of the scientific literature can be found at http://mkt.s.designsforhealth.com/techsheets/Creatine-Benefits-and-Supportive-Abstracts.pdf.

51. Arnold et al., "PGC-1α and Myokines in the Aging Muscle—a Mini-Review."

52. Marion Pauly, Beatrice Chabi, Francois Favier, Franki Vanterpool, et al., "Combined Strategies for Maintaining Skeletal Muscle Mass and Function in Aging: Myostatin Inactivation and AICAR-Associated Oxidative Metabolism Induction," *Journals of Gerontology. Series A, Biological Sciences and Medical Sciences* 70, no. 9 (2015): 1077–87. doi: 10.1093/gerona/glu147. PMID: 25227129; and to read about the role(s) of myostatin in inhibiting muscle growth and regeneration, see Gilles Carnac, Barbara Vernus, and Anne Bonnieu, "Myostatin in the Pathophysiology of Skeletal Muscle," *Current Genomics* 8, no. 7 (2007): 415–22. https://doi.org/10.2174/138920207783591672.

53. https://www.wired.com/2008/10/the-gene-for-jamaican-sprinting-success-no-not-really/.

54. Zudin Puthucheary, James R. Skipworth, Jai Rawal, Mike Loosemore, et al., "The ACE Gene and Human Performance: 12 Years On," *Sports Medicine* 41, no. 6 (2011): 433–48. doi: 10.2165/11588720-000000000-00000. PMID: 21615186.

CHAPTER 6. SKELETON

1. For a good, basic overview, see Alistair Farley, Charles Hendry, and Ella McLafferty, eds., *The Physiological Effects of Ageing* (Oxford: Wiley-Blackwell, 2011). Another is written by Jane A. Cauley, "Osteoporosis," in *The Epidemiology of Aging*, edited by Anne Newman and Jane A. Cauley, 499–522 (New York: Springer, 2012). For the current screening recommendations, see Jane A. Cauley, "Screening for Osteoporosis," *Journal of the American Medical Association* 319, no. 24 (2018): 2483–85. doi: 10.1001/jama.2018.5722. PMID: 29946707. The NIH site is https://www.bones.nih .gov/, and the Sheffield tool is available at https://www.sheffield.ac.uk/FRAX/tool.jsp.

2. Paula Mera, Kathrin Lauen, Matthieu Ferron, Cyril Confavreux, et al., "Osteocalcin Signaling in Myofibers Is Necessary and Sufficient for Optimum Adaptation to Exercise," *Cell Metabolism* 23, no. 6 (2016): 1078–92. doi: 10.1016/j. cmet.2016.05.004. PMID: 27304508. These findings were nicely summarized and extended in the accompanying editorial: Frank W. Booth, Gregory N. Ruegsegger, and T. Dylan Olver, "Exercise Has a Bone to Pick with Skeletal Muscle," *Cell Metabolism* 23, no. 6 (2016): 961–62. doi: 10.1016/j.cmet.2016.05.016. PMID: 27304494.

3. Paula Mera, Kathrin Lauen, Matthieu Ferron, Cyril Confavreux, et al., "Osteocalcin Signaling in Myofibers Is Necessary and Sufficient for Optimum Adaptation to Exercise," *Cell Metabolism* 23, no. 6 (2016): 1078–92.

4. Johannes Fessler, Russner Husic, Verena Schwetz, Elisabeth Lerchbaum et al., "Senescent T-Cells Promote Bone Loss in Rheumatoid Arthritis," *Frontiers in Immunology* 9 (2018): 95. doi: 10.3389/fimmu.2018.00095. PMID: 29472917.

5. Regina M. Martin and Pedro H. Correa, "Bone Quality and Osteoporosis Therapy," *Arquivos brasileiros de endocrinologia e metabologia* 54, no. 2 (2010): 186–99. doi: 10.1590/s0004-27302010000200015. PMID: 20485908.

6. https://ods.od.nih.gov/factsheets/Calcium-HealthProfessional/.

7. Mark J. Bolland, William Leung, Vicki Tai, Sonia Bastin, Greg D. Gamble, Andrew Grey, and Ian R. Reid, "Calcium Intake and Risk of Fracture: Systematic Review," *British Medical Journal* 351 (2015): h4580. doi: 10.1136/bmj.h4580. PMID: 26420387.

8. An early review of studies of supplementation was conducted by Benjamin M. Tang, Guy D. Eslick, Carol Nowson, Caroline Smith, and Alan Bensoussan, "Use of Calcium or Calcium in Combination with Vitamin D Supplementation to Prevent Fractures and Bone Loss in People Aged 50 Years and Older: A Meta-Analysis," *Lancet* 370, no. 9588 (2007): 657–66. doi: 10.1016/S0140-6736(07)61342-7. PMID: 17720017; the topic was revisited by Jia-Guo Zhao, Xien-Tie Zeng, Jia Wang, and Lin Liu, "Association between Calcium or Vitamin D Supplementation and Fracture Incidence in Community-Dwelling Older Adults: A Systematic Review and Meta-

Analysis," *Journal of the American Medical Association* 318, no. 24 (2017): 2466–82. doi: 10.1001/jama.2017.19344. PMID: 29279934.

9. Lynette M. Smith, J. Christopher Gallagher, Glenville Jones, and Martin Kaufmann, "Estimation of the Recommended Daily Allowance (RDA) for Vitamin D Intake Using Serum 25 Hydroxyvitamin D Level of 20ng/Ml as the End Point, May Vary According to the Analytical Measurement Technique Used," Endocrine Society Meeting, Presentation OR07-4. Summarized in a press release by the Endocrine Society, https://www.endocrine.org/news-and-advocacy/news-room/2017/new -measurement-technique-lowers-estimated-vitamin-d-recommended-daily-allowance.

10. The protective role of estrogen has been recognized for a long time; it was only after the WHI published its findings of increased cancer risk that HRT was stigmatized as protective against osteoporosis. Some of the earlier studies include N. S. Weiss, C. L. Ure, J. H. Ballard, A. R. Williams, and J. R. Daling, "Decreased Risk of Fractures of the Hip and Lower Forearm with Postmenopausal Use of Estrogen," *New England Journal of Medicine* 303, no. 21 (1980): 1195–98. doi: 10.1056/NEJM198011203032102. PMID: 7421945; and Karl Michaëlsson, John A. Baron, Bahman Y. Farahmand, Olof Johnell, Cecilia Magnusson, Per-Gunnar Persson, Ingemar Persson, and Sverker Ljunghall, "Hormone Replacement Therapy and Risk of Hip Fracture: Population Based Case-Control Study," The Swedish Hip Fracture Study Group, *British Medical Journal (clinical research ed.)* 316, no. 7148 (1998): 1858–63, https://doi.org/10.1136/bmj.316.7148.1858. Many other studies are summarized in the excellent book by Avrum Bluming and Carol Travis, *Estrogen Matters: Why Taking Hormones in Menopause Can Improve Women's Well-Being and Lengthen Their Lives—Without Raising the Risk of Breast Cancer* (New York: Little Brown Spark, 2018).

11. Again, many studies have highlighted the need to continue hormone therapy to protect against osteoporotic fractures. Two of these are D. Grady, S. M. Rubin, D. B. Petitti, C. S. Fox, D. Black, B. Ettinger, L. Ernster, and S. R. Cummings, "Hormone Therapy to Prevent Disease and Prolong Life in Postmenopausal Women," *Annals of Internal Medicine* 117, no. 12 (1992): 1016–37. doi: 10.7326/0003-4819-117-12-1016. PMID: 1443971; and N. F. Col, L. A. Bowlby, and K. McGarry, "The Role of Menopausal Hormone Therapy in Preventing Osteoporotic Fractures: A Critical Review of the Clinical Evidence," *Minerva Medica* 96, no. 5 (2005): 331–42. PMID: 16227948.

12. Writing Group for the PEPI, "Effects of Hormone Therapy on Bone Mineral Density: Results from the Postmenopausal Estrogen/Progestin Interventions (PEPI) Trial," *Journal of the American Medical Association* 276, no. 17 (1996): 1389–96. PMID: 8892713.

13. Testosterone and other "male" hormones contribute to bone density, described by Ekrim Tok, Devrim Ertunc, Utkum Oz, Handan Camdeviren, Gulay Ozdemir, and Dilek Saffet, "The Effect of Circulating Androgens on Bone Mineral Density in Postmenopausal Women," *Maturitas* 48, no. 3 (2004): 235–42. doi: 10.1016/j.maturitas.2003.11.007. PMID: 15207889. Testosterone specifically increased bone density as shown by B. E. Miller, M. J. De Souza, K. Slade, and A. A. Luciano, "Sublingual Administration of Micronized Estradiol and Progesterone, with and without Micronized Testosterone: Effect on Biochemical Markers of Bone Metabolism and Bone Mineral

Density," *Menopause* 7, no. 5 (2000): 318–26. doi: 10.1097/00042192-200007050 -00006. PMID: 10993031.

14. One of the clinical trials for the MA was reported by Kenneth G. Saag, Jeffrey Petersen, Maria Luisa Brandi, Andrew C. Karaplis, et al., "Romosozumab or Alendronate for Fracture Prevention in Women with Osteoporosis," *New England Journal of Medicine* 377, no. 15 (2017): 1417–27. doi: 10.1056/NEJMoa170832. The journal website also provides a brief video describing the results with some useful graphics: https://www.nejm.org/doi/full/10.1056/NEJMoa1708322; the *New York Times* also has a cogent summary, https://www.nytimes.com/2019/04/09/health/ osteoporosis-evenity-bone-amgen.html.

15. Two convincing studies of supplemental collagen: first, in rats, by Elisia de Almeida Jackix, Florencia Cúneo, Jamie Amaya-Farfan, Juvenal V. de Assunção, and Kesia D. Quintaes, "A Food Supplement of Hydrolyzed Collagen Improves Compositional and Biodynamic Characteristics of Vertebrae in Ovariectomized Rats," *Journal of Medicinal Food* 13, no. 6 (2010): 1385–90. doi: 10.1089/jmf.2009.0256. PMID: 20874246; and second, in humans: Suresh Kumar, Fumahito Sugihara, Keiji Suzuki, Naoki Inoue, and Siriam Venkateswarathirukumara, "A Double-Blind, Placebo-Controlled, Randomised, Clinical Study on the Effectiveness of Collagen Peptide on Osteoarthritis," *Journal of the Science of Food and Agriculture* 95, no. 4 (2015): 702–7. doi: 10.1002/jsfa.6752. PMID: 24852756. The labeling study was done by Mari Watanabe-Kamiyama, Munishigi Shimizu, Shin Kamiyama, Yasuki Taguchi, et al., "Absorption and Effectiveness of Orally Administered Low Molecular Weight Collagen Hydrolysate in Rats," *Journal of Agriculture and Food Chemistry* 58, no. 2 (2010): 835–41. doi: 10.1021/jf9031487. PMID: 19957932.

16. Unfortunately, most of the scientific literature on this topic is quite technical. The annual review piece by Robling, Castillo, and Turner, "Biomechanical and Molecular Regulation of Bone Remodeling," gives a thorough description of how load and stress affect bone. This is a little less mathematical: Engin Ozcivici, Yen K. Luu, Ben Adler, Yi-Jian Qin, Janet Rubin, Stefan Judex, and Clinton T. Rubin, "Mechanical Signals as Anabolic Agents in Bone," *Nature Reviews. Rheumatology* 6, no. 1 (2010): 50–59. doi: 10.1038/nrrheum.2009.239. PMID: 20046206.

17. Ryan E. Tomlinson and Matthew J. Silva, "Skeletal Blood Flow in Bone Repair and Maintenance," *Bone Research* 1, no. 4 (2013): 311–22. doi: 10.4248/ BR201304002. PMID: 26273509.

18. Kanniiram Alagiakrishnan, Angela Juby, David Hanley, Wayne Tymchak, and Anne Sclater A, "Role of Vascular Factors in Osteoporosis," *Journals of Gerontology. Series A, Biological Sciences and Medical Sciences* 58, no. 4 (2003): 362–26. doi: 10.1093/ gerona/58.4.m362. PMID: 12663699.

19. Described in Ozcivici et al., "Mechanical Signals as Anabolic Agents in Bone."

20. For an overview, see H. C. Heitkamp, "Training with Blood Flow Restriction. Mechanisms, Gain in Strength and Safety," *Journal of Sports Medicine and Physical Fitness* 55, no. 5 (2015): 446–56. PMID: 25678204; for a case study, see Jeremy P. Loenneke, Kaelin C. Young, Jacob M. Wilson, and J. C. Andersen, "Rehabilitation of an Osteochondral Fracture using Blood Flow Restricted Exercise: A Case Review,"

Journal of Bodywork and Movement Therapies 17, no. 1 (2013): 42–45. doi: 10.1016/j .jbmt.2012.04.006. PMID: 23294682.

21. A good summary of the causes of OA is by C. K. Kwoh (2012), "Epidemiology of Osteoarthritis," in *The Epidemiology of Aging*, edited by Anne Newman and Jane A. Cauley, 523–36 (New York: Springer, 2012).

22. Kumar et al., "A Double-Blind, Placebo-Controlled, Randomised, Clinical Study on the Effectiveness of Collagen Peptide on Osteoarthritis."

23. Two reviews with similar findings, one by a U.S. agency: Sidney J. Newberry, John D. Fitzgerald, Margaret A. Maglione, Claire E. O'Hanlon, Mareeka Booth, Aneesa Motala, Martha Timmer, Roberta Shanman, and Paul G. Shekelle, "Systematic Review for Effectiveness of Hyaluronic Acid in the Treatment of Severe Degenerative Joint Disease (DJD) of the Knee [Internet]," Rockville (MD): Agency for Healthcare Research and Quality (US) 2015, PMID: 26866204; a second from Canada: Mohit Bhandari, Raveendhara R. Bannur, Eric M. Babins, Johanna Martel-Pelletier, Moin Khan, Jean-Pierre Raynauld, Reynata Frankovich, Deanna Mcleod, Tahira Devji, Mark Phillips, et al., "Intra-Articular Hyaluronic Acid in the Treatment of Knee Osteoarthritis: A Canadian Evidence-Based Perspective," *Therapeutic Advances in Musculoskeletal Disease* 9, no. 9 (2017): 231–46, https://doi.org/10.1177/1759720X17729641; and a clinical trial by Bahar Dernek, Tihar M. Duymus, Pinar K. Koseoglu, Tugba Aydin, Falma N Kesiktas, Cihan Aksoy, and Serhat Mutlu, "Efficacy of Single-Dose Hyaluronic Acid Products with Two Different Structures in Patients with Early-Stage Knee Osteoarthritis," *Journal of Physical Therapy Science* 28, no. 11 (2016): 3036–40, https:// doi.org/10.1589/jpts.28.3036.

24. For clinical evaluations of stem cells in these joints, see Rodrigo Mardones, Claudio M. Jofré, L. Tobar, and Jose J. Minguell, "Mesenchymal Stem Cell Therapy in the Treatment of Hip Osteoarthritis," *Journal of Hip Preservation Surgery* 4, no. 2 (2017): 159–63. doi: 10.1093/jhps/hnx011. PMID: 28630737; Fareydoun Davatchi, Bahar Sadeghi Abdollahi, Mandana Mohyeddin, and Beyrooz Nikbin. "Mesenchymal Stem Cell Therapy for Knee Osteoarthritis: 5 Years Follow-up of Three Patients," *International Journal of Rheumatic Diseases* 19, no. 3 (2016): 219–25. doi: 10.1111/1756 -185X.12670. PMID: 25990685. And my brief, nontechnical evaluation of stem cell therapies for knee OA: Beth Bennett, "Stem Cells to Treat Osteoarthritis," *Trail Runner* 2018, https://trailrunnermag.com/training/stem-the-joint-aging-tide.html.

25. Jeffrey, Kiernan, Sally Hu, Mark D. Grynpas, John E. Davies, and William L. Stanford, "Systemic Mesenchymal Stromal Cell Transplantation Prevents Functional Bone Loss in a Mouse Model of Age-Related Osteoporosis," *Stem Cells and Translational Medicine* 5, no. 5 (2016): 683–93. doi: 10.5966/sctm.2015-0231. PMID: 26987353.

26. https://stemcells.nih.gov/info/basics/7.htm.

27. To read about the utility and uses of MSC, see Hassan Afizah and James H. Hui, "Mesenchymal Stem Cell Therapy for Osteoarthritis," *Journal of Clinical Orthopaedics and Trauma* 7, no. 3 (2016): 177–82. doi: 10.1016/j.jcot.2016.06.006. PMID: 27489413; for even more on the MSC, see Roberto Berebichez-Fridman, Ricardo Gómez-García, Julio Granados-Montiel, Enrique Berebichez-Fastlicht, Anell Olivos-Meza, Julio Granados, Cristain Velasquillo, and Clemente Ibarra, "The Holy Grail

of Orthopedic Surgery: Mesenchymal Stem Cell—Their Current Uses and Potential Applications," *Stem Cells International* (2017): 2638305. doi: 10.1155/2017/2638305. PMID: 28698718. The problem of rejection of stem cells from allogeneic sources is described by Valeria Sordi and Lorenzo Piemonti, "Therapeutic Plasticity of Stem Cells and Allograft Tolerance," *Cytotherapy* 13, no. 6 (2011): 647–60. doi: 10.3109/14653249.2011.583476. PMID: 21554176.

28. Byron A. Tompkins, Darcy L. DiFede, Aisha Khan, Ana Marie Landin, et al., "Allogeneic Mesenchymal Stem Cells Ameliorate Aging Frailty: A Phase II Randomized, Double-Blind, Placebo-Controlled Clinical Trial," *Journals of Gerontology. Series A, Biological Sciences and Medical Sciences* 72, no. 11 (2017): 1513–22. doi: 10.1093/gerona/glx137. PMID: 28977399.

29. Hassan and Hui, "Mesenchymal Stem Cell Therapy for Osteoarthritis."

30. https://vcel.com/about-vericel/.

31. For a clinical trial evaluating the MAC treatment, see Mats Brittberg, David Recker, John Ilgenfritz, and Daniel B. F. Saris, SUMMIT Extension Study Group, "Matrix-Applied Characterized Autologous Cultured Chondrocytes Versus Microfracture: Five-Year Follow-up of a Prospective Randomized Trial," *American Journal of Sports Medicine* 46, no. 6 (2018): 1343–51. doi: 10.1177/0363546518756976. PMID: 29565642; I'm not endorsing this procedure, but the company has a nifty video on its website showing the role of knee cartilage in joint protection and their procedure: https://www.maci.com/patients/how-maci-works/the-maci-procedure.html. For a comparative look at some of the past treatments including MAC and microfracture, see Ajaykumar Shanmugaraj, Ryan P. Coughlin, Gabriel N. Kuper, Seper Ekhtiari, Nicole Simunovic, Volker Musahl, and Olufemi R. Ayeni, "Changing Trends in the Use of Cartilage Restoration Techniques for the Patellofemoral Joint: A Systematic Review," *Knee Surgery, Sports Traumatology, Arthroscopy* 27, no. 3 (2019): 854–67. doi: 10.1007/s00167-018-5139-4. PMID: 30232541. To read about microfractures, see J. Richard Steadman, Karen K. Briggs, Juan J. Rodrigo, Mininder S. Kocher, et al., "Outcomes of Microfracture for Traumatic Chondral Defects of the Knee: Average 11-year Follow-Up," *Arthroscopy* 19, no. 5 (2003): 477–84. doi: 10.1053/jars.2003.50112. PMID: 12724676.

32. Ok Hee Jeon, Chaekyu Kim, Sona Rathod, Jae Wook Chung, et al., "Local Clearance of Senescent Cells Attenuates the Development of Post-Traumatic Osteoarthritis and Creates a Pro-Regenerative Environment," *Nature Medicine* 23 (2017): 775–81. https://doi.org/10.1038/nm.4324.

33. Caressa Lietman, Brian Wu, Sarah Lechner, Andrew Shinar, et al., "Inhibition of Wnt/β-Catenin Signaling Ameliorates Osteoarthritis in a Murine Model of Experimental Osteoarthritis," *JCI Insight* 3, no. 3 (2018): e96308. doi: 10.1172/jci .insight.96308. PMID: 29415892, https://insight.jci.org/articles/view/96308.

34. Lee H. Riley and Suzanne M. Jan de Beur, *White Paper on Back Pain and Osteoporosis* (Berkeley, CA: UC Berkeley School of Public Health, 2020).

35. Stuart McGill, *Back Mechanic: The Step-by-Step McGill Method to Manage Back Pain* (Gravenhurst, Ontario: Backfitpro, 2015), www.backfitpro.com.

CHAPTER 7. CARDIOVASCULAR SYSTEM

1. Good statistics from both of these sources, though NIH probably updates frequently: https://www.nia.nih.gov/health/heart-health-and-aging; and P. A. Heidenreich, J. G. Trogdon, O. A. Khavjou, J. Butler, K. Dracup, M. D. Ezekowitz, E. A. Finkelstein, Y. Hong, S. C. Johnston, A. Khera, et al., "Forecasting the Future of Cardiovascular Disease in the United States: A Policy Statement from the American Heart Association," *Circulation* 123, no. 8 (2011): 933–44. doi: 10.1161/CIR.0b013e31820a55f5. PMID: 21262990.

2. Marja Steenman and Gilles Lande, "Cardiac Aging and Heart Disease in Humans," *Biophysical Reviews* 9, no. 2 (2017): 131–37, https://doi.org/10.1007/s12551-017-0255-9.

3. Goro Katsuumi, Ippei Shimizu, Yoko Yoshida, and Tohru Minamino, "Vascular Senescence in Cardiovascular and Metabolic Diseases," *Frontiers in Cardiovascular Medicine* 5 (2018): 18. doi: 10.3389/fcvm.2018.00018. PMID: 29556500.

4. Steenman and Lande, "Cardiac Aging and Heart Disease in Humans." You can see a good illustration of the fibrosis process in Alison K. Schroer and W. David Merryman, "Mechanobiology of Myofibroblast Adhesion in Fibrotic Cardiac Disease," *Journal of Cell Science* 128, no. 10 (2015): 1865–75. doi: 10.1242/jcs.162891. PMID: 25918124; and the misfolding that produces amyloid at the Cleveland Clinic website, https://consultqd.clevelandclinic.org/antibody-treatment-holds-promise-in-treating-patients-with-relapsed-or-refractory-light-chain-amyloidosis/.

5. Huiji Li, Sven Horke, and Ulrich Förstermann, "Oxidative Stress in Vascular Disease and its Pharmacological Prevention," *Trends in Pharmacological Science* 34, no. 6 (2013): 313–19. doi: 10.1016/j.tips.2013.03.007. PMID: 23608227.

6. John R. Mercer, "Mitochondrial Bioenergetics and Therapeutic Intervention in Cardiovascular Disease," *Pharmacology and Therapeutics* 141, no. 1 (2014): 13–20. doi: 10.1016/j.pharmthera.2013.07.011. PMID: 23911986. A lovely illustration of this damage is in Yuliya Mikhed, Andreas Daiber, and Sebastian Steven, "Mitochondrial Oxidative Stress, Mitochondrial DNA Damage and Their Role in Age-Related Vascular Dysfunction," *International Journal of Molecular Sciences* 16, no. 7 (2015): 15918–53. doi: 10.3390/ijms160715918. PMID: 26184181.

7. For a readable (and entertaining) treatise on the effects of chronic stress, see Robert Sapolsky, *Why Zebras Don't Get Ulcers*, 3rd ed. (New York: Henry Holt, 2004).

8. Natalie E. de Picciotto, Lindsey B. Gano, Lawrence C. Johnson, Christopher R. Martens, Amy L. Sindler, Kaatherine F. Mills, Shin-Ichiro Imai, and Douglas R. Seals DR, "Nicotinamide Mononucleotide Supplementation Reverses Vascular Dysfunction and Oxidative Stress with Aging in Mice," *Aging Cell* 15, no. 3 (2016): 522–30. doi: 10.1111/acel.12461. PMID: 26970090.

9. For a thorough review of how the body regulates cholesterol and how this regulation wanes with age, see A. E. Morgan, K. M. Mooney, S. J. Wilkinson, N. A. Pickles, and M. T. McAuley, "Cholesterol Metabolism: A Review of How Ageing Disrupts the Biological Mechanisms Responsible for its Regulation," *Ageing Research Reviews* 27

(2016): 108–24. doi: 10.1016/j.arr.2016.03.008. PMID: 27045039; the microbial action is described by Susan A. Joyce, John MacSharry, Patrick G. Casey, Michael Kinsella, Eileen F. Murphy, Fergus Shanahan, Colin Hill, and Cormac G. M. Gahan, "Regulation of Host Weight Gain and Lipid Metabolism by Bacterial Bile Acid Modification in the Gut," *Proceedings of the National Academy of Sciences* 111, no. 20 (2014): 7421–26. doi: 10.1073/pnas.1323599111. The role of oxidation damage is thoroughly described by Florian Kleefeldt, Uwe Rueckschloss, and Suleyman Ergün, "CEACAM1 Promotes Vascular Aging Processes," *Aging* 12, no. 4 (2020): 3121–23, https://doi.org/10.18632/aging.102868; and for a digestion of the technical articles, read about various aspects of cholesterol metabolism on my blog, www.Senesc-sense.com.

　　10. Matthew J. Rossman, Jessica R. Santos-Parker, Chelsea A. C. Steward, Nina Z. Bispham, Lauren M. Cuevas, Hannah L. Rosenberg, Kayla A. Woodward, Michael Chonchol, Rachel A. Gioscia-Ryan, Michael P. Murphy, and Douglas R. Seals, "Chronic Supplementation with a Mitochondrial Antioxidant (MitoQ) Improves Vascular Function in Healthy Older Adults," *Hypertension* 71, no. 6 (2018): 1056–63. doi: 10.1161/HYPERTENSIONAHA.117.10787. PMID: 29661838.

　　11. Katsuumi et al., "Vascular Senescence in Cardiovascular and Metabolic Diseases."

　　12. Emma J. Akers, Stephen J. Nicholls, and Belinda A. Di Bartolo, "Plaque Calcification: Do Lipoproteins Have a Role?," *Arteriosclerosis, Thrombosis and Vascular Biology* 39, no. 10 (2019): 1902–10. doi: 10.1161/ATVBAHA.119.311574. PMID: 31462089; these authors provide illuminating illustrations of the process at https://www.ahajournals.org/doi/10.1161/ATVBAHA.119.311574; the effect of statins on infections is discussed by Elizabeth Sapey, Jaimin M. Patel, Hannah L. Greenwood, Georgia M. Walton, et al., "Pulmonary Infections in the Elderly Lead to Impaired Neutrophil Targeting, Which Is Improved by Simvastatin," *American Journal of Respiratory and Critical Care Medicine* 196, no. 10 (2017): 1325–36, https://doi.org/10.1164/rccm.201704-0814OC.

　　13. Helene Girouard and Costantino Iadecola, "Neurovascular Coupling in the Normal Brain and in Hypertension, Stroke, and Alzheimer Disease," *Journal of Applied Physiology* 100, no. 1 (2006): 328–35. doi: 10.1152/japplphysiol.00966.2005. PMID: 16357086.

　　14. For a very readable and comprehensive overview of why aerobic exercise is beneficial for the CV system and the rest of the body, see Douglas R. Seals, "Edward F. Adolph Distinguished Lecture: The Remarkable Anti-Aging Effects of Aerobic Exercise on Systemic Arteries," *Journal of Applied Physiology* 117, no. 5 (2014): 425–39. doi: 10.1152/japplphysiol.00362.2014. PMID: 24855137; for a good, brief overview, see the (short) editorial introducing an entire journal volume on the issue by Sulin Cheng and Lijuan Mao, "Physical Activity Continuum throughout the Lifespan: Is Exercise Medicine or What?," *Journal of Sport and Health Science* 5, no. 2 (2016): 127–28, https://doi.org/10.1016/j.jshs.2016.03.005.

　　15. S. Taddei, F. Galetta, A. Virdis, L. Ghiadoni, et al., "Physical Activity Prevents Age-Related Impairment in Nitric Oxide Availability in Elderly Athletes," *Circulation* 101, no. 25 (2000): 2896–901. doi: 10.1161/01.cir.101.25.2896. PMID: 10869260.

16. To read about differential responses of older women to aerobic exercise, see Kari L. Moreau, Brian L. Stauffer, Wendy M. Kohrt, and D. R. Seals, "Essential Role of Estrogen for Improvements in Vascular Endothelial Function with Endurance Exercise in Postmenopausal Women," *Journal of Clinical Endocrinology and Metabolism* 98, no. 11 (2013): 4507–15, https://doi.org/10.1210/jc.2013-2183; M. Yoshizawa, S. Maeda, A. Miyaki, M. Misono, et al., "Effect of 12 Weeks of Moderate-Intensity Resistance Training on Arterial Stiffness: A Randomised Controlled Trial in Women Aged 32–59 Years," *British Journal of Sports Medicine* 43, no. 8 (2009): 615–18. doi: 10.1136/bjsm.2008.052126. PMID: 18927168; finally, for a really deep dive into what estrogen does to muscle, see Deborah L. Enns and Peter M. Tiidus, "The Influence of Estrogen on Skeletal Muscle: Sex Matters," *Sports Medicine* 40, no. 1 (2010): 41–58. doi: 10.2165/11319760-000000000-00000. PMID: 20020786.

17. Raphael F. P. Castellan and Marco Meloni, "Mechanisms and Therapeutic Targets of Cardiac Regeneration: Closing the Age Gap," *Frontiers in Cardiovascular Medicine* 5 (2018): 7. doi: 10.3389/fcvm.2018.00007. PMID: 29459901.

18. Shey-Shing Sheu, Danhanjaya Nauduri, and M. W. Anders, "Targeting Antioxidants to Mitochondria: A New Therapeutic Direction," *Biochimica Biophysica Acta* 1762, no. 2 (2006): 256–65. doi: 10.1016/j.bbadis.2005.10.007. PMID: 16352423.

19. Seals, "The Remarkable Anti-Aging Effects of Aerobic Exercise on Systemic Arteries."

20. For clinical trials, see Rossman et al., "Chronic Supplementation with a Mitochondrial Antioxidant (MitoQ) Improves Vascular Function in Healthy Older Adults," and Li, "Oxidative Stress in Vascular Disease and its Pharmacological Prevention"; for an extensive discussion of mitochondrial structure and function and its role in CVD, see Mercer, "Mitochondrial Bioenergetics and Therapeutic Intervention in Cardiovascular Disease."

21. Another reason to read the great review by Seals, "The Remarkable Anti-Aging Effects of Aerobic Exercise on Systemic Arteries."

22. Adriana Buitrago-Lopez, Jean Sanderson, Laura Johnson, Samantha Warnakula, Angela Wood, Emanuele Di Angelantonio, and Oscar H. Franco, "Chocolate Consumption and Cardiometabolic Disorders: Systematic Review and Meta-Analysis," *British Medical Journal* 343 (2011): d4488. doi: 10.1136/bmj.d4488.

23. Eric van der Veer, Cynthia Ho, Caroline O'Neil, Nicole Barbosa, et al., "Extension of Human Cell Lifespan by Nicotinamide Phosphoribosyltransferase," *Journal of Biological Chemistry* 282, no. 15 (2007): 10841–45. doi: 10.1074/jbc.C700018200. PMID: 17307730.

24. Katsuumi et al., "Vascular Senescence in Cardiovascular and Metabolic Diseases."

25. Russell H. Knutsen, Scott C. Beeman, Thomas J. Broekelmann, Delong Liu, et al., "Minoxidil Improves Vascular Compliance, Restores Cerebral Blood flow, and Alters Extracellular Matrix Gene Expression in a Model of Chronic Vascular Stiffness," *American Journal of Physiology, Heart and Circulatory Physiology* 315, no. 1 (2018): H18–32. doi: 10.1152/ajpheart.00683.2017. PMID: 29498532; Marion Coquand-Gandit, Marie-Paul Jacob, Wassim Fhayli, Beatriz Romero, et al., "Chronic Treatment

with Minoxidil Induces Elastic Fiber Neosynthesis and Functional Improvement in the Aorta of Aged Mice," *Rejuvenation Research* 20, no. 3 (2017): 218–30. doi: 10.1089/rej.2016.1874. PMID: 28056723.

26. Lisa A. Lesniewski, Douglas R. Seals, Ashley E. Walker, Grant D. Henson, et al., "Dietary Rapamycin Supplementation Reverses Age-Related Vascular Dysfunction and Oxidative Stress, while Modulating Nutrient-Sensing, Cell Cycle, and Senescence Pathways," *Aging Cell* 16, no. 1 (2017): 17–26. doi: 10.1111/acel.12524. PMID: 27660040.

27. Kate McKeage, David Murdoch, and Karen Goa, "The Sirolimus-Eluting Stent: A Review of Its Use in the Treatment of Coronary Artery Disease," *American Journal of Cardiovascular Drugs* 3, no. 3 (2003): 211–30. doi: 10.2165/00129784-200303030-00007. PMID: 14727933.

28. For the human trial, see Christopher R. Martens, Blaire A. Denman, Melissa R. Mazzo, Michael L. Armstrong, et al., "Chronic Nicotinamide Riboside Supplementation is Well-Tolerated and Elevates NAD⁺ in Healthy Middle-Aged and Older Adults," *Nature Communications* 9, no. 1 (2018): 1286. doi: 10.1038/s41467-018-03421-7. PMID: 29599478; for information from a startup retailing NR, see www.truniagen.com/science; recall that I don't endorse any commercial product.

29. See the NIH site on stem cells, https://stemcells.nih.gov.

30. Yuan Fang, Zheng Wei, Bin Chen, Tianye Pan, Shiang Gu, Peng Liu, Daqiao Guo, Xin Xu, Jinhao Jiang, et al., "Five-Year Study of the Efficacy of Purified CD34+ Cell Therapy for Angiitis-Induced No-Option Critical Limb Ischemia," *Stem Cells Translational Medicine* 7, no. 8 (2018): 583–90. doi: 10.1002/sctm.17-0252. PMID: 29709112.

31. J. Michael Gaziano, Howard D. Sesso, William G. Christen, Vadim Bubes, Joan P. Smith, Jean MacFadyen, Miriam Schvartz, JoAnn E. Manson, Robert J. Glynn, and Julie E. Buring, "Multivitamins in the Prevention of Cancer in Men: The Physicians' Health Study II Randomized Controlled Trial," *Journal of the American Medical Association* 308, no. 18 (2012): 1871–80. doi: 10.1001/jama.2012.14641. PMID: 23162860.

32. Michael Gregor, *How Not to Die* (New York: Flatiron Books, 2015). For a good, but technical, review of the evidence supporting the low-carb diet, see Richard D. Feinman, *Nutrition in Crisis* (White River Junction, VT: Chelsea Green, 2019). For a review of the protein issue, see Sara B. Seidelmann, Brian Claggett, Susan Cheng, Mir Henglin, et al., "Dietary Carbohydrate Intake and Mortality: A Prospective Cohort Study and Meta-Analysis," *Lancet Public Health* 3, no. 9 (2018): e419–28. doi: 10.1016/S2468-2667(18)30135-X. PMID: 30122560; these authors found a slightly protective effect of low-carb diets. However, a press release from the European Society for Cardiology reported work by M. Banach showing the opposite effect (https://www.escardio.org/The-ESC/Press-Office/Press-releases/Low-carbohydrate-diets-are-unsafe-and-should-be-avoided). I should note that both of these studies (and many other similar analyses) rely on meta-analyses of observational studies whose weaknesses I discussed in chapter 1.

33. Sadeq Hasan Al-Sheraji, Amin Ismail, Mohd Yazid Manap, Shuhaimi Mustafa, Rokiah Mohd Yusof, and Fouad Abdulrahman Hassan, "Hypocholesterolaemic Effect of Yoghurt Containing Bifidobacterium pseudocatenulatum G4 or Bifidobacterium

longum BB536," *Food Chemistry* 135, no. 2 (2012): 356–61. doi.org/10.1016/j.food chem.2012.04.120; a highly readable general introduction to the gut microbiome is Erica D. Sonnenburg and Justin Sonnenburg, *The Good Gut: Taking Control of Your Weight, Your Mood, and Your Long-Term Health* (New York: Penguin, 2015).

34. The largest observational study examined almost two million individual medical records: Steven Bell, Marina Daskalopoulou, Eleni Rapsomaniki, Julie George, Annie Britton, Martin Bobak, Juan P. Casas, Caroline E. Dale, Spiros Denaxas, Anoop Shah, and Harry Hemingway, "Association between Clinically Recorded Alcohol Consumption and Initial Presentation of 12 Cardiovascular Diseases: Population Based Cohort Study Using Linked Health Records," *British Medical Journal* 356 (2017): j909. doi: 10.1136/bmj.j909. PMID: 28331015.

35. GBD Alcohol Collaborators, "Alcohol Use and Burden for 195 Countries and Territories, 1990–2016: A Systematic Analysis for the Global Burden of Disease Study," *Lancet* 382, no. 10152 (2016): 1015–35.

36. Philip J. Barter, H. Bria Brewer Jr., M. John Chapman, Charles H. Hennekens, Daniel J. Rader, and Alan R. Tall, "Cholesteryl Ester Transfer Protein: A Novel Target for Raising HDL and Inhibiting Atherosclerosis," *Arteriosclerosis, Thrombosis and Vascular Biology* 23, no. 2 (2003): 160–67. doi: 10.1161/01.atv.0000054658.91146.64. PMID: 12588754.

37. Morgan et al., "Cholesterol Metabolism."

38. Raffaele De Caterina, Philippa J. Talmud, Piera A. Merlini, . . . Gruppo Italiano Aterosclerosi, "Strong Association of the APOA5-1131T>C Gene Variant and Early-Onset Acute Myocardial Infarction," *Atherosclerosis* 214, no. 2 (2011): 397–403. doi: 10.1016/j.atherosclerosis.2010.11.011. PMID: 21130994.

39. Morgan et al., "Cholesterol Metabolism."

40. Philippa J. Talmud, David M. Flavell, Khalid Alfakih, Jackie A. Cooper, et al., "The Lipoprotein Lipase Gene Serine 447 Stop Variant Influences Hypertension-Induced Left Ventricular Hypertrophy and Risk of Coronary Heart Disease," *Clinical Science (London)* 112, no. 12 (2007): 617–24. doi: 10.1042/CS20060344. PMID: 17291198.

CHAPTER 8. THE BRAIN AND COGNITIVE DECLINE

1. For more information on fMRI, see https://web.csulb.edu/~cwallis/482/fmri/fmri.html.

2. In this excellent book, Oliver Sacks, *The Man Who Mistook His Wife for a Hat and Other Clinical Tales* (New York: Touchstone, 1970), a neurologist, describes the unusual case histories of some of his patients.

3. There is a lot of confusing information on memory and how it works. For a good overview of this and other brain topics, see http://thebrain.mcgill.ca/flash/a/a_07/a_07_p/a_07_p_tra/a_07_p_tra.html#3.

4. For an engaging book by a neuroscientist covering many of the neurological aspects of aging, read Daniel J. Levitin, *Successful Aging* (New York: Random House,

2020). In addition to addressing the physiology and potential solutions to many of the problems of age, he incorporates many positive aspects. This is also true of another interesting book written by a neurologist who focuses on the increasing ability of the aging brain to recognize and use patterns: Elkhonen Goldberg, *The Wisdom Paradox: How Your Mind Can Grow Stronger as Your Brain Grows Older* (London: Free Press, 2005).

5. M. M. Esiri, "Ageing and the Brain," *Journal of Pathology* 211, no. 2 (2007): 181–87. doi: 10.1002/path.2089. PMID: 17200950.

6. Alistair Farley, Charles Hendry, and Ella McLafferty, eds., *The Physiological Effects of Ageing* (Oxford: Wiley-Blackwell, 2011).

7. Esiri, "Ageing and the Brain."

8. Riqiang Yan, Qingyuan Fan, John Zhoum, and Robert Vassar, "Inhibiting BACE1 to Reverse Synaptic Dysfunctions in Alzheimer's Disease," *Neuroscience and Biobehavioral Reviews* 65 (2016): 326–40. doi.org/10.1016/j.neubiorev.2016.03.025.

9. Atsushi Aoyagi, Carlo Condello, Jan Stöhr, Weizhou Yue, et al., "Aβ and Tau Prion-Like Activities Decline with Longevity in the Alzheimer's Disease Human Brain," *Science and Translational Medicine* 11, no. 490 (2019): eaat8462. doi: 10.1126/scitranslmed.aat8462. PMID: 31043574.

10. Candice E. Van Skike and Veronica Galvan, "A Perfect sTORm: The Role of the Mammalian Target of Rapamycin (mTOR) in Cerebrovascular Dysfunction of Alzheimer's Disease: A Mini-Review," *Gerontology* 64, no. 3 (2018): 205–11. doi: 10.1159/000485381. PMID: 29320772.

11. Jean C. Cruz Hernández, Oliver Bracko, Calvin J. Kersbergen, Victorine Muse, et al., "Neutrophil Adhesion in Brain Capillaries Reduces Cortical Blood Flow and Impairs Memory Function in Alzheimer's Disease Mouse Models," *Nature Neuroscience* 22, no. 3 (2019): 413–20. doi: 10.1038/s41593-018-0329-4. PMID: 30742116.

12. Dmitri Leonoudakis, Anand Rane, Suzanne Angeli, Gordon J. Lithgow, Julie K. Andersen, and Shankar J. Chinta, "Anti-Inflammatory and Neuroprotective Role of Natural Product Securinine in Activated Glial Cells: Implications for Parkinson's Disease," *Mediators of Inflammation* (2017): 8302636. doi: 10.1155/2017/8302636. PMID.

13. Esiri, "Ageing and the Brain."

14. Sten Orrenius, Vladimir Gogvadze, and Boris Zhivotovsky, "Calcium and Mitochondria in the Regulation of Cell Death," *Biochemical and Biophysical Research Communications* 460, no. 1 (2015): 72–81. doi: 10.1016/j.bbrc.2015.01.137. PMID: 25998735.

15. Robert Dantzer, "Cytokine, Sickness Behavior, and Depression," *Immunology and Allergy Clinics of North America* 29, no. 2 (2010): 247–64, https://doi.org/10.1016/j.iac.2009.02.002.

16. Kie Honjo, Robert van Reekum, and Nikolaas P. Verhoeff, "Alzheimer's Disease and Infection: Do Infectious Agents Contribute to Progression of Alzheimer's Disease?," *Alzheimers and Dementia* 5, no. 4 (2009): 348–60. doi: 10.1016/j.jalz.2008.12.001. PMID: 19560105.

17. On the effect of rapamycin, see Van Skike and Veronica Galvan, "A Perfect sTORm." To read about many interventions to the TOR system that may affect AD, see Nicholas G. Norwitz and Henry Querfurth, "mTOR Mysteries: Nuances and

Questions about the Mechanistic Target of Rapamycin in Neurodegeneration," *Frontiers in Neuroscience* 14 (2020): 775–85. doi: 10.3389/fnins.2020.00775.

18. An entire issue of the *Journal of Sport and Health Science* was dedicated to this topic; the introductory editorial gives a good overview of the articles: Yu-Kai Chang and Jennifer L. Etnier, "Acute Exercise and Cognitive Function: Emerging Research Issues," *Journal of Sport and Health Science* 4 (2015): 1–3; the visual system is specifically addressed by Vicki Chrysostomou, Sandra Galic S, Peter van Wijngaarden P, et al., "Exercise Reverses Age-Related Vulnerability of the Retina to Injury by Preventing Complement-Mediated Synapse Elimination via a BDNF-Dependent Pathway," *Aging Cell* 15, no. 6 (2016): 1082–91. doi: 10.1111/acel.12512. PMID: 27613664.

19. David A. Raichlen and Gene E. Alexander, "Why Your Brain Needs Exercise," *Scientific American*, January 2020.

20. We have a growing body of literature on the role of diet and dementia. A good introduction is presented by Steven Masley, *The Better Brain Solution* (New York: Knopf, 2018); to read about specific foods, see Marshall G. Miller, Nopporn Thangthaeng N, Shibu M. Poulose SM, and Barbara Shukitt-Hale, "Role of Fruits, Nuts, and Vegetables in Maintaining Cognitive Health," *Experimental Gerontology* 94 (2017): 24–28. doi: 10.1016/j.exger.2016.12.014. PMID: 28011241; and Anne M. Minihane, Sophie Vinoy, Wendy R. Russell, Athanasia Baka, et al., "Low-Grade Inflammation, Diet Composition and Health: Current Research Evidence and Its Translation," *British Journal of Nutrition* 114, no. 7 (2015): 999–1012. doi: 10.1017/S0007114515002093. PMID: 26228057. For evidence showing the effect of the ketogenic diet in animals, see Andrew J. Murray, Nicholas S. Knight, Mark A. Cole, Lowri E. Cochlin, et al., "Novel Ketone Diet Enhances Physical and Cognitive Performance," *FASEB Journal* 30, no. 12 (2016): 4021–32. doi: 10.1096/fj.201600773R. PMID: 27528626. And for the human studies, see Lilianne R. Mujica-Parodi, Anar Amgalan, Syed Fahad Sultan, et al., "Diet Modulates Brain Network Stability, a Biomarker for Brain Aging, in Young Adults," *Proceedings of the National Academy of Sciences US* 117, no. 11 (2020): 6170–77. doi: 10.1073/pnas.1913042117. For a novel, diet-based approach to reversing type 2 diabetes, look at the research papers by the clinical group Virta, https://www.virtahealth.com/research.

21. Cecilia Samieri, Martha-Claire Morris, David A. Bennett, Claudine Berr, et al., "Fish Intake, Genetic Predisposition to Alzheimer Disease, and Decline in Global Cognition and Memory in 5 Cohorts of Older Persons," *American Journal of Epidemiology* 187, no. 5 (2018): 933–40. doi: 10.1093/aje/kwx330. PMID: 29053784.

22. M. C. Morris, "The Role of Nutrition in Alzheimer's Disease: Epidemiological Evidence," *European Journal of Neurology* 16, suppl. 1 (2009): 1–7. doi: 10.1111/j.1468-1331.2009.02735.x. PMID: 19703213.

23. Institute of Medicine, *Cognitive Aging: Progress in Understanding and Opportunities for Action* (Washington, DC: National Academies Press, 2015).

24. Gwenelle Douaud, Helga Refsum, Celeste A. de Jager, Robin Jacoby, Thomas E. Nichols, Steven M. Smith, and A. David Smith, "Preventing Alzheimer's Disease-Related Gray Matter Atrophy by B-Vitamin Treatment," *Proceedings of the*

National Academy of Sciences USA 110, no. 23 (2013): 9523–28. doi: 10.1073/pnas.1301816110. PMID: 23690582.

25. Esiri, "Ageing and the Brain."

26. See the mouse study by Vladimir Ilievski, Paulina K. Zuchowska, Stefan J. Green, et al., "Chronic Oral Application of a Periodontal Pathogen Results in Brain Inflammation, Neurodegeneration and Amyloid Beta Production in Wild Type Mice," *PLoS One* 13, no. 10 (2018): e0204941. doi: 10.1371/journal.pone.0204941. PMID: 30281647. The Phase I clinical trial results in human volunteers were reported in 2018, https://www.businesswire.com/news/home/20181024005522/en/Cortexyme -Announces-Phase-1-Data-Demonstrating-COR388Inh.

27. P. Lina Santaguida, Tatyan A. Shamliyan, and David R. Goldman, "Cholinesterase Inhibitors and Memantine in Adults with Alzheimer Disease," *American Journal of Medicine* 129, no. 10 (2016): 1044–47.

28. Dale E. Bredesen, "Reversal of Cognitive Decline: A Novel Therapeutic Program," *Aging* 6, no. 9 (2014): 707–17. doi: 10.18632/aging.100690. PMID: 25324467.

29. This group has developed an interactive website, www.alzu.org/, where you can learn about AD. In addition, this site has information about ongoing clinical trials and links to clinics that do in-depth individualized assessments. For development of the risk factors, see Matthew W. Schelke, Peter Attia, Daniel J. Palenchar, Bob Kaplan, et al., "Mechanisms of Risk Reduction in the Clinical Practice of Alzheimer's Disease Prevention," *Frontiers in Aging Neuroscience* 10 (2018): 96. doi: 10.3389/fnagi.2018.00096. PMID: 29706884.

30. UBI: https://www.unitedneuroscience.com/pipeline/.

31. Katherine P. Riley, David A. Snowdon, Mark F. Desrosiers, and William R. Markesbery, "Early Life Linguistic Ability, Late Life Cognitive Function, and Neuropathology: Findings from the Nun Study," *Neurobiology of Aging* 26, no. 3 (2005): 341–47. doi: 10.1016/j.neurobiolaging.2004.06.019. PMID: 15639312.

32. David J. Simons, Walter R. Boot, Neil Charness, Susan E. Gathercole, Christopher F. Chabris, David Z. Hambrick, and Elizabeth A. Stine-Morrow, "Do 'Brain-Training' Programs Work?," *Psychological Science in the Public Interest* 17, no. 3 (2016): 103–86. doi: 10.1177/1529100616661983. PMID: 27697851.

33. Alan L. Pelletier, Ledy Rojas-Roldan, and Janis Coffin, "Vision Loss in Older Adults," *American Family Physician* 94, no. 3 (2016): 219–26. PMID: 27479624.

34. Good overview and detailed information on treatment and prevention at https://www.macular.org/.

35. Good overview and detailed information on treatment and prevention at https://www.aao.org/eye-health/diseases/what-is-glaucoma.

36. Good overview and detailed information on treatment and prevention at https://nei.nih.gov/health/diabetic/retinopathy.

37. https://nei.nih.gov/health/cataract/cataract_facts.

38. Farley, *The Physiological Effects of Ageing.*

39. Elizabeth H. Rickenbach, David M. Almeida, Teresa E. Seeman, and Margie E. Lachman, "Daily Stress Magnifies the Association between Cognitive Decline and

Everyday Memory Problems: An Integration of Longitudinal and Diary Methods," *Psychology and Aging* 29, no. 4 (2014): 852–62, https://doi.org/10.1037/a0038072.

40. Julie L. Bienias, Laurel A. Beckett, David A. Bennett, Robert S. Wilson, and Denis A. Evans, "Design of the Chicago Health and Aging Project (CHAP)," *Journal of Alzheimers Disease* 5, no. 5 (2003): 349–55. doi: 10.3233/jad-2003-5501. PMID: 14646025.

41. Farley, *The Physiological Effects of Ageing.*

42. For a more in-depth discussion of some of these genes, see https://www.alzfo rum.org/news/conference-coverage/new-genetics-frontiers-finding-modifiers-making -sense-pathways.

43. https://www.foundmyfitness.com.

CHAPTER 9. INTERVENTIONS PART 1: ACTIONS YOU CAN TAKE

1. For a good review of the many options, see the review by Thomas J. LaRocca, Christopher R. Martens, and Douglas R. Seals, "Nutrition and Other Lifestyle Influences on Arterial Aging," *Ageing Research Reviews* 39 (2017): 106–19. doi: 10.1016/j. arr.2016.09.002. PMID: 27693830; PMCID.

2. Joshua Most, Valeria Tosti, Leanne M. Redman, and Luigi Fontan, "Calorie Restriction in Humans: An Update," *Ageing Research Reviews* 39 (2017): 36–45. doi: 10.1016/j.arr.2016.08.005. PMID: 27544442.

3. A thorough review of human studies of CR is provided by Most et al., "Calorie Restriction in Humans." A number of reviews of human aging studies are analyzed with respect to CR—for example, Priya Balasubramanian, Porsha R. Howell, and Rozalyn M. Anderson, "Aging and Caloric Restriction Research: A Biological Perspective with Translational Potential," *EBioMedicine* 21 (2017): 37–44. doi: 10.1016/j. ebiom.2017.06.015; Daniele Lettieri-Barbato, Esmerelda Giovannetti, and Katya Aquilano, "Effects of Dietary Restriction on Adipose Mass and Biomarkers of Healthy Aging in Human," *Aging (Albany NY)* 8, no. 12 (2016): 3341–55. doi: 10.18632/ag ing.101122; and a great review of CR and other intervention on specific age-related disorders by Ines Figueira, Adelaide Fernandes, Aleksandra Mladenovic Djordjevic, Andre Lopez-Contreras, et al., "Interventions for Age-Related Diseases: Shifting the Paradigm," *Mechanisms of Ageing and Development* 160 (2016): 69–92. doi: 10.1016/j .mad.2016.09.009. PMID: 27693441. For a really deep trip into mechanisms, see Christopher B. Newgard and Jeffrey E. Pessin, "Recent Progress in Metabolic Signaling Pathways Regulating Aging and Life Span," *Journals of Gerontology. Series A, Biological Sciences and Medical Sciences* 69, suppl. 1 (2014): S21–27. doi: 10.1093/gerona/ glu058. PMID: 24833582; PMCID: PMC4022126. For a detailed, if dense, analysis of the monkey studies, see Julie A. Mattison, Ricki J. Colman, T. Mark Beasley, David B. Allison, Joseph W. Kenmitz, George S. Roth, Donald K. Ingram, et al., "Caloric Restriction Improves Health and Survival of Rhesus Monkeys," *Nature Communications*, January 17 (2017): 14063. doi: 10.1038/ncomms14063.

4. Dr. Valter Longo is a longtime proponent of these alternatives to CR. His book, *The Longevity Diet* (New York: Avery Press, 2018), describes them in accessible detail. For a more academic review, see Valter D. Longo and Satchem Panda, "Fasting, Circadian Rhythms, and Time-Restricted Feeding in Healthy Lifespan," *Cell Metabolism* 23, no. 6 (2016): 1048–59. On the anticancer benefits, see Alessio Nencioni, Irene Caffa, Salvatore Cortellino, and Valter D. Longo, "Fasting and Cancer: Molecular Mechanisms and Clinical Application," *Nature Reviews. Cancer* 18, no. 11 (2018), 707–19, https://doi.org/10.1038/s41568-018-0061-0.

5. M. Ristow and S. Schmeisser, "Extending Life Span by Increasing Oxidative Stress," *Free Radical Biology and Medicine* 51, no. 2 (2011): 327–36. doi: 10.1016/j.freeradbiomed.2011.05.010. PMID: 21619928; also reviewed by Christopher R. Martens and Douglas R. Seals, "Practical Alternatives to Chronic Caloric Restriction for Optimizing Vascular Function with Ageing," *Journal of Physiology* 594, no. 24 (2016): 7177–95. doi: 10.1113/JP272348. PMID: 27641062.

6. Martens and Seals,. "Practical Alternatives to Chronic Caloric Restriction."

7. Ristow and Schmeisser. "Extending Life Span by Increasing Oxidative Stress"; and Stephanie E. Wohlgemuth, Arnold Y. Seo, Emmanuelle Marzetti, Hazel A. Lees, and Christian Leeuwenburgh, "Skeletal Muscle Autophagy and Apoptosis during Aging: Effects of Calorie Restriction and Life-Long Exercise," *Experimental Gerontolology* 45, no. 2 (2010): 138–48. doi: 10.1016/j.exger.2009.11.002. PMID: 19903516.

8. For a historical overview and summary of what happens in the cell during this process, see Vikramit Lahiri and Daniel J. Konski, "Eat Yourself to Live: Autophagy's Role in Health and Disease," *The Scientist*, March (2018); also see Wohlgemuth et al., "Skeletal Muscle Autophagy and Apoptosis during Aging."

9. Yuan Zhang, Yang Xie, Eric O. Berglund, Katie C. Coate, Tian T. He, Takeshi Katafuchi, Guanghua Xiao, et al., "The Starvation Hormone, Fibroblast Growth Factor-21, Extends Lifespan in Mice," *eLife* 1 (2012): e00065. https://doi.org/10.7554/eLife.00065.

10. There is a lot of really interesting, recent work on variable feeding routines, starting with Longo's work cited in note 4. If you want to try TRF, see Dr. Satcham Panda's website. His lab has developed an app for tracking your consumption data and adding it to their growing data set (http://www.mycircadianclock.org/).

11. Gretchen Reynolds, who writes an exercise column for the *New York Times*, has done a great job of summarizing recent research on the benefits of various types of exercise. In addition, she takes a good stab at answering the questions of what kind and how much, in Gretchen Reynolds, *The First 20 Minutes: Surprising Science Reveals How We Can Exercise Better, Train Smarter, Live Longer* (New York: Penguin Group, 2012). Here's a link to her articles: https://muckrack.com/gretchen-reynolds/articles. For a thorough, though technical, review of the role of mitochondrial activity in exercise, see Hai Bo, Ning Jiang, LiJi Li, and Yong Zhang, "Mitochondrial Redox Metabolism in Aging: Effect of Exercise Interventions," *Journal of Sport and Health Science* 2, no. 2 (2013): 67–74. A more recent issue of this journal focused on the medicinal aspect of exercise; the accompanying editorial summarizes some of the relevant papers: Sulin Cheng and Lijuan Mao, "Physical Activity Continuum throughout the Lifespan: Is

Exercise Medicine or What?," *Journal of Sport and Health Science* 5, no. 2 (2016): 127–28, https://doi.org/10.1016/j.jshs.2016.03.005. An excellent review of the role of mitochondria in sarcopenia and many of the targeted interventions toward this organelle is in Paul M. Coen, Robert V. Musci, J. Matthew Hinkley, and Benjamin F. Miller, "Mitochondria as a Target for Mitigating Sarcopenia," *Frontiers in Physiology* 9 (2019): 1883. doi: 10.3389/fphys.2018.01883. PMID: 30687111.

12. You can read the full study by Serge C. Harb, Paul C. Cremer, Yuping Wu, Bo Xu, Leslie Cho, Veno Menon, and Wael A. Jaber, "Estimated Age Based on Exercise Stress Testing Performance Outperforms Chronological Age in Predicting Mortality," *European Journal of Preventive Cardiology* 13 (2019): 2047487319826400. doi: 10.1177/2047487319826400. PMID: 30760022, or a synopsis in a press release from the publisher, the European Society for Cardiology, at https://www.escardio.org/The -ESC/Press-Office/Press-releases/What-s-age-got-to-do-with-it.

13. C. Scott Bickel, James M. Cross, and Marcas M. Bamman, "Exercise Dosing to Retain Resistance Training Adaptations in Young and Older Adults," *Medicine and Science in Sports and Exercise* 43, no. 7 (2011): 1177–87. doi: 10.1249/MSS.0b013e318207c15d.

14. Sammi R. Chekroud, Ralitza Gueorguieva, Amanda B. Zheutlin, Martin Paulus, Harlan M. Krumholz, John H. Krystal, and Adam M. Chekroud, "Association between Physical Exercise and Mental Health in 1–2 Million Individuals in the USA between 2011 and 2015: A Cross-Sectional Study," *Lancet Psychiatry* 5, no. 9 (2018): 739–46. doi: 10.1016/S2215-0366(18)30227-X. PMID: 30099000.

15. Jari Laukkanen and his group have looked at many health end points in their twenty-year study population of more than two thousand Finnish men ages 42–60 years. Some of their publications include the following: Tanjanalina Laukkanen, Hassan Khan, Francesco Zaccardi, and Jari A. Laukkanen, "Association between Sauna Bathing and Fatal Cardiovascular and All-Cause Mortality Events," *JAMA Internal Medicine* 175, no. 4 (2015): 542–48. doi: 10.1001/jamainternmed.2014.8187. PMID: 25705824; Tanjanalina Laukkanen, Setor Kunutsor, Jussi Kauhanen, and Jari A. Laukkanen, "Sauna Bathing Is Inversely Associated with Dementia and Alzheimer's Disease in Middle-Aged Finnish Men," *Age and Ageing* 46, no. 2 (2017): 245–49. doi: 10.1093/ageing/afw212. PMID: 27932366; also see Jari A. Laukkanen and Tanjanalina Laukkanen, "Sauna Bathing and Systemic Inflammation," *European Journal of Epidemiology* 33, no. 3 (2018): 351–53. doi: 10.1007/s10654-017-0335-y. PMID: 29209938. And finally, for updates on this and many other topics related to aging therapies, see Rhonda Patrick's comprehensive and searchable website, https://www.foundmyfitness.com.

16. Read about the role of HSP in Ling Yang, Danilo Licastro, Edda Cava, Nicola Veronese, et al., "Long-Term Calorie Restriction Enhances Cellular Quality-Control Processes in Human Skeletal Muscle," *Cell Reports* 14, no. 3 (2016): 422–28. doi: 10.1016/j.celrep.2015.12.042. PMID: 26774472; the mouse study is reported by Yuki Tamura, Yataka Matsunaga, Yu Kitaoka, and Hideo Hatta, "Effects of Heat Stress Treatment on Age-Dependent Unfolded Protein Response in Different Types of Skeletal Muscle," *Journals of Gerontology. Series A, Biological Sciences and Medical Sciences* 72, no. 3 (2017): 299–308. doi: 10.1093/gerona/glw063. PMID: 27071782.

17. M. Kox, L. T. van Eijk, J. Zwaag, J. van den Wildenberg, F. Sweep, J. G. van der Hoeven, and P. Pickkers, "Voluntary Activation of the Sympathetic Nervous System and Attenuation of the Innate Immune Response in Humans," *Intensive Care Medicine Experimental* 2, suppl. 1 (2014), https://doi.org/10.1186/2197-425X-2-S1-O2; also see Leo Pruimboom, and Frits A. J. Muskiet, "Intermittent Living; The Use of Ancient Challenges as a Vaccine against the Deleterious Effects of Modern Life—A Hypothesis," *Medical Hypotheses* 120 (2018): 28–42. doi: 10.1016/j.mehy.2018.08.002. PMID: 30220336.

18. A good start is one of the early books on this topic by Edward A. Charlesworth and Ronald C. Nathan, *Stress Management* (New York: Ballantine Books Trade Paperback, 2012). For a deep dive into the physiology and an entertaining read, see Robert Sapolsky, *Why Zebras Don't Get Ulcers*, 3rd ed. (New York: Henry Holt, 2004). Again, I refer the interested reader to Rhonda Patrick's comprehensive and searchable site, https://www.foundmyfitness.com.

19. For this and many other examples of the importance of sleep, as well as suggestions on how to sleep better, see Matthew Walker, *Why We Sleep: Unlocking the Power of Sleep and Dreams* (New York: Scribner, 2017). The cognitive behavioral therapy is outlined in Colleen Ehrnstrom and Alisha L. Brosse, *End the Insomnia Struggle: A Step-by-Step Guide to Help You Get to Sleep and Stay Asleep* (Oakland, CA: New Harbinger Publications, 2016). Finally, James Nestor, *Breath: The New Science of a Lost Art* (New York: Penguin Random House, 2020) addresses the issue of breathing, an important component of sleep as well as exercise and relaxation.

CHAPTER 10. INTERVENTIONS PART 2:
DRUGS AND SUPPLEMENTS YOU CAN TAKE

1. A. Ward, P. Bates, R. Fisher, L. Richardson, and C. F. Graham, "Disproportionate Growth in Mice with Igf-2 Transgenes," *Proceedings of the National Academy of Sciences of the United States of America* 91, no. 22 (1994): 10365–69, https://doi.org/10.1073/pnas.91.22.10365.

2. There aren't many easy reads on rapamycin and mTOR. Some informative but technical papers include Matthieu Laplante and David M. Sabatini, "mTOR Signaling at a Glance," *Journal of Cell Science* 122, pt. 20 (2009): 3589–94. doi: 10.1242/jcs.051011. PMID: 19812304; Zhen Yu, Rong Wang, Wilson C. Fok, Alexander Coles, Adam B. Salmon, and Viviana I. Pérez, "Rapamycin and Dietary Restriction Induce Metabolically Distinctive Changes in Mouse Liver," *Journals of Gerontology. Series A, Biological Sciences and Medical Sciences* 70, no. 4 (2015): 410–20. doi: 10.1093/gerona/glu053. PMID: 24755936; Brina K. Kennedy and Dudley W. Lamming, "The Mechanistic Target of Rapamycin: The Grand ConducTOR of Metabolism and Aging," *Cell Metabolism* 23, no. 6 (2016): 990–1003. doi: 10.1016/j.cmet.2016.05.009. PMID: 27304501; and Lisa A. Lesniewski, Douglas R. Seals, Ashley E. Walker, Grant D. Henson, et al., "Dietary Rapamycin Supplementation Reverses Age-Related Vascular Dysfunction and Oxidative Stress, while Modulating Nutrient-sensing, Cell Cycle, and Senescence Pathways," *Aging Cell* 16, no. 1 (2017): 17–26. doi: 10.1111/

acel.12524. PMID: 27660040. In addition, a number of scientists have written (and illustrated) on mTOR and other concepts in the aging field at the antiaging site https://www.anti-agingfirewalls.com.

3. To read more about the clinical trial currently underway, see Nur Barzilai, Jill P. Crandall, Stephen B. Kritchevsky, and Mark A. Espeland, "Metformin as a Tool to Target Aging," *Cell Metabolism* 23, no. 6 (2016): 1060–65, https://doi.org/10.1016/j.cmet.2016.05.011; for a brief overview, see https://healthyagingproject.org/2016/04/healthy-aging-drug-on-the-horizon/; for the potential downside effect of metformin on the benefits from aerobic exercise, see Adam R. Konopka, Jaime L. Laurin JL, Hayden M. Schoenberg HM, Justin J. Reid JJ, William M. Castor WM, Christopher A. Wolff CA, Robert V. Musci RV, et al., "Metformin Inhibits Mitochondrial Adaptations to Aerobic Exercise Training in Older Adults," *Aging Cell* 18, no. 1 (2019): e12880. doi: 10.1111/acel.12880. PMID: 30548390. For updates on this topic, see Dr. Rhonda Patrick's excellent website, https://www.foundmyfitness.com/search.

4. Lee A. Witters, "The Blooming of the French Lilac," *Journal of Clinical Investigation* 108, no. 8 (2001): 1105–7, https://doi.org/10.1172/JCI14178.

5. Charles N. Serhan, "Novel Pro-Resolving Lipid Mediators in Inflammation Are Leads for Resolution Physiology," *Nature* 510, no. 7503 (2014): 92–101, https://doi.org/10.1038/nature13479. A slightly less technical explanation is at https://en.wikipedia.org/wiki/Specialized_pro-resolving_mediators. For a compelling review of these compounds and their dietary source in fish, see Bruce D. Levy, "Resolvins and Protectins: Natural Pharmacophores for Resolution Biology," *Prostaglandins, Leukotrienes, and Essential Fatty Acids* 82, nos. 4–6 (2010): 327–32. doi: 10.1016/j.plefa.2010.02.003. PMID: 20227865. The eosinophil experiments are described by Daniel Brigger, Carsten Riether, Robin van Brummelen, Kira I. Mosher, et al., "Eosinophils Regulate Adipose Tissue Inflammation and Sustain Physical and Immunological Fitness in Old Age," *Nature Metabolism* 2, no. 8 (2020): 688–702. doi: 10.1038/s42255-020-0228-3. PMID: 32694825.

6. The longevity effects of ibuprofen are described by Chong He, Scott K. Tsuchiyama, Quynh T. Nguyen, Ekaterina N. Plyusnina, et al., "Enhanced Longevity by Ibuprofen, Conserved in Multiple Species, Occurs in Yeast through Inhibition of Tryptophan Import," *PLoS Genetics* 10, no. 12 (2014): e1004860. doi: 10.1371/journal.pgen.1004860. PMID: 25521617; the ability of some NSAIDS to affect AMP is discussed by Tanya S. King, Otto Q. Russe, Christine V. Möser, Nerea Ferreiró, et al., "AMP-Activated Protein Kinase Is Activated by Non-Steroidal Anti-inflammatory Drugs," *European Journal of Pharmacology* 762 (2015): 299–305. doi: 10.1016/j.ejphar.2015.06.001. PMID: 26049010.

7. Matthew J. Rossman, Jessica R. Santos-Parker, Chelsea A. C. Steward, Nina Z. Bispham, Lauren M. Cuevas, Hannah L. Rosenberg, Kayla A. Woodward, Michael Chonchol, Rachel A. Gioscia-Ryan, Michael P. Murphy, and Douglas R. Seals, "Chronic Supplementation with a Mitochondrial Antioxidant (MitoQ) Improves Vascular Function in Healthy Older Adults," *Hypertension* 71, no. 6 (2018): 1056–63. doi: 10.1161/HYPERTENSIONAHA.117.10787. PMID: 29661838. On the newer compounds, see https://www.ncbi.nlm.nih.gov/pubmed/18205623).

8. Early experimental evidence for reversing cross-link damage was provided by M. E. Cooper, V. Thallas, J. Forbes, E. Scalbert, S. Sastra, I. Darby, T. Soulis, "The Cross-Link Breaker, N-phenacylthiazolium Bromide Prevents Vascular Advanced Glycation End-Product Accumulation," *Diabetologia* 43, no. 5 (2000): 660–64. doi: 10.1007/s001250051355. PMID: 10855541; a thorough but technical summary of how these compounds work and their prospects is in Ryoji Nagai, David B. Murray, Thomas O. Metz, and John W. Baynes, "Chelation: A Fundamental Mechanism of Action of AGE Inhibitors, AGE Breakers, and Other Inhibitors of Diabetes Complications," *Diabetes* 61, no. 3 (2012): 549–59. doi: 10.2337/db11-1120. PMID: 22354928. Read about the human cell study in Brian S. Bradke and Deepak Vashishth, "N-Phenacylthiazolium Bromide Reduces Bone Fragility Induced by Nonenzymatic Glycation," *PLoS One* 9, no. 7 (2014): e103199. doi: 10.1371/journal.pone.0103199. PMID: 25062024. For a great overview of AGEs and AGE breakers, see the Legendary Pharmaceutical site, www.legendarypharma.com/glycation.html.

9. The study showing that niacin reduced glycation can be found in K. M. Abdullah, Faizan A. Qais, Iqban Ahmad, and Imrana Naseem, "Inhibitory Effect of Vitamin B_3 against Glycation and Reactive Oxygen Species Production in HSA: An in vitro Approach," *Archives of Biochemistry and Biophysics* 627 (2017): 21–29. doi: 10.1016/j.abb.2017.06.009. PMID: 28624351.

10. Michael B. Stout, Frederic J. Steyn, Michael J. Jurczak, Joao-Paulo G. Camporez, Yi Zhu, John R. Hawse, Diana Jurk, et al., "17α-Estradiol Alleviates Age-Related Metabolic and Inflammatory Dysfunction in Male Mice without Inducing Feminization," *Journals of Gerontology. Series A, Biological Sciences and Medical Sciences* 72, no. 1 (2017): 3–15. doi: 10.1093/gerona/glv309. PMID: 26809497

11. For a good review of recent findings on NAD⁺ and other age-related events, see Judith Campisi, Pankaj Kapahi, Gordon J. Lithgow, Simon Melov, John C. Newman, and Eric Verdin, "From Discoveries in Ageing Research to Therapeutics for Healthy Ageing," *Nature* 571, no. 7764 (2019): 183–92. doi: 10.1038/s41586-019-1365-2; for a good overview of sirtuins and their role in cells, see https://www.elysiumhealth.com/en-us/knowledge/science-101/why-sirtuins-are-important-for-aging; and for development and testing of NRH, Judith Giroud-Gerbetant, Migali Joffraud, Maria P. Giner, Angelique Cercillieux, Simona Bartova, Mikhail V. Makarov, Ruben Zapata-Pérez, et al., "A Reduced Form of Nicotinamide Riboside Defines a New Path for NAD⁺ Biosynthesis and Acts as an Orally Bioavailable NAD⁺ Precursor," *Molecular Metabolism* 30 (2019): 192–202. doi: 10.1016/j.molmet.2019.09.013. PMID: 31767171.

12. A recent book by David Sinclair, *Lifespan: Why We Age—and Why We Don't Have To* (New York: Atria Books, 2019), covers all you want to know about sirtuins, as well as theories of aging and potential remedies. A couple of sample papers on sirtuins: Carlos Cantó and Johan Auwerx, "Targeting Sirtuin 1 to Improve Metabolism: All You Need Is NAD(+)?," *Pharmacological Reviews* 64, no. 1 (2012): 166–87, https://doi.org/10.1124/pr.110.003905; Xiao Tian, Denis Firsanov, Zhihui Zhang, Yang Cheng, Lingfeng Luo, Gregory Tombline, Ruiyue Tan, et al., "SIRT6 Is Responsible for More Efficient DNA Double-Strand Break Repair in Long-Lived Species," *Cell* 177, no. 3 (2019): 622–38.e22. doi: 10.1016/j.cell.2019.03.043. PMID: 31002797.

13. Jessica Stockinger, Nicholas Maxwell, Dylan Shapiro, Rafael deCabo, and Gregorio Valdez, "Caloric Restriction Mimetics Slow Aging of Neuromuscular Synapses and Muscle Fibers," *Journals of Gerontology. Series A, Biological Sciences and Medical Sciences* 73, no. 1 (2017): 21–28. doi: 10.1093/gerona/glx023. PMID: 28329051.

14. James M. Smoliga, Joseph A. Baur, and Heather A. Hausenblas, "Resveratrol and Health—a Comprehensive Review of Human Clinical Trials," *Molecular Nutrition and Food Research* 55, no. 8 (2011): 1129–41. doi: 10.1002/mnfr.201100143. PMID: 21688389.

15. As for mTOR, it's difficult to find an easy read on NAD$^+$ (nicotinamide adenine dinucleotide). The Firewalls on Aging blog, http://www.anti-agingfirewalls.com/?s=NAD, has many short summaries of technical papers along with great diagrams, but they aren't simple to digest. For a simplified overview, see the Elyssium article at https://www.elysiumhealth.com/en-us/knowledge/science-101/everything-you-need-to-know-about-nicotinamide-adenine-dinucleotide-nad. For more technical papers, this group tested the compound in mice to good effect: Natalie E. de Picciotto, Lindsey B. Gano, Lawrence C. Johnson, Christopher R. Martens, et al., "Nicotinamide Mononucleotide Supplementation Reverses Vascular Dysfunction and Oxidative Stress with Aging in Mice," *Aging Cell* 15, no. 3 (2016): 522–30. doi: 10.1111/acel.12461. PMID: 26970090; for evidence showing that NR is the most readily absorbed and converted precursor to NAD, read Samuel A. Trammell, Mark S. Schmidt, Benjamin J. Weidemann, Philip Redpath, et al., "Nicotinamide Riboside Is Uniquely and Orally Bioavailable in Mice and Humans," *Nature Communications* 7 (2016): 12948. doi: 10.1038/ncomms12948. PMID: 27721479. The research showing that supplementation with NR produced good outcome in older people is presented by Christopher R. Martens, Blaire A. Denman, Melissa R. Mazzo, Michael L. Armstrong, et al., "Chronic Nicotinamide Riboside Supplementation Is Well-Tolerated and Elevates NAD$^+$ in Healthy Middle-Aged and Older Adults," *Nature Communications* 9, no. 1 (2018): 1286. doi: 10.1038/s41467-018-03421-7. PMID: 29599478, and this paper has a fairly readable summary in the introduction. The changes that occur with age in NAD$^+$ are described by James Clement, Matthew Wong, Anne Poljak, Perminder Sachdev, et al., "The Plasma NAD$^+$ Metabolome Is Dysregulated in 'Normal' Aging," *Rejuvenation Research* 22, no. 2 (2019): 121–30. doi: 10.1089/rej.2018.2077. PMID: 30124109. A potentially worrying finding is presented by Charles Brenner and Amy C. Boileau, "Pterostilbene Raises Low Density Lipoprotein Cholesterol in People," *Clinical Nutrition* 38, no. 1 (2019): 480–81. doi: 10.1016/j.clnu.2018.10.007. PMID: 30482564.

16. Ryan W. Dellinger, Santiago R. Santos, Mark Morris, Mal Evans, Dan Alminana, Leonard Guarente, and Eric Marcotulli, "Repeat Dose NRPT (Nicotinamide Riboside and Pterostilbene) Increases NAD$^+$ Levels in Humans Safely and Sustainably: A Randomized, Double-Blind, Placebo-Controlled Study," *NPJ Aging and Mechanisms of Disease* 3 (2017): 17. doi: 10.1038/s41514-017-0016-9. PMID: 29184669; and for an overview of Elyssium, the manufacturer of Basis, and a brief summary of the science, read https://www.fastcompany.com/3041800/one-of-the-worlds-top-aging-researchers-has-a-pill-to-keep-you-feeling-young. But keep in mind that this study was developed and run by some of the same scientists who developed the intervention.

17. https://siwatherapeutics.com/home/. Same caveat as above.

18. The nanocapsules were developed by Daniel Muñoz-Espín, Miguel Rovira, Irene Galiana, Cristina Giménez, Beatriz Lozano-Torres, Marta Paez-Ribes, Susana Llanos, et al., "A Versatile Drug Delivery System Targeting Senescent Cells," (2018). doi: 10.15252/emmm.201809355. PMID: 30012580; this and other senolytics strategies are reviewed by Cayetano von Kobbe, "Targeting Senescent Cells: Approaches, Opportunities, Challenges," *Aging* 11, no. 24 (2019): 12844–61. doi: 10.18632/aging.102557.

19. https://www.oisinbio.com/#the-approach, information from yet another biotech company, so be aware of the potential for bias.

20. https://unitybiotechnology.com/pipeline/; these so-called pro-apoptotic drugs were the first to be developed against senescent cells because of the observation that those cells did not commit suicide (i.e., apoptosis) when they should have. Much more detail on the history of this development and some of the earlier drugs in James L. Kirkland and Tamar Tchkonia, "Cellular Senescence: A Translational Perspective," *EBioMedicine* 21 (2017): 21–28. doi: 10.1016/j.ebiom.2017.04.013. PMID: 28416161. For a slightly less technical overview, see the commentary by Jan M. van Deursen, "Senolytic Therapies for Healthy Longevity," *Science* 364, no. 6441 (2019): 636–37. doi: 10.1126/science.aaw1299; and if you like video presentations, James Kirkland, one of the early researchers in the senolytics field, gives an excellent overview of the field at https://www.youtube.com/watch?v=7wiZb-QdVX4.

21. Von Kobbe, "Targeting Senescent Cells."

22. The first report that parabiosis reverses muscle aging was made by Irina M. Conboy, Michael J. Conboy, Amy J. Wagers, Eric R. Girma, Irving L. Weissman, and Thomas A. Rando, "Rejuvenation of Aged Progenitor Cells by Exposure to a Young Systemic Environment," *Nature* 433, no. 7027 (2005): 760–64. doi: 10.1038/nature03260. PMID: 15716955; the studies on the effects on learning and memory were done by Saul A. Villeda, Kristofer Plambeck, Jinte Middeldorp, Joseph M. Castellano, et al., "Young Blood Reverses Age-Related Impairments in Cognitive Function and Synaptic Plasticity in Mice," *Nature Medicine* 20, no. 6 (2014): 659–63. doi: 10.1038/nm.3569. PMID: 24793238; you can hear about it in an excellent TED talk by Tony Wyss-Coray, https://www.ted.com/talks/tony_wyss_coray_how_young_blood_might_help_reverse_aging_yes_really.

23. You can read about the clinical trial at the government website, https://clinicaltrials.gov/ct2/show/NCT02803554; and the company website, https://www.ambrosiaplasma.com. A second company, Alkahest, is investigating the effects specifically in Alzheimer's disease: http://www.alkahest.com/science/drug-discovery/.

24. Kotaro Azuma and Satoshi Inoue, "Vitamin K Benefits in Aging and Cancer," in *Aging Mechanisms*, edited by Nozomo Mori and Inhee Mook-Jung, 223–39 (Tokyo, Japan: Springer, 2015).

25. Matthew W. Schelke, Peter Attia, Daniel J. Palenchar, Bob Kaplan, et al., "Mechanisms of Risk Reduction in the Clinical Practice of Alzheimer's Disease Prevention," *Frontiers in Aging Neuroscience* 10 (2018): 96. doi: 10.3389/fnagi.2018.00096. PMID: 29706884.

26. For a complete discussion of glycation and inhibitory compounds, see Izabela Sadowska-Bartosz and Grzegorz Bartosz, "Effect of Glycation Inhibitors on Aging and Age-Related Diseases," *Mechanisms of Ageing and Development* 160 (2016): 1–18. doi: 10.1016/j.mad.2016.09.006. PMID: 27671971; to read about the green tea experiment, see Shan-Qing Zheng, Xiao-Bing Huang, Ti-Kun Xing, Ai-Jun Ding, et al., "Chlorogenic Acid Extends the Lifespan of *Caenorhabditis elegans* via Insulin/IGF-1 Signaling Pathway," *Journals of Gerontology. Series A, Biological Sciences and Medical Sciences* 72, no. 4 (2017): 464–72. doi: 10.1093/gerona/glw105. PMID: 27378235.

27. For a thorough review of this and other interventions, see Valter D. Longo, Adam Antebi, Andrzej Bartke, Nir Barzilai, Holly M. Brown-Borg, Calogero Caruso, Tyler J. Curiel, et al., "Interventions to Slow Aging in Humans: Are We Ready?," *Aging Cell* 14, no. 4 (2015): 497–510. doi: 10.1111/acel.12338. PMID: 25902704.

28. For an excellent and thorough book on cancer metabolism and the role of the ketogenic diet in slowing cancer growth, see Miriam Kalamian, *Keto for Cancer* (White River Junction, VT: Chelsea Green Press, 2017).

29. Alison E. DeVan, Lawrence C. Johnson, Forest A. Brooks, Trent D. Evans, et al., "Effects of Sodium Nitrite Supplementation on Vascular Function and Related Small Metabolite Signatures in Middle-Aged and Older Adults," *Journal of Applied Physiology* 120, no. 4 (2016): 416–25. doi: 10.1152/japplphysiol.00879.2015. PMID: 26607249; to read about the clinical trial, see clinicaltrials.gov/ct2/show/NCT02393742.

30. Jessica R. Santos-Parker, Talia R. Strahler, Candace J. Bassett, Nina Z. Bispham, et al., "Curcumin Supplementation Improves Vascular Endothelial Function in Healthy Middle-aged and Older Adults by Increasing Nitric Oxide Bioavailability and Reducing Oxidative Stress," *Aging (Albany NY)* 9, no. 1 (2017): 187–208. doi: 10.18632/aging.101149. PMID: 28070018.

31. Matthew W. Schelke, Peter Attia, Daniel J. Palenchar, Bob Kaplan, Monica Mureb, Christine A. Ganzer, Olivia Scheyer, et al., "Mechanisms of Risk Reduction in the Clinical Practice of Alzheimer's Disease Prevention," *Frontiers in Aging Neuroscience* 10 (2018): 96. doi: 10.3389/fnagi.2018.00096. PMID: 29706884.

32. Yao Dang, Yongpan An, Jinzhao He, Boyue Huang, Jie Zhu, Miaomiao Gao, Shun Zhang, et al., "Berberine Ameliorates Cellular Senescence and Extends the Lifespan of Mice via Regulating p16 and Cyclin Protein Expression," *Aging Cell* 19, no. 1 (2020), https://doi.org/10.1111/acel.13060; Rhonda Patrick is a researcher with an interest in nutraceuticals and longevity who blogs on many of these topics at the Found My Fitness website. Her piece on berberine contains many references and a good overview of the current knowledge: https://www.foundmyfitness.com/topics/berberine.

33. Cantó and Auwerx, "Targeting Sirtuin 1 to Improve Metabolism."

34. An excellent readable review of nutraceuticals and the cellular basis for their effects is presented by Thomas J. LaRocca, Christopher R. Martens, and Douglas R. Seals, "Nutrition and Other Lifestyle Influences on Arterial Aging," *Ageing Research Reviews* 39 (2017): 106–19. doi: 10.1016/j.arr.2016.09.002. PMID: 27693830; PMCID; this lab also maintains The Healthy Aging Project Website, featuring new research into healthy aging and links to a lot of good articles, ranging from technical

to popular: https://healthyagingproject.org. The Found My Fitness site has a number of articles on spermidine that are continually updated: https://www.foundmyfitness .com/search?q=spermidine.

35. https://www.nia.nih.gov/research/dab/interventions-testing-program-itp/ compounds-testing.

36. SNPedia is a fantastic resource for learning more about the various alleles of our genes. This entry, and the embedded links, can take you further into the story: https:// www.snpedia.com/index.php/MTHFR.

37. Matthew J. Yousefzadeh, Marissa J. Schafer, Nicole Noren Hooten, Elizabeth J. Atkinson, Michelle K. Evans, Darren J. Baker, Ellen K. Quarles, et al., "Circulating Levels of Monocyte Chemoattractant Protein-1 as a Potential Measure of Biological Age in Mice and Frailty in Humans," *Aging Cell* 17, no. 2 (2018): e12706. doi: 10.1111/acel.12706. PMID: 29290100.

38. The bird study is described by Valeria Marasco, Antoine Stier, Winnie Boner, Kate Griffiths, et al., "Environmental Conditions Can Modulate the Links among Oxidative Stress, Age, and Longevity," *Mechanisms of Ageing and Development* 164 (2017): 100–107. doi: 10.1016/j.mad.2017.04.012. PMID: 28487181. Human studies include Mille Løhr, Annie Jensen, Louise Eriksen, Morten Grønbæk, Steffen Loft, and Peter Møller, "Association between Age and Repair of Oxidatively Damaged DNA in Human Peripheral Blood Mononuclear Cells," *Mutagenesis* 30, no. 5 (2015): 695–700. doi: 10.1093/mutage/gev031. PMID: 25925070; Jorge P. Soares, Amelia M. Silva, Sandra Fonseca, Maria M. Oliveira, Francesco Peixoto, Isabel Gaivão, and Maria P. Mota, "How Can Age and Lifestyle Variables Affect DNA Damage, Repair Capacity and Endogenous Biomarkers of Oxidative Stress?," *Experimental Gerontolology* 62 (2015): 45–52. doi: 10.1016/j.exger.2015.01.001. PMID: 25576678; Douglas R. Seals and Simon Melov, "Translational Geroscience: Emphasizing Function to Achieve Optimal Longevity," *Aging* 6, no. 9 (2014): 718–30. doi: 10.18632/aging.100694. PMID: 25324468.

39. The original article describing the clock: Steve Horvath, "DNA Methylation Age of Human Tissues and Cell Types," *Genome Biology* 14, no. 10 (2013): R115–35. doi: 10.1186/gb-2013-14-10-r115. PMID: 24138928; the later work was done by Morgan E. Levine, Ake T. Lu, Austin Quach, Brian H. Chen, Theristocles L. Assimes, Stefania Bandinelli, Lifang Hou, et al., "An Epigenetic Biomarker of Aging for Lifespan and Healthspan," *Aging (Albany NY)* 10, no. 4 (2018): 573–91. doi: 10.18632/aging.101414. PMID: 29676998; the time to death clock is by Ake T. Lu, Austin Quach, James G. Wilson, Alex P. Reiner, Abraham Aviv, Kenneth Raj, Lifong Hou, et al., "DNA Methylation GrimAge Strongly Predicts Lifespan and Healthspan," *Aging (Albany NY)* 11, no. 2 (2019): 303–27. doi: 10.18632/aging.101684. PMID: 30669119.

40. Gregory M. Fahy, Robert T. Brooke, James P. Watson, Zinaida Good, Shreyas S. Vasanawala, Holden Maecker, Michael D. Leipold, et al., "Reversal of Epigenetic Aging and Immunosenescent Trends in Humans," *Aging Cell* (2019): 18(6):e13028. doi: 10.1111/acel.13028. Epub 2019 Sep 8. PMID: 31496122.

41. Elizabeth Blackburn and Elissa Epel, *The Telomere Effect* (New York: Grand Central Press, 2016), an excellent book, discusses many of the factors affecting

telomere length. A good review of additional caveats and technology is provided by Geraldine Aubert, Mark Hills, and Peter M. Lansdorp PM, "Telomere Length Measurement—Caveats and a Critical Assessment of the Available Technologies and Tools," *Mutation Research* 730, nos. 1–2 (2012): 59–67. doi: 10.1016/j .mrfmmm.2011.04.003. PMID: 21663926. The lifestyle study was done on a small cohort of patients with low-grade prostate cancer over a five-year period by Dean Ornish, Jue Lin, June M. Chan, Elissa Epel, Colleen Kemp, Gerdi Weidner, Ruth Marlin, et al., "Effect of Comprehensive Lifestyle Changes on Telomerase Activity and Telomere Length in Men with Biopsy-Proven Low-Risk Prostate Cancer: 5-Year Follow-up of a Descriptive Pilot Study," *Lancet Oncology* 14, no. 11 (2013): 1112–20. doi: 10.1016/S1470-2045(13)70366-8. PMID: 24051140.

42. You can find links to so-called bio-hacks at the Found My Fitness website, https://www.foundmyfitness.com/search?q=spermidine. Although I don't recommend specific authors, some of the more scientifically inclined include Dave Asprey, Tim Ferris, and Chris Kelly, whose website offers a lot of good material: https://nourish balancethrive.com.

43. For an excellent overview, see https://www.fightaging.org/self-experimentation/; for a specific example, see https://www.fightaging.org/archives/2018/05/how-to-plan -and-carry-out-a-simple-self-experiment-a-single-person-trial-of-a-mitochondrially -targeted-antioxidant.

Bibliography

Aagaard, P., C. Suetta, P. Caserotti, S. P. Magnusson, and M. Kjaer. "Role of the Nervous System in Sarcopenia and Muscle Atrophy with Aging: Strength Training as a Countermeasure." *Scandinavian Journal of Medicine and Science in Sports* 20, no. 1 (2010): 49–64. doi: 10.1111/j.1600-0838.2009.01084.x. PMID: 20487503.

Abdullah, K. M., Faizan A. Qais, Iqban Ahmad, and Imrana Naseem. "Inhibitory Effect of Vitamin B$_3$ against Glycation and Reactive Oxygen Species Production in HSA: An in vitro Approach." *Archives of Biochemestry and Biophysics* 627 (2017): 21–29. doi: 10.1016/j.abb.2017.06.009. PMID: 28624351.

Afizah, Hassan, and James H. Hui. "Mesenchymal Stem Cell Therapy for Osteoarthritis." *Journal of Clinical Orthopaedics and Trauma* 7, no. 3 (2016): 177–82. doi: 10.1016/j.jcot.2016.06.006. PMID: 27489413.

Akers, Emma J., Stephen J. Nicholls, and Belinda A. Di Bartolo. "Plaque Calcification: Do Lipoproteins Have a Role?" *Arteriosclerosis, Thrombosis and Vascular Biology* 39, no. 10 (2019): 1902–10. doi: 10.1161/ATVBAHA.119.311574. PMID: 31462089.

Alagiakrishnan, Kanniiram, Angela Juby, David Hanley, Wayne Tymchak, and Anne Sclater A. "Role of Vascular Factors in Osteoporosis." *Journals of Gerontology. Series A, Biological Sciences and Medical Sciences* 58, no. 4 (2003): 362–26. doi: 10.1093/gerona/58.4.m362. PMID: 12663699.

de Almeida Jackix, Elisia, Florencia Cúneo, Jamie Amaya-Farfan, Juvenal V. de Assunção, and Kesia D. Quintaes. "A Food Supplement of Hydrolyzed Collagen Improves Compositional and Biodynamic Characteristics of Vertebrae in Ovariectomized Rats." *Journal of Medicinal Food* 13, no. 6 (2010): 1385–90. doi: 10.1089/jmf.2009.0256. PMID: 20874246.

Al-Sheraji, Sadeq Hasan, Amin Ismail, Mohd Yazid Manap, Shuhaimi Mustafa, Rokiah Mohd Yusof, and Fouad Abdulrahman Hassan. "Hypocholesterolaemic Effect of

Yoghurt Containing Bifidobacterium pseudocatenulatum G4 or Bifidobacterium longum BB536." *Food Chemistry* 135, no. 2 (2012): 356–61. doi: org/10.1016/j .foodchem.2012.04.120.

Aoyagi, Atsushi, Carlo Condello, Jan Stöhr, Weizhou Yue, Brianna M. Rivera, Joanna C. Lee, Amanda L. Woerman, et al. "Aβ and Tau Prion-like Activities Decline with Longevity in the Alzheimer's Disease Human Brain." *Science and Translational Medicine* 11, no. 490 (2019): eaat8462. doi: 10.1126/scitranslmed.aat8462. PMID: 31043574.

Armstrong, Sue. *Borrowed Time: The Science of How and Why We Age.* London: Bloomsbury Sigma, 2019.

Arnold, Ann-Sophie, Anna Egger, and Christof Handschin. "PGC-1α and Myokines in the Aging Muscle—A Mini-Review." *Gerontology* 57, no. 1 (2011): 37–43. doi: 10.1159/000281883. PMID: 20134150.

Atherton, P. J., J. Babraj, K. Smith, J. Singh, M. J. Rennie, and H. Wackerhage. "Selective Activation of AMPK-PGC-1alpha or PKB-TSC2-mTOR Signaling Can Explain Specific Adaptive Responses to Endurance or Resistance Training-like Electrical Muscle Stimulation." *FASEB Journal* 19, no. 7 (2005): 786–88. doi: 10.1096/fj.04-2179fje. PMID: 15716393.

Attia, Peter. "Controversial Topic Affecting All Women—The Role of Hormone Replacement Therapy through Menopause and Beyond—The Compelling Case for Long-Term HRT and Dispelling the Myth That It Causes Breast Cancer." Podcasts. February 25, 2019. https://peterattiamd.com/caroltavris-avrumbluming/.

———. "Studying Studies: Part II—Observational Epidemiology." Topics. January 15, 2018. https://peterattiamd.com/ns002.

Aubert, Geraldine, Mark Hills, and Peter M. Lansdorp. "Telomere Length Measurement—Caveats and a Critical Assessment of the Available Technologies and Tools." *Mutation Research* 730, nos. 1–2 (2012): 59–67. doi: 10.1016/j.mrfmmm.2011.04.003. PMID: 21663926.

Azuma, Kotaro, and Satoshi Inoue. "Vitamin K Benefits in Aging and Cancer." In *Aging Mechanisms*, edited by Nozomo Mori and Inhee Mook-Jung, 223–39. Tokyo, Japan: Springer, 2015.

Balasubramanian, Priya, Chia-Weh Cheng, Federica Madia, Luigi Fontana, Mario Mirisola, Jaime Guevara-Aguirre, et al. "Low Protein Intake Is Associated with a Major Reduction in IGF-1, Cancer, and Overall Mortality in the 65 and Younger But Not Older Population." Cell Metabolism 19, no. 3 (2014): 407–17.

Barter, Philip J., H. Brian Brewer Jr., M. John Chapman, Charles H. Hennekens, Daniel J. Rader, and Alan R. Tall. "Cholesteryl Ester Transfer Protein: A Novel Target for Raising HDL and Inhibiting Atherosclerosis." *Arteriosclerosis, Thrombosis and Vascular Biology* 23, no. 2 (2003): 160–67. doi: 10.1161/01.atv.0000054658.91146.64. PMID: 12588754.

Bartke, Andrzej, and Nana Quainoo. "Impact of Growth Hormone-Related Mutations on Mammalian Aging." *Frontiers in Genetics* 9 (2018): 586. doi: 10.3389/fgene.2018.00586.

Bartke, Andrzej, and Westbrook Reyhan. "Metabolic Characteristics of Long-Lived Mice." *Frontiers in Genetics* 3 (2012): 288. doi: 10.3389/fgene.2012.00288.

Barzilai, Nur, Jill P. Crandall, Stephen B. Kritchevsky, and Mark A. Espeland. "Metformin as a Tool to Target Aging." *Cell Metabolism* 23, no. 6 (2016): 1060–65. https://doi.org/10.1016/j.cmet.2016.05.011.

Basisty, Nathan., Dao-Fu Dai, Ami Gagnidze, Lemuel Gitari, Jeanne Fredrickson, Yvonne Maina, Richard P. Beyer, Mary J. Emond, Edward J. Hsieh, Michael J. MacCoss, George M. Martin, and Peter S. Rabinovitch. "Mitochondrial-Targeted Catalase Is Good for the Old Mouse Proteome, But Not for the Young: 'Reverse' Antagonistic Pleiotropy?" *Aging Cell* 15, no. 4 (2016): 634–45. https://doi.org/10.1111/acel.12472.

Bell, Steven, Marina Daskalopoulou, Eleni Rapsomaniki, Julie George, Annie Britton, Martin Bobak, Juan P. Casas, Caroline E. Dale, Spiros Denaxas, Anoop Shah, and Harry Hemingway. "Association between Clinically Recorded Alcohol Consumption and Initial Presentation of 12 Cardiovascular Diseases: Population Based Cohort Study Using Linked Health Records." *British Medical Journal* 356 (2017): j909. doi: 10.1136/bmj.j909. PMID: 28331015.

Bennett, Beth. "Stem Cells to Treat Osteoarthritis." Trail Runner, 2018. https://trailrunnermag.com/training/stem-the-joint-aging-tide.html.

———. What Exactly Is Osteoporosis? Blog post, February 28, 2019. http://senesc-sense.com/what-exactly-is-osteoporosis/.

Berebichez-Fridman, Roberto, Ricardo Gómez-García, Julio Granados-Montiel, Enrique Berebichez-Fastlicht, Anell Olivos-Meza, Julio Granados, Cristain Velasquillo, and Clemente Ibarra. "The Holy Grail of Orthopedic Surgery: Mesenchymal Stem Cells—Their Current Uses and Potential Applications." *Stem Cells International* (2017): 2638305. doi: 10.1155/2017/2638305. PMID: 28698718.

Besse-Patin, A., E. Montastier, C. Vinel, I. Castan-Laurell, K. Louche, C. Dray, D. Daviaud, L. Mir, M. A. Marques, C. Thalamas, et al. "Effect of Endurance Training on Skeletal Muscle Myokine Expression in Obese Men: Identification of Apelin as a Novel Myokine." *International Journal of Obesity (London)* 38, no. 5 (2014): 707–13. doi: 10.1038/ijo.2013.158. PMID: 23979219.

Bhandari, Mohit, Raveendhara R. Bannur, Eric M. Babins, Johanna Martel-Pelletier, Moin Khan, Jean-Pierre Raynauld, Reynata Frankovich, Deanna Mcleod, Tahira Devji, Mark Phillips, et al. "Intra-articular Hyaluronic Acid in the Treatment of Knee Osteoarthritis: A Canadian Evidence-Based Perspective." *Therapeutic Advances in Musculoskeletal Disease* 9, no. 9 (2017): 231–46. https://doi.org/10.1177/1759720X17729641.

Bickel, C. Scott, James M. Cross, and Marcas M. Bamman. "Exercise Dosing to Retain Resistance Training Adaptations in Young and Older Adults." *Medicine and Science in Sports and Exercise* 43, no. 7 (2011): 1177–87. doi: 10.1249/MSS.0b013e318207c15d.

Bienias, Julie L., Laurel A. Beckett, David A. Bennett, Robert S. Wilson, and Denis A. Evans. "Design of the Chicago Health and Aging Project (CHAP)." *Journal of Alzheimers Disease* 5, no. 5 (2003): 349–55. doi: 10.3233/jad-2003-5501. PMID: 14646025.

Blackburn, Elizabeth, and Elissa Epel. *The Telomere Effect.* New York: Grand Central Press, 2016.

Blagosklonny, Mikhail V. "Aging and Immortality: Quasi-Programmed Senescence and Its Pharmacologic Inhibition." *Cell Cycle* 5, no. 18 (2006): 2087–2102. doi: 10.4161/cc.5.18.3288. PMID: 17012837.

Bluming, Avrum, and Carol Tavris. *Estrogen Matters: Why Taking Hormones in Menopause Can Improve Women's Well-Being and Lengthen Their Lives—Without Raising the Risk of Breast Cancer.* New York: Little Brown Spark, 2018.

Bo, Hai, Ning Jiang, LiJi Li, and Yong Zhang. "Mitochondrial Redox Metabolism in Aging: Effect of Exercise Interventions." *Journal of Sport and Health Science* 2, no. 2 (2013): 67–74.

Bolland, Mark J., MJ William Leung, Vicki Tai, Sonia Bastin, Greg D. Gamble, Andrew Grey, and Ian R. Reid. "Calcium Intake and Risk of Fracture: Systematic Review." *British Medical Journal* 351 (2015): h4580. doi: 10.1136/bmj.h4580. PMID: 26420387.

Booth, Frank W., Gregory N. Ruegsegger, and T. Dylan Olver. "Exercise Has a Bone to Pick with Skeletal Muscle." *Cell Metabolism* 23, no. 6 (2016): 961–62. doi: 10.1016/j.cmet.2016.05.016. PMID: 27304494.

Booth, Frank W., and K. A. Zwetsloot. "Basic Concepts about Genes, Inactivity and Aging." *Scandinavian Journal of Medicine and Science in Sports* 20, no. 1 (2010): 1–4. doi: 10.1111/j.1600-0838.2009.00972.x. PMID: 19602189.

Boroni, Mariana, Alessandra Zonari, Carolina Reis de Oliveira, Kallie Alkatib, Edgar Andres Ochoa Cruz, Lear E. Brace, and Juliana Lott de Carvalho. "Highly Accurate Skin-Specific Methylome Analysis Algorithm as a Platform to Screen and Validate Therapeutics for Healthy Aging." *Clinical Epigenetics* 12 (2020): article no. 105. doi.org/10.1186/s13148-020-00899-1.

Bradke, Brian S., and Deepak Vashishth. "N-Phenacylthiazolium Bromide Reduces Bone Fragility Induced by Nonenzymatic Glycation." *PLoS One* 9, no 7 (2014): e103199. doi: 10.1371/journal.pone.0103199. PMID: 25062024.

Bredesen, Dale E. "Reversal of Cognitive Decline: A Novel Therapeutic Program." *Aging* 6, no. 9 (2014): 707–17. doi: 10.18632/aging.100690. PMID: 25324467.

Brenner, Charles, and Amy C. Boileau. "Pterostilbene Raises Low Density Lipoprotein Cholesterol in People." *Clinical Nutrition* 38, no. 1 (2019): 480–81. doi: 10.1016/j.clnu.2018.10.007. PMID: 30482564.

Brigger, Daniel, Carsten Riether, Robin van Brummelen, Kira I. Mosher, Alicia Shiu, Zhaoqing Ding, Noemi Zbären, et al. "Eosinophils Regulate Adipose Tissue Inflammation and Sustain Physical and Immunological Fitness in Old Age." *Nature Metabolism* 2, no. 8 (2020): 688–702. doi: 10.1038/s42255-020-0228-3. PMID: 32694825.

Brioche, T., R. A. Kireev, S. Cuesta, A. Gratas-Delamarche, J. A. Tresguerres, M. C. Gomez-Cabrera, and J. Viña. "Growth Hormone Replacement Therapy Prevents Sarcopenia by a Dual Mechanism: Improvement of Protein Balance and of Antioxidant Defenses." *Journals of Gerontology. Series A, Biological Sciences and Medical Sciences* 69, no. 10 (2014): 1186–98. doi: 10.1093/gerona/glt187. PMID: 24300031.

Brittberg, Mats, David Recker, John Ilgenfritz, and Daniel B. F. Saris; SUMMIT Extension Study Group. "Matrix-Applied Characterized Autologous Cultured Chondrocytes Versus Microfracture: Five-Year Follow-up of a Prospective Randomized Trial." *American Journal of Sports Medicine* 46, no. 6 (2018): 1343–51. doi: 10.1177/0363546518756976. PMID: 29565642.

Bucci, Laura, Stell L. Yani, Christina Fabbri, Astrid Y. Bijlsma, Andrea B. Maier, Carol G. Meskers, Marco V. Narici, David A. Jones, Jamie S. McPhee, . . . and Stefano Salvioli. "Circulating Levels of Adipokines and IGF-1 Are Associated with Skeletal Muscle Strength of Young and Old Healthy Subjects." *Biogerontology* 14, no. 3 (2013): 261–72. doi: 10.1007/s10522-013-9428-5. PMID: 23666343.

Buettner, Dan. *The Blue Zones: 9 Lessons for Living Longer*, 2nd ed. Washington, DC: National Geographic Partners, 2012.

Buitrago-Lopez, Adriana, Jean Sanderson, Laura Johnson, Samantha Warnakula, Angela Wood, Emanuele Di Angelantonio, and Oscar H. Franco. "Chocolate Consumption and Cardiometabolic Disorders: Systematic Review and Meta-analysis." *British Medical Journal* 343 (2011): d4488. doi: 10.1136/bmj.d4488.

Burd, Nicholas A., Stefan H. Gorissen, and Luc J. van Loon. "Anabolic Resistance of Muscle Protein Synthesis with Aging." *Exercise and Sport Sciences Review* 41, no. 3 (2013): 169–73. doi: 10.1097/JES.0b013e318292f3d5. PMID: 23558692.

Butler-Browne, Gillian, Jamie McPhee, Vincent Mouly, and Anton Ottavi. "Understanding and Combating Age-Related Muscle Weakness: MYOAGE Challenge." *Biogerontology* 14, no. 3 (2013): 229–30. https://doi.org/10.1007/s10522-013-9438-3.

Butler-Browne, Gillian, Vincent Mouly, Anne Bigot, and Capucine Trollet. "How Muscles Age and How Exercise Can Slow It." *The Scientist*, September 2018. https://www.the-scientist.com/features/how-muscles-age--and-how-exercise-can-slow-it-64708.

Campisi, Judith, Pankaj Kapahi, Gordon J. Lithgow, Simon Melov, John C. Newman, and Eric Verdin. "From Discoveries in Ageing Research to Therapeutics for Healthy Ageing." *Nature* 571, no. 7764 (2019): 183–92. doi: 10.1038/s41586-019-1365-2.

Cantó, Carlos, and Johan Auwerx. "Targeting Sirtuin 1 to Improve Metabolism: All You Need Is NAD(+)?" *Pharmacological Reviews* 64, no. 1 (2012): 166–87. https://doi.org/10.1124/pr.110.003905.

Carnac, Gilles, Barbara Vernus, and Anne Bonnieu. "Myostatin in the Pathophysiology of Skeletal Muscle." *Current Genomics* 8, no. 7 (2007): 415–22. https://doi.org/10.2174/138920207783591672.

Carnio, Silvia, Francesca LoVerso, Martin A. Baraibar, Emaneula Longa, Muzamil M. Khan, Manuela Maffei, Marcus Reischl, MonicaCanepari, Stefan Loefler, Helmut Kern, et al. "Autophagy Impairment in Muscle Induces Neuromuscular Junction Degeneration and Precocious Aging." *Cell Reports* 8, no. 5 (2014): 1509–21. doi: 10.1016/j.celrep.2014.07.061. PMID: 25176656.

Cartee, Gregory D., Russell T. Hepple, Marcus M. Bamman, and Juleen R. Zierath. "Exercise Promotes Healthy Aging of Skeletal Muscle." *Cell Metabolism* 23, no. 6 (2016): 1034–47. doi: 10.1016/j.cmet.2016.05.007. PMID: 27304505.

Case, Christopher C., John Mandrola, and Lennard Zinn. *The Haywire Heart: How Too Much Exercise Can Kill You, and What You Can Do to Protect Your Heart.* Boulder, CO: VeloPress, 2017.

Castellan, Raphael F. P., and Marco Meloni. "Mechanisms and Therapeutic Targets of Cardiac Regeneration: Closing the Age Gap." *Frontiers in Cardiovascular Medicine* 5 (2018): 7. doi: 10.3389/fcvm.2018.00007. PMID: 29459901.

Cauley, Jane A. "Osteoporosis." In *The Epidemiology of Aging*, edited by Anne Newman and Jane A. Cauley, 499–522. New York: Springer, 2012.

———. "Screening for Osteoporosis." *Journal of the American Medical Association* 319, no. 24 (2018): 2483–85. doi: 10.1001/jama.2018.5722. PMID: 29946707.

Chai, Ruth J., Jana Vukovic, Sarah Dunlop, Miranda D. Grounds, and Thea Shavlakadze. "Striking Denervation of Neuromuscular Junctions without Lumbar Motoneuron Loss in Geriatric Mouse Muscle." *PLoS One* 6, no. 12 (2011): e28090. doi: 10.1371/journal.pone.0028090. PMID: 22164231.

Chang, Yu-Kai, and Jennifer L. Etnier. "Acute Exercise and Cognitive Function: Emerging Research Issues." *Journal of Sport and Health Science* 4 (2015): 1–3.

Charlesworth, Edward A., and Ronald C. Nathan. *Stress Management.* New York: Ballantine Books Trade Paperback, 2012.

Chekroud, Sammi R., Ralitza Gueorguieva, Amanda B. Zheutlin, Martin Paulus, Harlan M. Krumholz, John H. Krystal, and Adam M. Chekroud. "Association between Physical Exercise and Mental Health in 1·2 Million Individuals in the USA between 2011 and 2015: A Cross-Sectional Study." *Lancet Psychiatry* 5, no. 9 (2018): 739–46. doi: 10.1016/S2215-0366(18)30227-X. PMID: 30099000.

Cheng, Sulin, and Lijuan Mao. "Physical Activity Continuum throughout the Lifespan: Is Exercise Medicine or What?" *Journal of Sport and Health Science* 5, no. 2 (2016): 127–28. https://doi.org/10.1016/j.jshs.2016.03.005.

Chrysostomou, Vicki, Sandra Galic S, Peter van Wijngaarden P, Ian A. Trounce IA, Gregory Steinberg GR, and Jonathan G. Crowston. "Exercise Reverses Age-Related Vulnerability of the Retina to Injury by Preventing Complement-Mediated Synapse Elimination via a BDNF-dependent Pathway." *Aging Cell* 15, no. 6 (2016): 1082–91. doi: 10.1111/acel.12512. PMID: 27613664.

Chung, Hae Young, Mateo Cesari, Stephen Anton, Emmaneuelle Marzetti, Silvia Giovannini, Arnold Y. Seo, Christy Carter, Byung Pal Yu, Christian Leeuwenburgh. "Molecular Inflammation: Underpinnings of Aging and Age-Related Diseases." *Ageing Research Reviews* 8, no. 1 (2009): 18–30. doi: 10.1016/j.arr.2008.07.002. PMID: 18692159.

Clark, Richard V., Ann C. Walker, Susan Andrews, Phillip Turnbull, Jeffrey A. Wald, and Mindy H. Magee. "Safety, Pharmacokinetics and Pharmacological Effects of the Selective Androgen Receptor Modulator, GSK2881078, in Healthy Men and Postmenopausal Women." *British Journal of Clinical Pharmacology* 83, no. 10 (2017): 2179–94. doi: 10.1111/bcp.13316. PMID: 28449232.

Clement, James, Matthew Wong, Anne Poljak, Perminder Sachdev, and Nady Braidy. "The Plasma NAD+ Metabolome Is Dysregulated in 'Normal' Aging." *Rejuvenation Research* 22, no. 2 (2019): 121–30. doi: 10.1089/rej.2018.2077. PMID: 30124109.

Coen, Paul M., Robert V. Musci, J. Matthew Hinkley, and Benjamin F. Miller. "Mitochondria as a Target for Mitigating Sarcopenia." *Frontiers in Physiology* 9 (2019): 1883. doi: 10.3389/fphys.2018.01883. PMID: 30687111.

Col, N. F., L. A. Bowlby, and K. McGarry. "The Role of Menopausal Hormone Therapy in Preventing Osteoporotic Fractures: A Critical Review of the Clinical Evidence." *Minerva Medica* 96, no. 5 (2005): 331–42. PMID: 16227948.

Conboy, Irina M., Michael J. Conboy, Amy J. Wagers, Eric R. Girma, Irving L. Weissman, and Thomas A. Rando. "Rejuvenation of Aged Progenitor Cells by Exposure to a Young Systemic Environment." *Nature* 433, no. 7027 (2005): 760–64. doi: 10.1038/nature03260. PMID: 15716955.

Cooper, M. E., V. Thallas, J. Forbes, E. Scalbert, S. Sastra, I. Darby, T. Soulis. "The Cross-Link Breaker, N-phenacylthiazolium Bromide Prevents Vascular Advanced Glycation End-Product Accumulation." *Diabetologia* 43, no. 5 (2000): 660–64. doi: 10.1007/s001250051355. PMID: 10855541.

Coquand-Gandit, Marion, Marie-Paul Jacob, Wassim Fhayli, Beatriz Romero, Miglena Georgieva, Stephanie Bouillot, Eric Estève, Jean-Pierre Andrieu, Sandrine Brasseur, Sophie Bouyon, et al. "Chronic Treatment with Minoxidil Induces Elastic Fiber Neosynthesis and Functional Improvement in the Aorta of Aged Mice." *Rejuvenation Research* 20, no. 3 (2017): 218–30. doi: 10.1089/rej.2016.1874. PMID: 28056723.

Cruz Hernández, Jean C., Oliver Bracko, Calvin J. Kersbergen, Victorine Muse, Muhammed Haft-Javaherian, Maxine Berg, Laibaic Park, Lindsey Vinarcsik, . . . and Chris B. Schaffer. "Neutrophil Adhesion in Brain Capillaries Reduces Cortical Blood Flow and Impairs Memory Function in Alzheimer's Disease Mouse Models." *Nature Neuroscience* 22, no. 3 (2019): 413–20. doi: 10.1038/s41593-018-0329-4. PMID: 30742116.

Dang, Yao, Yongpan An, Jinzhao He, Boyue Huang, Jie Zhu, Miaomiao Gao, Shun Zhang, et al. "Berberine Ameliorates Cellular Senescence and Extends the Lifespan of Mice via Regulating p16 and Cyclin Protein Expression." *Aging Cell* 19, no. 1 (2020). https://doi.org/10.1111/acel.13060.

Dantzer, Robert. "Cytokine, Sickness Behavior, and Depression." *Immunology and Allergy Clinics of North America* 29, no. 2 (2010): 247–64. https://doi.org/10.1016/j.iac.2009.02.002.

Davatchi, Fareydoun, Bahar Sadeghi Abdollahi, Mandana Mohyeddin, and Beyrooz Nikbin. "Mesenchymal Stem Cell Therapy for Knee Osteoarthritis: 5 Years Follow-up of Three Patients." *International Journal of Rheumatic Diseases* 19, no. 3 (2016): 219–25. doi: 10.1111/1756-185X.12670. PMID: 25990685.

Davidson, R. A. "Source of Funding and Outcome of Clinical Trials." *Journal of General Internal Medicine* 1, no. 3 (1986): 155–58. doi: 10.1007/BF02602327. PMID: 3772583.

De Caterina, Raffaele, Philippa J. Talmud, Piera A. Merlini, Luisa Foco, Roberta Pastorino, David Altshuler, Francesco Mauri, . . . and Gruppo Italiano Aterosclerosi. "Strong Association of the APOA5-1131T>C Gene Variant and Early-Onset Acute Myocardial Infarction." *Atherosclerosis* 214, no. 2 (2011): 397–403. doi: 10.1016/j.atherosclerosis.2010.11.011. PMID: 21130994.

Dellinger, Ryan W., Santiago R. Santos, Mark Morris, Mal Evans, Dan Alminana, Leonard Guarente, and Eric Marcotulli. "Repeat Dose NRPT (Nicotinamide Riboside and Pterostilbene) Increases NAD⁺ Levels in Humans Safely and Sustainably: A Randomized, Double-Blind, Placebo-Controlled Study." *NPJ Aging and Mechanisms of Disease* 3 (2017): 17. doi: 10.1038/s41514-017-0016-9. PMID: 29184669.

Del Rosso, James Q., and Leon H. Kurcik. "Spotlight on the Use of Nitric Oxide in Dermatology: What Is It? What Does It Do? Can It Become an Important Addition to the Therapeutic Armamentarium for Skin Disease?" *Journal of Drugs in Dermatology* 16, no. 1 (2017): s4–10. PMID: 28095537.

Denison, Haley J., Cyrus Cooper, Alvin A. Sayer, and Sian M. Robinson. "Prevention and Optimal Management of Sarcopenia: A Review of Combined Exercise and Nutrition Interventions to Improve Muscle Outcomes in Older People." *Clinical Interventions in Aging* 10 (2015): 859–69. doi: 10.2147/CIA.S55842. PMID: 25999704.

Dernek, Bahar, Tihar M. Duymus, Pinar K. Koseoglu, Tugba Aydin, Falma N. Kesiktas, Cihan Aksoy, and Serhat Mutlu. "Efficacy of Single-Dose Hyaluronic Acid Products with Two Different Structures in Patients with Early-Stage Knee Osteoarthritis." *Journal of Physical Therapy Science* 28, no. 11 (2016): 3036–40. https://doi.org/10.1589/jpts.28.3036.

DeVan, Alison E., Lawrence C. Johnson, Forest A. Brooks, Trent D. Evans, Jamie N. Justice, Charmion Cruickshank-Quinn, Nichole Reisdorph, et al. "Effects of Sodium Nitrite Supplementation on Vascular Function and Related Small Metabolite Signatures in Middle-Aged and Older Adults." *Journal of Applied Physiology* 120, no. 4 (2016): 416–25. doi: 10.1152/japplphysiol.00879.2015. PMID: 26607249.

Douaud, Gwenelle, Helga Refsum, Celeste A. de Jager, Robin Jacoby, Thomas E. Nichols, Steven M. Smith, and A. David Smith. "Preventing Alzheimer's Disease-Related Gray Matter Atrophy by B-Vitamin Treatment." *Proceedings of the National Academy of Sciences USA* 110, no. 23 (2013): 9523–28. doi: 10.1073/pnas.1301816110. PMID: 23690582.

Edström, Erik, Mikael Altun, Esbjorn Bergman, Hans Johnson, Susanna Kullberg, Vania Ramírez-León, and Brun Ulfhake. "Factors Contributing to Neuromuscular Impairment and Sarcopenia during Aging." *Physiology and Behavior* 92, nos. 1–2 (2007): 129–35. doi: 10.1016/j.physbeh.2007.05.040. PMID: 17585972.

Ehrnstrom, Colleen, and Alisha L. Brosse. *End the Insomnia Struggle: A Step-by-Step Guide to Help You Get to Sleep and Stay Asleep.* Oakland, CA: New Harbinger Publications, 2016.

Enns, Deborah L., and Peter M. Tiidus. "The Influence of Estrogen on Skeletal Muscle: Sex Matters." *Sports Medicine* 40, no. 1 (2010): 41–58. doi: 10.2165/11319760-000000000-00000. PMID: 20020786.

Esiri, M. M. "Ageing and the Brain." *Journal of Pathology* 211, no. 2 (2007): 181–87. doi: 10.1002/path.2089. PMID: 17200950.

Fahy, Gregory M., Robert T. Brooke, James P. Watson, Zinaida Good, Schreyas S. Vasanawala, Holden Maecker, Michael D. Leipold MD, David T. S. Lin, Michael S. Kobor MS, and Steve Horvath. Reversal of epigenetic aging and immunosenescent trends in humans. Aging Cell. 2019 Dec;18(6):e13028. doi: 10.1111/acel.13028. Epub 2019 Sep 8. PMID: 31496122; PMCID: PMC6826138.

Fang, Yuan, Zheng Wei, Bin Chen, Tianye Pan, Shiang Gu, Peng Liu, Daqiao Guo, Xin Xu, Jinhao Jiang, et al. "Five-Year Study of the Efficacy of Purified CD34+ Cell Therapy for Angitis-Induced No-Option Critical Limb Ischemia." *Stem Cells Translational Medicine* 7, no. 8 (2018): 583–90. doi: 10.1002/sctm.17-0252. PMID: 29709112.

Farley, Alistair, Charles Hendry, and Ella McLafferty, eds. *The Physiological Effects of Ageing.* Oxford: Wiley-Blackwell, 2011.

Feinman, Richard D. *Nutrition in Crisis* (White River Junction, VT: Chelsea Green, 2019).

Fessler, Johannes, Russner Husic, Verena Schwetz, Elizabeth Lerchbaum, Felix Aberer, Patrizia Fasching, Anja Ficjan, Barbera Obermayer-Pietsch, Christina Duftner, . . . and Christian Dejaco. "Senescent T-Cells Promote Bone Loss in Rheumatoid Arthritis." *Frontiers in Immunology* 9 (2018): 95. doi: 10.3389/fimmu.2018.00095. PMID: 29472917.

Figueira, Ines, Adelaide Fernandes, Aleksandra Mladenovic Djordjevic, Andre Lopez-Contreras, Caterina M. Henriques, Colin Selman, Elisabeta Ferreiro, Efstafios S. Gonos, Jose L. Trejo, Juhi Misra, et al. "Interventions for Age-Related Diseases: Shifting the Paradigm." *Mechanisms of Ageing and Development* 160 (2016): 69–92. doi: 10.1016/j.mad.2016.09.009. PMID: 27693441.

Franceschi, Claudio, and Judith Campisi. "Chronic Inflammation (Inflammaging) and Its Potential Contribution to Age-Associated Diseases." *Journals of Gerontology. Series A, Biological Sciences and Medical Sciences* 69, suppl. 1 (2014): S4–9. doi: 10.1093/gerona/glu057. PMID: 24833586.

Gaziano, J. Michael, Howard D. Sesso, William G. Christen, Vadim Bubes, Joan P. Smith, Jean MacFadyen, Miriam Schvartz, JoAnn E. Manson, Robert J. Glynn, and Julie E. Buring. "Multivitamins in the Prevention of Cancer in Men: The Physicians' Health Study II Randomized Controlled Trial." *Journal of the American Medical Association* 308, no. 18 (2012): 1871–80. doi: 10.1001/jama.2012.14641. PMID: 23162860.

GBD Alcohol Collaborators. "Alcohol Use and Burden for 195 Countries and Territories, 1990–2016: A Systematic Analysis for the Global Burden of Disease Study." *Lancet* 382, no. 10152 (2016): 1015–35.

Gifford, Bill. *Spring Chicken: Stay Young Forever (or Die Trying).* Waterville, MA: Thorndike Press, 2015.

Girouard, Helene, and Costantino Iadecola. "Neurovascular Coupling in the Normal Brain and in Hypertension, Stroke, and Alzheimer Disease." *Journal of Applied Physiology* 100, no. 1 (2006): 328–35. doi: 10.1152/japplphysiol.00966.2005. PMID: 16357086.

Giroud-Gerbetant, Judith, Migali Joffraud, Maria P. Giner, Angelique Cercillieux, Simona Bartova, Mikhail V. Makarov, Ruben Zapata-Pérez, et al. "A Reduced Form of Nicotinamide Riboside Defines a New Path for NAD⁺ Biosynthesis and Acts as an Orally Bioavailable NAD⁺ Precursor." *Molecular Metabolism* 30 (2019): 192–202. doi: 10.1016/j.molmet.2019.09.013. PMID: 31767171.

Gkogkolou, Paraskevi, and Markus Böhm. "Advanced Glycation End Products: Key Players in Skin Aging?" *Dermato-Endocrinology* 4, no. 3 (2012): 259–70. doi: 10.4161/derm.22028. PMID: 23467327.

Goldberg, Elkhonen. *The Wisdom Paradox: How Your Mind Can Grow Stronger as Your Brain Grows Older.* London: Free Press, 2005.

Gomes, Ana P., Nathan L. Price, Alvin J. Ling, Javin J. Moslehi, Magdalena K. Montgomery, Luis Rajman, James P. White, Joao S. Teodoro, Christianna D. Wrann, Basil P. Hubbard, et al. "Declining NAD(+) Induces a Pseudohypoxic State Disrupting Nuclear-Mitochondrial Communication during Aging." *Cell* 155, no. 7 (2013): 1624–38. doi: 10.1016/j.cell.2013.11.037. PMID: 24360282.

Gonzalez-Freire, Marta, Rafael de Cabo, Stephanie A. Studenski, and Luigi Ferrucci. "The Neuromuscular Junction: Aging at the Crossroad between Nerves and Muscle." *Frontiers in Aging Neuroscience* 6 (2014): 208. https://doi.org/10.3389/fnagi.2014.00208. PMID: 25157231.

Gouspillou, Gilles, Nicolas Sgarioto, Sofia Kapchinsky, Fennigje Purves-Smith, Brandon Norris, Charlotte H. Pion, Sebastein Barbat-Artigas, Francois Lemieux, Tanya Taivassalo, et al. "Increased Sensitivity to Mitochondrial Permeability Transition and Myonuclear Translocation of Endonuclease G in Atrophied Muscle of Physically Active Older Humans." *FASEB Journal* 28, no. 4 (2014): 1621–33. doi: 10.1096/fj.13-242750. PMID: 24371120.

Grady, D., S. M. Rubin, D. B. Petitti, C. S. Fox, D. Black, B. Ettinger, L. Ernster, and S. R. Cummings. "Hormone Therapy to Prevent Disease and Prolong Life in Postmenopausal Women." *Annals of Internal Medicine* 117, no. 12 (1992): 1016–37. doi: 10.7326/0003-4819-117-12-1016. PMID: 1443971.

Gregor, Michael. *How Not to Die.* New York: Flatiron Books, 2015.

Harb, Serge C., Paul C. Cremer, Yuping Wu, Bo Xu, Leslie Cho, Veno Menon, and Wael A. Jaber. "Estimated Age Based on Exercise Stress Testing Performance Outperforms Chronological Age in Predicting Mortality." *European Journal of Preventive Cardiology* 13 (2019): 2047487319826400. doi: 10.1177/2047487319826400. PMID: 30760022.

Hayflick, Leonard. "Biological Aging Is No Longer an Unsolved Problem." *Annals of the New York Academy of Sciences* 100, no. 4 (2007): 1–13. doi: 10.1196/annals.1395.001. PMID: 17460161.

He, Chong, Scott K. Tsuchiyama, Quynh T. Nguyen, Ekaterina N. Plyusnina, Samuel R. Terrill, Sara Sahibzada, Bhumil Patel, et al. "Enhanced Longevity by Ibuprofen, Conserved in Multiple Species, Occurs in Yeast through Inhibition of Tryptophan Import." *PLoS Genetics* 10, no. 12 (2014): e1004860. doi: 10.1371/journal.pgen.1004860. PMID: 25521617.

Heidenreich, P. A., J. G. Trogdon, O. A. Khavjou, J. Butler, K. Dracup, M. D. Ezekowitz, E. A. Finkelstein, Y. Hong, S. C. Johnston, A. Khera, et al. "Forecasting the Future of Cardiovascular Disease in the United States: A Policy Statement from the American Heart Association." *Circulation* 123, no. 8 (2011): 933–44. doi: 10.1161/CIR.0b013e31820a55f5. PMID: 21262990.

Heitkamp, H. C. "Training with Blood Flow Restriction. Mechanisms, Gain in Strength and Safety." *Journal of Sports Medicine and Physical Fitness* 55, no. 5 (2015): 446–56. PMID: 25678204.

Hepple, Russell T. "Impact of Aging on Mitochondrial Function in Cardiac and Skeletal Muscle." *Free Radical Biology and Medicine* 98 (2016): 177–86. doi: 10.1016/j .freeradbiomed.2016.03.017. PMID: 27033952.

Hepple, Russell T., David J. Baker, Jan J. Kaczor, and Daniel J. Krause. "Long-Term Caloric Restriction Abrogates the Age-Related Decline in Skeletal Muscle Aerobic Function." *FASEB Journal* 19 no. 10 (2005): 1320–22. doi: 10.1096/fj.04-3535fje. PMID: 15955841.

Higgins, M. W. "The Framingham Heart Study: Review of Epidemiological Design and Data, Limitations and Prospects." *Progress in Clinical and Biological Research* 147, no. 1 (1984): 51–64. PMID: 6739495.

Honjo, Kie, Robert van Reekum, and Nikolaas P. Verhoeff. "Alzheimer's Disease and Infection: Do Infectious Agents Contribute to Progression of Alzheimer's Disease?" *Alzheimers and Dementia* 5, no. 4 (2009): 348–60. doi: 10.1016/j.jalz.2008.12.001. PMID: 19560105.

Horstman, Astrid M., E. Lichar Dillon, Randall J. Urban, and Melissa Sheffield-Moore. "The Role of Androgens and Estrogens on Healthy Aging and Longevity." *Journals of Gerontology. Series A, Biological Sciences and Medical Sciences* 67, no. 11 (2012): 1140–52. doi: 10.1093/gerona/gls068. PMID: 22451474.

Horvath, Steve. "DNA Methylation Age of Human Tissues and Cell Types." *Genome Biology* 14, no. 10 (2013): R115–35. doi: 10.1186/gb-2013-14-10-r115. PMID: 24138928.

Hulbert, A. J. "Metabolism and Longevity: Is There a Role for Membrane Fatty Acids?" *Integrative and Comparative Biology* 50, no. 5 (2010): 808–17. doi: 10.1093/icb/ icq007. PMID: 21558243.

Ilievski, Vladimir, Paulina K. Zuchowska, Stefan J. Green, Peter T. Toth, Michael E. Ragozzino, Khuong Le, and Haider Aljewari, et al. "Chronic Oral Application of a Periodontal Pathogen Results in Brain Inflammation, Neurodegeneration and Amyloid Beta Production in Wild Type Mice." *PLoS One* 13, no. 10 (2018): e0204941. doi: 10.1371/journal.pone.0204941. PMID: 30281647.

Institute of Medicine. *Cognitive Aging: Progress in Understanding and Opportunities for Action.* Washington, DC: National Academies Press, 2015.

Inui, Shigeki, and Satoshi Itami. "Androgen Actions on the Human Hair Follicle: Perspectives." *Experimental Dermatology* 22, no. 3 (2013): 168–71. doi: 10.1111/ exd.12024. PMID: 23016593.

Jeon, Ok Hee, Chaekyu Kim, Sona Rathod, Jae Wook Chung, Do Hun Kim, and Jennifer H. Elisseef. "Local Clearance of Senescent Cells Attenuates the Development of Post-Traumatic Osteoarthritis and Creates a Pro-Regenerative Environment." *Nature Medicine* 23 (2017): 775–81. https://doi.org/10.1038/nm.4324.

Ji, Li Li, Chounghung Kang, and Yang Zhang. "Exercise-Induced Hormesis and Skeletal Muscle Health." *Free Radical Biology and Medicine* 98 (2016): 113–22. doi: 10.1016/j.freeradbiomed.2016.02.025. PMID: 26916558.

Jones, Roanne R., Valeria Castelletto, Che J. Connon, and Ian W. Hamley. "Collagen Stimulating Effect of Peptide Amphiphile C_{16}–KTTKS on Human Fibroblasts." *Molecular Pharmaceutics* 10, no. 3 (2013): 1063–69. doi: 10.1021/mp300549d. PMID: 23320752.

Joyce, Susan A., John MacSharry, Patrick G. Casey, Michael Kinsella, Eileen F. Murphy, Fergus Shanahan, Colin Hill, and Cormac G. M. Gahan. "Regulation of Host Weight Gain and Lipid Metabolism by Bacterial Bile Acid Modification in the Gut." *Proceedings of the National Academy of Sciences* 111, no. 20 (2014): 7421–26. doi: 10.1073/pnas.1323599111.

Kalamian, Miriam. *Keto for Cancer*. White River Junction, VT: Chelsea Green Press, 2017.

Kang, Chounghun, and Li Li Ji. "Role of PGC-1α in Muscle Function and Aging." *Journal of Sport Health Science* 2, no. 2 (2013): 81–86. doi: org/10.1016/j.jshs.2013.03.005.

Katsuumi, Goro, Ippei Shimizu, Yoko Yoshida, and Tohru Minamino. "Vascular Senescence in Cardiovascular and Metabolic Diseases." *Frontiers in Cardiovascular Medicine* 5 (2018): 18. doi: 10.3389/fcvm.2018.00018. PMID: 29556500.

Kennedy, Brina K., and Dudley W. Lamming. "The Mechanistic Target of Rapamycin: The Grand ConducTOR of Metabolism and Aging." *Cell Metabolism* 23, no. 6 (2016): 990–1003. doi: 10.1016/j.cmet.2016.05.009. PMID: 27304501.

Kiernan, Jeremy, Sally Hu, Mark D. Grynpas, John E. Davies, and William L. Stanford. "Systemic Mesenchymal Stromal Cell Transplantation Prevents Functional Bone Loss in a Mouse Model of Age-Related Osteoporosis." *Stem Cells and Translational Medicine* 5, no. 5 (2016): 683–93. doi: 10.5966/sctm.2015-0231. PMID: 26987353.

King, Tanya S., Otto Q. Russe, Christine V. Möser, Nerea Ferreiró, Katherina L. Kynast, Claudia Knothe, Katrin Olbrich, et al. "AMP-Activated Protein Kinase Is Activated by Non-Steroidal Anti-inflammatory Drugs." *European Journal of Pharmacology* 762 (2015): 299–305. doi: 10.1016/j.ejphar.2015.06.001. PMID: 26049010.

Kirkland, James L., and Tamar Tchkonia. "Cellular Senescence: A Translational Perspective." *EBioMedicine* 21 (2017): 21–28. doi: 10.1016/j.ebiom.2017.04.013. PMID: 28416161.

Klarsfeld, Andre, and Frederic Revah. *The Biology of Death*. Ithaca, NY: Cornell University Press, 2004.

Kleefeldt, Florian, Uwe Rueckschloss, and Suleyman Ergün. "CEACAM1 Promotes Vascular Aging Processes." *Aging* 12, no. 4 (2020): 3121–23. https://doi.org/10.18632/aging.102868.

Know, Lee. *The Future of Mitochondria in Medicine: The Key to Understanding Disease, Chronic Illness, Aging, and Life Itself*. White River Junction, VT: Chelsea Green Press, 2018.

Knutsen, Russell H., Scott C. Beeman, Thomas J. Broekelmann, Delong Liu, Kit ManTsang, Attila Kovacs, Li Ye, Joshua R. Danback, Anderson Watson, Amanda Wardlaw, et al. "Minoxidil Improves Vascular Compliance, Restores Cerebral Blood flow, and Alters Extracellular Matrix Gene Expression in a Model of Chronic Vascular Stiffness." *American Journal of Physiology, Heart and Circulatory Physiology* 315, no. 1 (2018): H18–32. doi: 10.1152/ajpheart.00683.2017. PMID: 29498532.

Konopka, Adam R., Jaime L. Laurin JL, Hayden M. Schoenberg HM, Justin J. Reid JJ, William M. Castor WM, Christopher A. Wolff CA, Robert V. Musci RV, et al. "Metformin Inhibits Mitochondrial Adaptations to Aerobic Exercise Training in Older Adults." *Aging Cell* 18, no. 1 (2019): e12880. doi: 10.1111/acel.12880. PMID: 30548390.

Konopka, Adam R., Miranda K. Suer, Christopher A. Wolff, and Matthew P. Harber. "Markers of Human Skeletal Muscle Mitochondrial Biogenesis and Quality Control: Effects of Age and Aerobic Exercise Training." *Journals of Gerontology. Series A, Biological Sciences and Medical Sciences* 69, no. 4 (2014): 371–78. doi: 10.1093/gerona/glt107. PMID: 23873965.

Kox, M., L. T. van Eijk, J. Zwaag, J. van den Wildenberg, F. Sweep, J. G. van der Hoeven, and P. Pickkers. "Voluntary Activation of the Sympathetic Nervous System and Attenuation of the Innate Immune Response in Humans." *Intensive Care Medicine Experimental* 2, suppl. 1 (2014): https://doi.org/10.1186/2197-425X-2-S1-O2.

Kumar, Suresh, Fumahito Sugihara, Keiji Suzuki, Naoki Inoue, and Siriam Venkateswarathirukumara. "A Double-Blind, Placebo-Controlled, Randomised, Clinical Study on the Effectiveness of Collagen Peptide on Osteoarthritis." *Journal of the Science of Food and Agriculture* 95, no. 4 (2015): 702–7. doi: 10.1002/jsfa.6752. PMID: 24852756.

Kwoh, C. Kent. "Epidemiology of Osteoarthritis." In *The Epidemiology of Aging*, edited by A. B. Newman and J. A. Cauley, 523–36. New York: Springer Science, 2012. doi: 10.1007/978-94-007-5061-6_16.

La Colla, Annabella, Lucia Pronsato, Lorena Milanesi, and Andrea Vasconsuelo. "17β-Estradiol and Testosterone in Sarcopenia: Role of Satellite Cells." *Ageing Research Reviews* 24, pt. B (2015): 166–77. doi: 10.1016/j.arr.2015.07.011. PMID: 26247846.

Lahiri, Vikramit, and Daniel J. Konski. "Eat Yourself to Live: Autophagy's Role in Health and Disease." *The Scientist*, March 2018. https://www.the-scientist.com/features/eat-yourself-to-live-autophagys-role-in-health-and-disease-30024.

Lane, Nick. *Life Ascending: The Ten Great Inventions of Evolution.* New York: Norton, 2009.

———. *Power, Sex and Suicide.* Oxford: Oxford University Press, 2005.

Laplante, Matthieu, and David M. Sabatini. "mTOR Signaling at a Glance." *Journal of Cell Science* 122, pt. 20 (2009): 3589–94. doi: 10.1242/jcs.051011. PMID: 19812304.

LaRocca, Thomas J., Christopher R. Martens, and Douglas R. Seals. "Nutrition and Other Lifestyle Influences on Arterial Aging." *Ageing Research Reviews* 39 (2017): 106–19. doi: 10.1016/j.arr.2016.09.002. PMID: 27693830; PMCID.

Laukkanen, Jari A., and Tanjanalina Laukkanen. "Sauna Bathing and Systemic Inflammation." *European Journal of Epidemiology* 33, no. 3 (2018): 351–53. doi: 10.1007/s10654-017-0335-y. PMID: 29209938.

Laukkanen, Tanjanalina, Hassan Khan, Francesco Zaccardi, and Jari A. Laukkanen. "Association between Sauna Bathing and Fatal Cardiovascular and All-Cause Mortality Events." *JAMA Internal Medicine* 175, no. 4 (2015): 542–28. doi: 10.1001/jamainternmed.2014.8187. PMID: 25705824.

Laukkanen, Tanjanalina, Setor Kunutsor, Jussi Kauhanen, and Jari A. Laukkanen. "Sauna Bathing Is Inversely Associated with Dementia and Alzheimer's Disease in Middle-Aged Finnish Men." *Age and Ageing* 46, no. 2 (2017): 245–49. doi: 10.1093/ageing/afw212. PMID: 27932366.

Lei, Mingqing, Linus J. Schumacher, Yung-Chin Lai, Weng Tao Juan, Chao-Yuan Yeh, Ping Wu, Ting-Xin Jiang, Ruth E. Baker, Randall Bruce Widelitz, Li Yang, and Cheng Ming Chuong. "Self-Organization Process in Newborn Skin Organoid Formation Inspires Strategy to Restore Hair Regeneration of Adult Cells." *Proceedings of the National Acadamy of Sciences U.S.A.* 114, no. 34 (2017): E7101–10. doi: 10.1073/pnas.1700475114. PMID: 28798065.

Leonoudakis, Dmitri, Anand Rane, Suzanne Angeli, Gordon J. Lithgow, Julie K. Andersen, and Shankar J. Chinta. "Anti-Inflammatory and Neuroprotective Role of Natural Product Securinine in Activated Glial Cells: Implications for Parkinson's Disease." *Mediators of Inflammation* (2017): 8302636. doi: 10.1155/2017/8302636. PMID.

Lesniewski, Lisa A., Douglas R. Seals, Ashley E. Walker, Grant D. Henson, Marc W. Blimline, Daniel W. Trott, Gary C. Bosshardt, Thomas J. LaRocca, Brooke R. Lawson, Melanie C. Zigler, and Anthony J. Donato. "Dietary Rapamycin Supplementation Reverses Age-Related Vascular Dysfunction and Oxidative Stress, while Modulating Nutrient-Sensing, Cell Cycle, and Senescence Pathways." *Aging Cell* 16, no. 1 (2017): 17–26. doi: 10.1111/acel.12524. PMID: 27660040.

Lettieri-Barbato, Daniele, Esmerelda Giovannetti, and Katya Aquilano. "Effects of Dietary Restriction on Adipose Mass and Biomarkers of Healthy Aging in Human." *Aging (Albany NY)* 8, no. 12 (2016): 3341–55. doi: 10.18632/aging.101122.

Levine, Morgan E., Ake T. Lu, Austin Quach, Brian H. Chen, Theristocles L. Assimes, Stefania Bandinelli, Lifang Hou, et al. "An Epigenetic Biomarker of Aging for Lifespan and Healthspan." *Aging (Albany NY)* 10, no. 4 (2018): 573–91. doi: 10.18632/aging.101414. PMID: 29676998.

Levine, Morgan E., Jorge A. Suarez, Sebasttian Brandhorst, Priya Balasubramanian, Chia-Weh Cheng, Federica Madia, Luigi Fontana, Mario Mirisola, Jaime Guevara-Aguirre, . . . and Valter Longo. "Low Protein Intake Is Associated with a Major Reduction in IGF-1, Cancer, and Overall Mortality in the 65 and Younger But Not Older Population." *Cell Metabolism* 19, no. 3 (2014): 407–17. https://doi.org/10.1016/j.cmet.2014.02.006.

Levitin, Daniel. *Successful Aging: A Neuroscientist Explores the Power and Potential of Our Lives.* New York: Dutton, 2020.

Levy, Bruce D. "Resolvins and Protectins: Natural Pharmacophores for Resolution Biology." *Prostaglandins, Leukotrienes, and Essential Fatty Acids* 82, nos. 4–6 (2010): 327–32. doi: 10.1016/j.plefa.2010.02.003. PMID: 20227865.

Li, Huiji, Sven Horke, and Ulrich Förstermann. "Oxidative Stress in Vascular Disease and Its Pharmacological Prevention." *Trends in Pharmacological Science* 34, no. 6 (2013): 313–19. doi: 10.1016/j.tips.2013.03.007. PMID: 23608227.

Lietman, Caressa, Brian Wu, Sarah Lechner, Andrew Shinar, Madgur Sehgal, Evganar Rossomacha, Poulani Datta, Anirudh Sharma, Rajiv Gandhi, Mohitt Kapoor, and Pampi P. Young. "Inhibition of Wnt/β-catenin Signaling Ameliorates Osteoarthritis in a Murine Model of Experimental Osteoarthritis." *JCI Insight* 3, no. 3 (2018): e96308. doi: 10.1172/jci.insight.96308. PMID: 29415892.

Loenneke, Jeremy P., Kaelin C. Young, Jacob M. Wilson, and J. C. Andersen. "Rehabilitation of an Osteochondral Fracture Using Blood Flow Restricted Exercise: A Case Review." *Journal of Bodywork and Movement Therapies* 17, no. 1 (2013): 42–45. doi: 10.1016/j.jbmt.2012.04.006. PMID: 23294682.

Løhr, Mille, Annie Jensen, Louise Eriksen, Morten Grønbæk, Steffen Loft, and Peter Møller. "Association between Age and Repair of Oxidatively Damaged DNA in Human Peripheral Blood Mononuclear Cells." *Mutagenesis* 30, no. 5 (2015): 695–700. doi: 10.1093/mutage/gev031. PMID: 25925070.

Longo, Valter, *The Longevity Diet*. New York: Avery Books, 2016.

Longo, Valter D., Adam Antebi, Andrzej Bartke, Nir Barzilai, Holly M. Brown-Borg, Calogero Caruso, Tyler J. Curiel, et al. "Interventions to Slow Aging in Humans: Are We Ready?" *Aging Cell* 14, no. 4 (2015): 497–510. doi: 10.1111/acel.12338. PMID: 25902704.

Longo, Valter D., and Satchem Panda. "Fasting, Circadian Rhythms, and Time-Restricted Feeding in Healthy Lifespan." *Cell Metabolism* 23, no. 6 (2016): 1048–59.

Lu, Ake T., Austin Quach, James G. Wilson, Alex P. Reiner, Abraham Aviv, Kenneth Raj, Lifong Hou, et al. "DNA Methylation GrimAge Strongly Predicts Lifespan and Healthspan." *Aging (Albany NY)* 11, no. 2 (2019): 303–27. doi: 10.18632/aging.101684. PMID: 30669119.

Marasco, Valeria, Antoine Stier, Winnie Boner, Kate Griffiths, Britt Heidinger, and Pat Monaghan. "Environmental Conditions Can Modulate the Links among Oxidative Stress, Age, and Longevity." *Mechanisms of Ageing and Development* 164 (2017): 100–107. doi: 10.1016/j.mad.2017.04.012. PMID: 28487181.

Mardones, Rodrigo, Claudio M. Jofré, L. Tobar, and Jose J. Minguell. "Mesenchymal Stem Cell Therapy in the Treatment of Hip Osteoarthritis." *Journal of Hip Preservation Surgery* 4, no. 2 (2017): 159–63. doi: 10.1093/jhps/hnx011. PMID: 28630737.

Martens, Christopher R., Blaire A. Denman, Melissa R. Mazzo, Michael L. Armstrong, Nicole Reisdorph, Matthew B. McQueen, Michel Chonchol, and Douglas R. Seals. "Chronic Nicotinamide Riboside Supplementation is Well-Tolerated and Elevates NAD+ in Healthy Middle-Aged and Older Adults." *Nature Communications* 9, no. 1 (2018): 1286. doi: 10.1038/s41467-018-03421-7. PMID: 29599478.

Martens, Christopher R., and Douglas R. Seals. "Practical Alternatives to Chronic Caloric Restriction for Optimizing Vascular Function with Ageing." *Journal of Physiology* 594, no. 24 (2016): 7177–95. doi: 10.1113/JP272348. PMID: 27641062.

Martin, Regina M., and Pedro H. Correa. "Bone Quality and Osteoporosis Therapy." *Arquivos brasileiros de endocrinologia e metabologia* 54, no. 2 (2010): 186–99. doi: 10.1590/s0004-27302010000200015. PMID: 20485908.

Masley, Steven. *The Better Brain Solution*. New York: Knopf, 2018.

Mattison, Julie A., Ricki J. Colman, T. Mark Beasley, David B. Allison, Joseph W. Kenmitz, George S. Roth, Donald K. Ingram, et al. "Caloric Restriction Improves Health and Survival of Rhesus Monkeys." *Nature Communications* (January 17, 2017): 14063. doi: 10.1038/ncomms14063.

McGill, Stuart. *Back Mechanic: The Step-by-Step McGill Method to Manage Back Pain.* Gravenhurst, Ontario: Backfitpro Inc. (www.backfitpro.com), 2015.

McGregor, Robin A., David Cameron-Smith, and Sally D. Poppitt. "It Is Not Just Muscle Mass: A Review of Muscle Quality, Composition and Metabolism during Ageing as Determinants of Muscle Function and Mobility in Later Life." *Longevity & Healthspan* 3, no. 1 (2014): 9–17. https://doi.org/10.1186/2046-2395-3-9.

McGuff, Doug, and John Little. *Body by Science.* New York: McGraw-Hill, 2009.

McKeage, Kate, David Murdoch, and Karen Goa. "The Sirolimus-Eluting Stent: A Review of Its Use in the Treatment of Coronary Artery Disease." *American Journal of Cardiovascular Drugs* 3, no. 3 (2003): 211–30. doi: 10.2165/00129784-200303030-00007. PMID: 14727933.

Melov, Simon, Mark A. Tarnopolsky, Kenneth Beckma, Kristin Felkey, and Alan Hubbard. "Resistance Exercise Reverses Aging in Human Skeletal Muscle." *PloS One* 2, no. 5 (2007): e465. https://doi.org/10.1371/journal.pone.0000465. PMID: 17520024.

Mera, Paula, Kathrin Lauen, Matthieu Ferron, Cyril Confavreux, Jienwin Wei, Marta Galán-Díez, Alain Lacampagne, Sarah J. Mitchell, Julie A. Mattison, . . . and Gerard Karsenty. "Osteocalcin Signaling in Myofibers Is Necessary and Sufficient for Optimum Adaptation to Exercise." *Cell Metabolism* 23, no. 6 (2016): 1078–92. doi: 10.1016/j.cmet.2016.05.004. PMID: 27304508.

Mercer, John R. "Mitochondrial Bioenergetics and Therapeutic Intervention in Cardiovascular Disease." *Pharmacology and Therapeutics* 141, no. 1 (2014): 13–20. doi: 10.1016/j.pharmthera.2013.07.011. PMID: 23911986.

Michaëlsson, Karl, John A. Baron, Bahman Y. Farahmand, Olof Johnell, Cecilia Magnusson, Per-Gunnar Persson, Ingemar Persson, and Sverker Ljunghall. "Hormone Replacement Therapy and Risk of Hip Fracture: Population Based Case-Control Study." The Swedish Hip Fracture Study Group. *British Medical Journal (Clinical research ed.)* 316, no. 7148 (1998): 1858–63. https://doi.org/10.1136/bmj.316.7148.1858.

Mikhed, Yuliya, Andreas Daiber, and Sebasatien Steven. "Mitochondrial Oxidative Stress, Mitochondrial DNA Damage and Their Role in Age-Related Vascular Dysfunction." *International Journal of Molecular Sciences* 16, no. 7 (2015): 15918–53. doi: 10.3390/ijms160715918. PMID: 26184181.

Miller, B. E., M. J. De Souza, K. Slade, and A. A. Luciano. "Sublingual Administration of Micronized Estradiol and Progesterone, with and without Micronized Testosterone: Effect on Biochemical Markers of Bone Metabolism and Bone Mineral Density." *Menopause* 7, no. 5 (2000): 318–26. doi: 10.1097/00042192-200007050-00006. PMID: 10993031.

Miller, Marshall G., Nopporn Thangthaeng, Shibu M. Poulose, and Barbara Shukitt-Hale. "Role of Fruits, Nuts, and Vegetables in Maintaining Cognitive Health." *Experimental Gerontology* 94 (2017): 24–28. doi: 10.1016/j.exger.2016.12.014. PMID: 28011241.

Minetto, Marco A., Ales Holobar, Alberto Botter, and Dario Farina. "Origin and Development of Muscle Cramps." *Exercise and Sport Sciences Review* 41, no. 1 (2013): 3–10. doi: 10.1097/JES.0b013e3182724817. PMID: 23038243.

Minihane, Anne M., Sophie Vinoy, Wendy R. Russell, Athanasia Baka, Helen M. Roche, Kieren M. Tuohy, Jessica L. Teeling, Ellen E. Blaak, Michael Fenech, David Vauzour, et al. "Low-Grade Inflammation, Diet Composition and Health: Current Research Evidence and Its Translation." *British Journal of Nutrition* 114, no. 7 (2015): 999–1012. doi: 10.1017/S0007114515002093. PMID: 26228057.

Mittledorf, Joshua, and Dorian Sagan. *Cracking the Aging Code: The New Science of Growing Old—And What It Means for Staying Young.* New York: Macmillan, 2016.

Moreau, Kari. L., Brian L. Stauffer, Wendy M. Kohrt, and D. R. Seals. "Essential Role of Estrogen for Improvements in Vascular Endothelial Function with Endurance Exercise in Postmenopausal Women." *Journal of Clinical Endocrinology and Metabolism* 98, no. 11 (2013): 4507–15. https://doi.org/10.1210/jc.2013-2183.

Morgan, A. E., K. M. Mooney, S. J. Wilkinson, N. A. Pickles, and M. T. McAuley. "Cholesterol Metabolism: A Review of How Ageing Disrupts the Biological Mechanisms Responsible for Its Regulation." *Ageing Research Reviews* 27 (2016): 108–24. doi: 10.1016/j.arr.2016.03.008. PMID: 27045039.

Morley, John E. "Pharmacologic Options for the Treatment of Sarcopenia." *Calcified Tissue International* 98, no. 4 (2016): 319–33. doi: 10.1007/s00223-015-0022-5. PMID: 26100650.

Morris, M. C. "The Role of Nutrition in Alzheimer's Disease: Epidemiological Evidence." *European Journal of Neurology* 16, suppl. 1 (2009): 1–7. doi: 10.1111/j.1468-1331.2009.02735.x. PMID: 19703213.

Most, Joshua, Valeria Tosti, Leanne M. Redman, and Luigi Fontan. "Calorie Restriction in Humans: An Update." *Ageing Research Reviews* 39 (2017): 36–45. doi: 10.1016/j.arr.2016.08.005. PMID: 27544442.

Mujica-Parodi, Lilianne R., Anar Amgalan, Syed Fahad Sultan, Botond Antal, Xiaofei Sun, Steven Skiena, Andrew Lithen, et al. "Diet Modulates Brain Network Stability, a Biomarker for Brain Aging, in Young Adults." *Proceedings of the National Academy of Sciences US* 117, no. 11 (2020): 6170–77. doi: 10.1073/pnas.1913042117.

Muñoz-Espín, Daniel, Miguel Rovira, Irene Galiana, Cristina Giménez, Beatriz Lozano-Torres, Marta Paez-Ribes, Susana Llanos, et al. "A Versatile Drug Delivery System Targeting Senescent Cells." doi: 10.15252/emmm.201809355. PMID: 30012580.

Murray, Andrew J., Nicholas S. Knight, Mark A. Cole, Lowri E. Cochlin, Emma Carter, Kieiri Tchabanenko, Tika Pichulik, et al. "Novel Ketone Diet Enhances Physical and Cognitive Performance." *FASEB Journal* 30, no. 12 (2016): 4021–32. doi: 10.1096/fj.201600773R. PMID: 27528626.

Nagai, Ryoji, David B. Murray, Thomas O. Metz, and John W. Baynes. "Chelation: A Fundamental Mechanism of Action of AGE Inhibitors, AGE Breakers, and Other Inhibitors of Diabetes Complications." *Diabetes* 61, no. 3 (2012): 549–59. doi: 10.2337/db11-1120. PMID: 22354928.

Nelke, Christopher, Ranier Dziewas, Jens Minnerup, Sven G. Meuth, Tobias Ruck. "Skeletal Muscle as Potential Central Link between Sarcopenia and Immune Senescence." *EBioMedicine* 49 (2019): 381–88. doi: 10.1016/j.ebiom.2019.10.034. PMID: 31662290; PMCID: PMC6945275.

Nencioni, Alessio, Irene Caffa, Salvatore Cortellino, and Valter D. Longo. "Fasting and Cancer: Molecular Mechanisms and Clinical Application." *Nature Reviews. Cancer* 18, no. 11 (2018): 707–19. https://doi.org/10.1038/s41568-018-0061-0.

Nestor, James. *Breath: The New Science of a Lost Art.* New York: Penguin Random House, 2020.

Newberry, Sidney J., John D. Fitzgerald, Margaret A. Maglione, Claire E. O'Hanlon, Mareeka Booth, Aneesa Motala, Martha Timmer, Roberta Shanman, and Paul G. Shekelle. "Systematic Review for Effectiveness of Hyaluronic Acid in the Treatment of Severe Degenerative Joint Disease (DJD) of the Knee [Internet]." Rockville, MD: Agency for Healthcare Research and Quality (US), 2015. PMID: 26866204.

Newgard, Christopher B., and Jeffrey E. Pessin. "Recent Progress in Metabolic Signaling Pathways Regulating Aging and Life Span." *Journals of Gerontology. Series A, Biological Sciences and Medical Sciences* 69, suppl. 1 (2014): S21–27. doi: 10.1093/gerona/glu058. PMID: 24833582; PMCID: PMC4022126.

Newman, John C., Sofiya Milman, Shahrukh K. Hashmi, Steve N. Austad, James L. Kirkland, Jeffrey B. Halter, and Nir Barzilai N. "Strategies and Challenges in Clinical Trials Targeting Human Aging." *Journals of Gerontology. Series A, Biological Sciences and Medical Sciences* 71, no. 11 (2016): 1424–34. doi: 10.1093/gerona/glw149. PMID: 27535968.

Norwitz, Nicholas G., and Henry Querfurth. "mTOR Mysteries: Nuances and Questions about the Mechanistic Target of Rapamycin in Neurodegeneration." *Frontiers in Neuroscience* 14 (2020): 775–85. doi: 10.3389/fnins.2020.00775.

Ocampo, Alejandro, Pradeep Reddy, Paloma Martinez-Redondo, Aida Platero-Luengo, Fumiyuki Hatanaka, Tomoaki Hishida, Mo Li, David Lam, Masakazu Kurita, Ergin Beyret, et al. "In Vivo Amelioration of Age-Associated Hallmarks by Partial Reprogramming." *Cell* 167, no. 7 (2016): 1719–33. doi: 10.1016/j.cell.2016.11.052.

O'Keefe, James H., Evan L. O'Keefe, and Carl J. Lavie. "The Goldilocks Zone for Exercise: Not Too Little, Not Too Much." *Missouri Medicine* 115, no. 2 (2018): 98–105. PMID: 30228692.

Ornish, Dean, Jue Lin, June M. Chan, Elissa Epel, Colleen Kemp, Gerdi Weidner, Ruth Marlin, et al. "Effect of Comprehensive Lifestyle Changes on Telomerase Activity and Telomere Length in Men with Biopsy-Proven Low-Risk Prostate Cancer: 5-Year Follow-up of a Descriptive Pilot Study." *Lancet Oncology* 14, no. 11 (2013): 1112–20. doi: 10.1016/S1470-2045(13)70366-8. PMID: 24051140.

Orrenius, Sten, Vladimir Gogvadze, and Boris Zhivotovsky. "Calcium and Mitochondria in the Regulation of Cell Death." *Biochemical and Biophysical Research Communications* 460, no. 1 (2015): 72–81. doi: 10.1016/j.bbrc.2015.01.137. PMID: 25998735.

Ozcivici, Engin, Yen K. Luu, Ben Adler, Yi-Jian Qin, Janet Rubin, Stefan Judex, and Clinton T. Rubin. "Mechanical Signals as Anabolic Agents in Bone." *Nature Reviews. Rheumatology* 6, no.1 (2010): 50–59. doi: 10.1038/nrrheum.2009.239. PMID: 20046206.

Partridge, Linda, Toren Finkel, Amita Sehgal, Pankaj Kapahi, Valter Longo, Rozalyn Anderson, Tim Spector, Heinrich Jasper, David A. Sinclair, Andrzej Bartke, et al. "Focus on Aging." *Cell Metabolism* 23 (2016): 951–56, a 2016.

Pasternak, Charles A. *The Molecules Within Us: Our Body in Health and Disease.* New York: Plenum Trade Books, 1998.

Pauly, Marion, Beatrice Chabi, Francois Favier, Franki Vanterpool, Stefan Matecki, Gilles Fouret, Beatrice Bonafos, Barbara Vernus, Christine Feillet-Coudray, Charles Coudray, et al. "Combined Strategies for Maintaining Skeletal Muscle Mass and Function in Aging: Myostatin Inactivation and AICAR-Associated Oxidative Metabolism Induction." *Journals of Gerontology. Series A, Biological Sciences and Medical Sciences* 70, no. 9 (2015): 1077–87. doi: 10.1093/gerona/glu147. PMID: 25227129.

Peake, Jonathon M., James F. Markworth, Kazunori Nosaka, Truls Raastad, Glenn D. Wadley, and Vernon G. Coffey. "Modulating Exercise-Induced Hormesis: Does Less Equal More?" *Journal of Applied Physiology* 119, no. 3 (2015): 172–89. doi: 10.1152/japplphysiol.01055.2014. PMID: 25977451.

Peffer, Melanie. *Biology Everywhere: How the Science of Life Matters to Everyday Life.* Greeley, CO: MKPEF4, 2020.

Pelletier, Alan L., Ledy Rojas-Roldan, and Janis Coffin. "Vision Loss in Older Adults." *American Family Physician* 94, no. 3 (2016): 219–26. PMID: 27479624.

Perkin, Oliver, Polly McGuigan, Dylan Thompson, and Keith Stokes. "A Reduced Activity Model: A Relevant Tool for the Study of Ageing Muscle." *Biogerontology* 17, no. 3 (2016): 435–47. https://doi.org/10.1007/s10522-015-9613-9.

de Picciotto, Natalie E., Lindsey B. Gano, Lawrence C. Johnson, Christopher R. Martens, Amy L. Sindler, Katherine F. Mills, Shin-Ichiro Imai, and Douglas R. Seals DR. "Nicotinamide Mononucleotide Supplementation Reverses Vascular Dysfunction and Oxidative Stress with Aging in Mice." *Aging Cell* 15, no. 3 (2016): 522–30. doi: 10.1111/acel.12461. PMID: 26970090.

Power, Geoffrey A., Brian H. Dalton, and Charles L. Rice. "Human Neuromuscular Structure and Function in Old Age: A Brief Review." *Journal of Sport and Health Science* 2, no. 4 (2011): 215–26. https://doi.org/10.1016/j.jshs.2013.07.001.

Powers, Scott K., and Edward T. Howley. *Exercise Physiology: Theory and Application to Fitness and Performance*, 9th ed. New York: McGraw-Hill, 2015.

Praetorius, Christian, Christine Grill, Simon N. Stacey, Alexander M. Metcalf, David U. Gorkin, Kathleen C. Robinson, Eric Van Otterloo, Rubin S. Q. Kim, Kristin Bergsteinsdottir, Margaret H. Ogmundsdottir, et al. "A Polymorphism in IRF4 Affects Human Pigmentation through a Tyrosinase-Dependent MITF/TFAP2A Pathway." *Cell* 155, no. 5 (2013): 1022–33. doi: 10.1016/j.cell.2013.10.022. PMID: 24267888.

Proske, Uwe, and Trevor J. Allen. "Damage to Skeletal Muscle from Eccentric Exercise." *Exercise and Sport Sciences Review* 33, no. 2 (2005): 98–104. doi: 10.1097/00003677-200504000-00007. PMID: 15821431.

Pruimboom, Leo, and Frits A. J. Muskiet. "Intermittent Living; The Use of Ancient Challenges as a Vaccine against the Deleterious Effects of Modern Life—A Hypothesis." *Medical Hypotheses* 120 (2018): 28–42. doi: 10.1016/j.mehy.2018.08.002. PMID: 30220336.

Puthucheary, Zudin, James R. Skipworth, Jai Rawal, Mike Loosemore, Ken Van Someren, and Hugh Montgomery. "The ACE Gene and Human Performance:

12 Years On." *Sports Medicine* 41, no. 6 (2011): 433–48. doi: 10.2165/11588720 -000000000-00000. PMID: 21615186.

Raichlen, David A., and Gene E. Alexander. "Why Your Brain Needs Exercise." *Scientific American*, January 2020.

Raison, Charles L., and Andrew H. Miller. "Pathogen-Host Defense in the Evolution of Depression: Insights into Epidemiology, Genetics, Bioregional Differences and Female Preponderance." *Neuropsychopharmacology: Official Publication of the American College of Neuropsychopharmacology* 42, no. 1 (2017): 5–27. doi: 10.1038/ npp.2016.194.

Ramamurthy B., and L. Larsson. "Detection of an Aging-related Increase in Advanced Glycation End Products in Fast- and Slow-Twitch Skeletal Muscles in the Rat." *Biogerontology* 14, no. 3 (2013): 293–301. doi: 10.1007/s10522-013-9430-y. PMID: 23681254.

Rennie, M. J., A. Selby, P. Atherton, K. Smith, V. Kumar, E. L. Glover, and S. M. Philips. "Facts, Noise and Wishful Thinking: Muscle Protein Turnover in Aging and Human Disuse Atrophy." *Scandinavian Journal of Medicine and Science in Sports* 20, no. 1 (2010): 5–9. doi: 10.1111/j.1600-0838.2009.00967.x. PMID: 19558380.

Reynolds, Gretchen. *The First 20 Minutes: Surprising Science Reveals How We Can Exercise Better, Train Smarter, Live Longer.* New York: Penguin Group, 2012.

Ricard-Blum, Sylvie. "The Collagen Family." *Cold Spring Harbor Perspectives in Biology* 3, no. 1 (2011): a004978. doi: 10.1101/cshperspect.a004978.

Rickenbach, Elizabeth H., David M. Almeida, Teresa E. Seeman, and Margie E. Lachman. "Daily Stress Magnifies the Association between Cognitive Decline and Everyday Memory Problems: An Integration of Longitudinal and Diary Methods." *Psychology and Aging* 29, no. 4 (2014): 852–62. https://doi.org/10.1037/ a0038072.

Riley, Katherine P., David A. Snowdon, Mark F. Desrosiers, and William R. Markesbery. "Early Life Linguistic Ability, Late Life Cognitive Function, and Neuropathology: Findings from the Nun Study." *Neurobiology of Aging* 26, no. 3 (2005): 341–47. doi: 10.1016/j.neurobiolaging.2004.06.019. PMID: 15639312.

Riley, Lee H., and Suzanne M. Jan de Beur. *White Paper on Back Pain and Osteoporosis.* Berkeley, CA: UC Berkeley School of Public Health, 2020.

Ristow, M., and S. Schmeisser. "Extending Life Span by Increasing Oxidative Stress." *Free Radical Biology and Medicine* 51, no. 2 (2011): 327–36. doi: 10.1016/j.freerad biomed.2011.05.010. PMID: 21619928.

Robinson, L. R., N. C. Fitzgerald, D. G. Doughty, N. C. Dawes, C. A. Berge, and D. L. Bissett. "Topical Palmitoyl Pentapeptide Provides Improvement in Photoaged Human Skin." *International Journal of Cosmetic Science* 27, no. 3 (2005): 155–60. doi: 10.1111/j.1467-2494.2005.00261.x. PMID: 18492182.

Robinson, Siân, Cyrus Cooper, and Avan Aihie Sayer. "Nutrition and Sarcopenia: A Review of the Evidence and Implications for Preventive Strategies." *Journal of Aging Research*, Article ID 510801 (2012). doi: org/10.1155/2012/510801.

Robling, Alexander G., Alesha B. Castillo, and Charles H. Turner. "Biomechanical and Molecular Regulation of Bone Remodeling." *Annual Review of Biomedical*

Engineering 8 (2006): 455–98. doi: 10.1146/annurev.bioeng.8.061505.095721. PMID: 16834564.

Rochon, James, Connie W. Bales, Eric Ravussin, Leanne M. Redman, John O. Holloszy, Susan B. Racette, Susan B. Roberts, Sai Kruppa Das, Sergei Romashkan, Katherine M. Galan, Evan C. Hadley, and William E Kraus. "CALERIE Study Group. Design and Conduct of the CALERIE Study: Comprehensive Assessment of the Long-Term Effects of Reducing Intake of Energy." *Journals of Gerontology. Series A, Biological Sciences and Medical Sciences* 66, no.1 (2011): 97–108. doi: 10.1093/gerona/glq168. Epub 2010 Oct 5. PMID: 20923909.

Rossman, Matthew J., Jessica R. Santos-Parker, Chelsea A. C. Steward, Nina Z. Bispham, Lauren M. Cuevas, Hannah L. Rosenberg, Kayla A. Woodward, Michael Chonchol, Rachel A. Gioscia-Ryan, Michael P. Murphy, and Douglas R. Seals. "Chronic Supplementation with a Mitochondrial Antioxidant (MitoQ) Improves Vascular Function in Healthy Older Adults." *Hypertension* 71, no. 6 (2018): 1056–63. doi: 10.1161/HYPERTENSIONAHA.117.10787. PMID: 29661838.

Rossouw, J. E., J. E. Manson, A. M. Kaunitz, and G. L. Anderson. "Lessons Learned from the Women's Health Initiative Trials of Menopausal Hormone Therapy." *Obstetrics and Gynecology* 121, no. 1 (2013): 172–76. doi: 10.1097/aog.0b013e31827a08c8. PMID: 23262943.

Roubenoff, Ronenn. "Sarcopenia: Effects on Body Composition and Function." *Journals of Gerontology. Series A, Biological Sciences and Medical Sciences* 58, no. 11 (2003): 1012–17. doi: 10.1093/gerona/58.11.m1012. PMID: 14630883.

Ruiz, Jonathon R., Xuemei Sui, Felipe Lobelo, James R. Morrow, Alan W. Jackson, Michael Sjöström, and Steven N. Blair. "Association between Muscular Strength and Mortality in Men: Prospective Cohort Study." *British Medical Journal* 337, no. 7661 (2008): a439. doi: 10.1136/bmj.a439. PMID: 18595904.

Saag, Kenneth G., Jeffrey Petersen, Maria Luisa Brandi, Andrew C. Karaplis, Mattias Lorentzon, Thierry Thomas, Judy Maddox, Michelle Fan, Paul D. Meisner, and Andreas Grauer. "Romosozumab or Alendronate for Fracture Prevention in Women with Osteoporosis." *New England Journal of Medicine* 377, no. 15 (2017): 1417–27. doi: 10.1056/NEJMoa1708322.

Sacks, Oliver. *The Man Who Mistook His Wife for a Hat and Other Clinical Tales.* New York: Touchstone Press, 1970.

Sadowska-Bartosz, Izabela, and Grzegorz Bartosz. "Effect of Glycation Inhibitors on Aging and Age-Related Diseases." *Mechanisms of Ageing and Development* 160 (2016): 1–18. doi: 10.1016/j.mad.2016.09.006. PMID: 27671971.

Samieri, Cecilia, Martha-Claire Morris, David A. Bennett, Claudine Berr, Phillippe Amouyel, Jean-Francois Dartigues, Christophe Tzourio, et al. "Fish Intake, Genetic Predisposition to Alzheimer Disease, and Decline in Global Cognition and Memory in 5 Cohorts of Older Persons." *American Journal of Epidemiology* 187, no. 5 (2018): 933–40. doi: 10.1093/aje/kwx330. PMID: 29053784.

Santaguida, P. Lina, Tatyan A. Shamliyan, and David R. Goldman. "Cholinesterase Inhibitors and Memantine in Adults with Alzheimer Disease." *American Journal of Medicine* 129, no. 10 (2016): 1044–47.

Santos-Parker, Jessica R., Talia R. Strahler, Candace J. Bassett, Nina Z. Bispham, Michel B. Chonchol, and Douglas R. Seals. "Curcumin Supplementation Improves Vascular Endothelial Function in Healthy Middle-Aged and Older Adults by Increasing Nitric Oxide Bioavailability and Reducing Oxidative Stress." *Aging (Albany NY)* 9, no. 1 (2017): 187–208. doi: 10.18632/aging.101149. PMID: 28070018.

Sapey, Elizabeth, Jaimin M. Patel, Hannah L. Greenwood, Georgia M. Walton, Jon Hazeldine, Charandeep Sadhra, Dhruv Parekh, Rachel Dancer, Peter Nightingale, Janet M. Lord, and David R. Thickett. "Pulmonary Infections in the Elderly Lead to Impaired Neutrophil Targeting, Which Is Improved by Simvastatin." *American Journal of Respiratory and Critical Care Medicine* 196, no. 10 (2017): 1325–36. https://doi.org/10.1164/rccm.201704-0814OC.

Sapolsky, Robert. *Why Zebras Don't Get Ulcers*, 3rd ed. New York: Henry Holt, 2004.

Schelke, Matthew W., Peter Attia, Daniel J. Palenchar, Bob Kaplan, Monica Mureb, Christine A. Ganzer, Olivia Scheyer, et al. "Mechanisms of Risk Reduction in the Clinical Practice of Alzheimer's Disease Prevention." *Frontiers in Aging Neuroscience* 10 (2018): 96. doi: 10.3389/fnagi.2018.00096. PMID: 29706884.

Schroer, Alison K., and W. David Merryman. "Mechanobiology of Myofibroblast Adhesion in Fibrotic Cardiac Disease." *Journal of Cell Science* 128, no. 10 (2015): 1865–75. doi: 10.1242/jcs.162891. PMID: 25918124.

Seals, Douglas R. "Edward F. Adolph Distinguished Lecture: The Remarkable Anti-Aging Effects of Aerobic Exercise on Systemic Arteries." *Journal of Applied Physiology* 117, no. 5 (2014): 425–39. doi: 10.1152/japplphysiol.00362.2014. PMID: 24855137.

Seals, Douglas R., Jamie N. Justice, and Thomas J. LaRocca. "Physiological Geroscience: Targeting Function to Increase Healthspan and Achieve Optimal Longevity." *Journal of Physiology* 594, no. 8 (2016): 2001–24. doi: 10.1113/jphysiol.2014.282665. PMID: 25639909.

Seals, Douglas R., and Simon Melov. "Translational Geroscience: Emphasizing Function to Achieve Optimal Longevity." *Aging* 6, no. 9 (2014): 718–30. doi: 10.18632/aging.100694. PMID: 25324468.

Seidelmann, Sara B., Brian Claggett, Susan Cheng, Mir Henglin, Amil Shah, Lynn M. Steffen, Aaron R. Folsom, Eric B. Rimm, Walter C. Willett, and Scott D. Solomon. "Dietary Carbohydrate Intake and Mortality: A Prospective Cohort Study and Meta-analysis." *Lancet Public Health* 3, no. 9 (2018): e419–28. doi: 10.1016/S2468-2667(18)30135-X. PMID: 30122560.

Serhan, Charles N. "Novel Pro-Resolving Lipid Mediators in Inflammation Are Leads for Resolution Physiology." *Nature* 510, no. 7503 (2014): 92–101. https://doi.org/10.1038/nature13479.

Shanmugaraj, Ajaykumar, Ryan P. Coughlin, Gabriel N. Kuper, Seper Ekhtiari, Nicole Simunovic, Volker Musahl, and Olufemi R. Ayeni. "Changing Trends in the Use of Cartilage Restoration Techniques for the Patellofemoral Joint: A Systematic Review." *Knee Surgery, Sports Traumatology, Arthroscopy* 27, no. 3 (2019): 854–67. doi: 10.1007/s00167-018-5139-4. PMID: 30232541.

Sheu, Shey-Shing, Danhanjaya Nauduri, and M. W. Anders. "Targeting Antioxidants to Mitochondria: A New Therapeutic Direction." *Biochimica Biophysica Acta* 1762, no. 2 (2006): 256–65. doi: 10.1016/j.bbadis.2005.10.007. PMID: 16352423.

Sierra, F. "Moving Geroscience into Uncharted Waters." *Journals of Gerontology. Series A, Biological Sciences and Medical Sciences* 71, no. 11 (2016): 1385–87. doi: 10.1093/gerona/glw087. PMID: 27535965.

Simons, David J., Walter R. Boot, Neil Charness, Susan E. Gathercole, Christopher F. Chabris, David Z. Hambrick, and Elizabeth A. Stine-Morrow. "Do 'Brain-Training' Programs Work?" *Psychological Science in the Public Interest* 17, no. 3 (2016): 103–86. doi: 10.1177/1529100616661983. PMID: 27697851.

Sinclair, David. *Lifespan: Why We Age—and Why We Don't Have To* (New York: Atria Books, 2019).

Smith, Lynette M., J. Christopher Gallagher, Glenville Jones, and Martin Kaufmann. "Estimation of the Recommended Daily Allowance (RDA) for Vitamin D Intake Using Serum 25 Hydroxyvitamin D Level of 20ng/Ml as the End Point, May Vary According to the Analytical Measurement Technique Used." Endocrine Society Meeting, Presentation OR07-4. https://plan.core-apps.com/tristar_endo17/abstract/f7e437ee5c2d999047a0315444cbbebb.

Smoliga, James M., Joseph A. Baur, and Heather A. Hausenblas. "Resveratrol and Health—a Comprehensive Review of Human Clinical Trials." *Molecular Nutrition and Food Research* 55, no. 8 (2011): 1129–41. doi: 10.1002/mnfr.201100143. PMID: 21688389.

Soares, Jorge P., Amelia M. Silva, Sandra Fonseca, Maria M. Oliveira, Francesco Peixoto, Isabel Gaivão, and Maria P. Mota. "How Can Age and Lifestyle Variables Affect DNA Damage, Repair Capacity and Endogenous Biomarkers of Oxidative Stress?" *Experimental Gerontology* 62 (2015): 45–52. doi: 10.1016/j.exger.2015.01.001. PMID: 25576678.

Sonnenburg, Erica D., and Justin Sonnenburg. *The Good Gut: Taking Control of Your Weight, Your Mood, and Your Long-Term Health.* New York: Penguin, 2015.

Sordi, Valeria, and Lorenzo Piemonti. "Therapeutic Plasticity of Stem Cells and Allograft Tolerance." *Cytotherapy* 13, no. 6 (2011): 647–60. doi: 10.3109/14653249.2011.583476. PMID: 21554176.

Soultoukis, George A., and Linda Partridge. "Dietary Protein, Metabolism, and Aging." *Annual Review of Biochemistry* 85 (2016): 5–34. doi: 10.1146/annurev-biochem-060815-014422. PMID: 27145842.

Steadman, J. Richard, Karen K. Briggs, Juan J. Rodrigo, Mininder S. Kocher, Thomas J. Gill, and William G. Rodkey. "Outcomes of Microfracture for Traumatic Chondral Defects of the Knee: Average 11-Year Follow-up." *Arthroscopy* 19, no. 5 (2003): 477–84. doi: 10.1053/jars.2003.50112. PMID: 12724676.

Steenman, Marja, and Gilles Lande. "Cardiac Aging and Heart Disease in Humans." *Biophysical Reviews* 9, no. 2 (2017): 131–37. https://doi.org/10.1007/s12551-017-0255-9.

Stockinger, Jessica, Nicholas Maxwell, Dylan Shapiro, Rafael deCabo, and Gregorio Valdez. "Caloric Restriction Mimetics Slow Aging of Neuromuscular Synapses and Muscle Fibers." *Journals of Gerontology. Series A, Biological Sciences and Medical Sciences* 73, no. 1 (2017): 21–28. doi: 10.1093/gerona/glx023. PMID: 28329051.

Stout, Michael B., Frederic J. Steyn, Michael J. Jurczak, Joao-Paulo G. Camporez, Yi Zhu, John R. Hawse, Diana Jurk, et al. "17α-Estradiol Alleviates Age-Related

Metabolic and Inflammatory Dysfunction in Male Mice without Inducing Feminization." *Journals of Gerontology. Series A, Biological Sciences and Medical Sciences* 72, no. 1 (2017): 3–15. doi: 10.1093/gerona/glv309. PMID: 26809497.

Sutter, Nathan B., Carlos D. Bustamante, Kevin Chase, Melissa M. Gray, Kayan Zhao, Lao Zhu, Badri Padhukasahasram, Eric Karlins, Sean Davis, Paul G. Jones, et al. "A Single IGF1 Allele Is a Major Determinant of Small Size in Dogs." *Science* 316, no. 5821 (2007): 112–15. doi: 10.1126/science.1137045. PMID: 17412960.

Taddei, S., F. Galetta, A. Virdis, L. Ghiadoni, G. Salvetti, F. Franzoni, C. Giusti, and A. Salvetti. "Physical Activity Prevents Age-related Impairment in Nitric Oxide Availability in Elderly Athletes." *Circulation* 101, no. 25 (2000): 2896–2901. doi: 10.1161/01.cir.101.25.2896. PMID: 10869260.

Talmud, Philippa J., David M. Flavell, Khalid Alfakih, Jackie A. Cooper, Anthony J. Balmforth, Mohan Sivananthan, Hugh E. Montgomery, Alistair S. Hall, and Steve E. Humphries. "The Lipoprotein Lipase Gene Serine 447 Stop Variant Influences Hypertension-Induced Left Ventricular Hypertrophy and Risk of Coronary Heart Disease." *Clinical Science (London)* 112, no. 12 (2007): 617–24. doi: 10.1042/CS20060344. PMID: 17291198.

Tamura, Yuki, Yataka Matsunaga, Yu Kitaoka, and Hideo Hatta. "Effects of Heat Stress Treatment on Age-Dependent Unfolded Protein Response in Different Types of Skeletal Muscle." *Journals of Gerontology. Series A, Biological Sciences and Medical Sciences* 72, no. 3 (2017): 299–308. doi: 10.1093/gerona/glw063. PMID: 27071782.

Tang, Benjamin M., Guy D. Eslick, Carol Nowson, Caroline Smith, and Alan Bensoussan. "Use of Calcium or Calcium in Combination with Vitamin D Supplementation to Prevent Fractures and Bone Loss in People Aged 50 Years and Older: A Meta-analysis." *Lancet* 370, no. 9588 (2007): 657–66. doi: 10.1016/S0140-6736(07)61342-7. PMID: 17720017.

Tezze, Caterina, Vanina Romanello, Maria A. Desbats, Gian P. Fadini, Mattia Albiero, Giulia Favaro, Stefano Ciciliot, Maria E. Soriano, Valeria Morbidoni, Cristina Cerqua, et al. "Age-Associated Loss of OPA1 in Muscle Impacts Muscle Mass, Metabolic Homeostasis, Systemic Inflammation, and Epithelial Senescence." *Cell Metabolism* 25, no. 6 (2017): 1374–89. e6. doi: 10.1016/j.cmet.2017.04.021. PMID: 28552492.

Tian, Xiao, Denis Firsanov, Zhihui Zhang, Yang Cheng, Lingfeng Luo, Gregory Tombline, Ruiyue Tan, et al. "SIRT6 Is Responsible for More Efficient DNA Double-Strand Break Repair in Long-Lived Species." *Cell* 177, no. 3 (2019): 622–38. e22. doi: 10.1016/j.cell.2019.03.043. PMID: 31002797.

Tok, Ekrim, Devrim Ertunc, Utkum Oz, Handan Camdeviren, Gulay Ozdemir, and Dilek Saffet. "The Effect of Circulating Androgens on Bone Mineral Density in Postmenopausal Women." *Maturitas* 48, no. 3 (2004): 235–42. doi: 10.1016/j.maturitas.2003.11.007. PMID: 15207889.

Tomlinson, Ryan E., and Matthew J. Silva. "Skeletal Blood Flow in Bone Repair and Maintenance." *Bone Research* 1, no. 4 (2013): 311–22. doi: 10.4248/BR201304002. PMID: 26273509.

Tompkins, Byron A., Darcy L. DiFede, Aisha Khan, Ana M. Landin, Ivonne H. Schulman, Marietsy V. Pujol, Alan W. Heldman, Roberto Miki, Pascal J. Goldschmidt-

Clermont, Bradley J. Goldstein, et al. "Allogeneic Mesenchymal Stem Cells Ameliorate Aging Frailty: A Phase II Randomized, Double-Blind, Placebo-Controlled Clinical Trial." *Journals of Gerontology. Series A, Biological Sciences and Medical Sciences* 72, no. 11 (2017): 1513–22. doi: 10.1093/gerona/glx137. PMID: 28977399.

Trammell, Samuel A., Mark S. Schmidt, Benjamin J. Weidemann, Philip Redpath, Frank Jaksch, Ryan W. Dellinger, Zhonggang Li, et al. "Nicotinamide Riboside Is Uniquely and Orally Bioavailable in Mice and Humans." *Nature Communications* 7 (2016): 12948. doi: 10.1038/ncomms12948. PMID: 27721479.

Valdez, Gregorio, Juan C. Tapia, Hiyuno Kang, Gregory D. Clemenson, F. H. Gage, Jeff W. Lichtman, and Joshua R. Sanes. "Attenuation of Age-Related Changes in Mouse Neuromuscular Synapses by Caloric Restriction and Exercise." *Proceedings of the National Academy of Sciences of the United States of America* 107, no. 33 (2010): 14863–68. https://doi.org/10.1073/pnas.1002220107.

van der Veer, Eric, Cynthia Ho, Caroline O'Neil, Nicole Barbosa, Robert Scott, Sean P. Cregan, and J. Geoffrey Pickering. "Extension of Human Cell Lifespan by Nicotinamide Phosphoribosyltransferase." *Journal of Biological Chemistry* 282, no. 15 (2007): 10841–45. doi: 10.1074/jbc.C700018200. PMID: 17307730.

Van Skike, Candice E., and Veronica Galvan. "A Perfect sTORm: The Role of the Mammalian Target of Rapamycin (mTOR) in Cerebrovascular Dysfunction of Alzheimer's Disease: A Mini-Review." *Gerontology* 64, no. 3 (2018): 205–11. doi: 10.1159/000485381. PMID: 29320772.

Villeda, Saul A., Kristofer Plambeck, Jinte Middeldorp, Joseph M. Castellano, Kira I. Mosher, Jian Luo, Lucas K. Smith, Gregor Bieri, et al. "Young Blood Reverses Age-Related Impairments in Cognitive Function and Synaptic Plasticity in Mice." *Nature Medicine* 20, no. 6 (2014): 659–63. doi: 10.1038/nm.3569. PMID: 24793238.

Visser, Marjolein, and Tamara B. Harris. "Body Composition and Aging." In *The Epidemiology of Aging*, edited by A. B. Newman and J. A. Cauley, 275–92. New York: Springer Science, 2012. doi: 10.1007/978-94-007-5061-6_16.

Vitale, Giovanni, Matteo Cesari, and Daniella Mari. "Aging of the Endocrine System and Its Potential Impact on Sarcopenia." *European Journal of Internal Medicine* 35 (2016): 10-15. doi: 10.1016/j.ejim.2016.07.017. PMID: 27484963.

von Deursen, Jan M. "Senolytic Therapies for Healthy Longevity," *Science* 364, no. 6441 (2019), 636–37.

von Kobbe, Cayetano. "Targeting Senescent Cells: Approaches, Opportunities, Challenges." *Aging* 11, no. 24 (2019): 12844–61. doi: 10.18632/aging.102557.

Wachter, Kenneth W., and Caleb E. Finch, eds. *Between Zeus and the Salmon*. Washington, DC: National Academy Press, 1997.

Walker, Matthew. *Why We Sleep: Unlocking the Power of Sleep and Dreams*. New York: Scribner, 2017.

Wallace, Douglas C. "A Mitochondrial Paradigm of Metabolic and Degenerative Diseases, Aging, and Cancer: A Dawn for Evolutionary Medicine." *Annual Review of Genetics* 39 (2005): 359–410. doi: 10.1146/annurev.genet.39.110304.095751.

Ward, A., P. Bates, R. Fisher, L. Richardson, and C. F. Graham. "Disproportionate Growth in Mice with Igf-2 Transgenes." *Proceedings of the National Academy of*

Sciences of the United States of America 91, no. 22 (1994): 10365–69. https://doi
.org/10.1073/pnas.91.22.10365.

Watanabe-Kamiyama, Mari, Munishigi Shimizu, Shin Kamiyama, Yasuki Taguchi,
Hideyuki Sone, Fumiki Morimatsu, Hitoshi Shirakawa, Yuji Furukawa, and Michio
Komai M. "Absorption and Effectiveness of Orally Administered Low Molecular
Weight Collagen Hydrolysate in Rats." *Journal of Agriculture and Food Chemistry* 58,
no. 2 (2010): 835–41. doi: 10.1021/jf9031487. PMID: 19957932.

Weaver, Ian C. G., Nadia Cervoni, Frances A. Champagne, Ana C D'Alessio, Shakti
Sharma, Jonathan R. Seckl, Sergiy Dymov, Moshe Szyf, Michael J. Meaney, et al.
"Epigenetic Programming by Maternal Behavior." *Nature Neuroscience* 7, no. 8
(2004): 847–54. doi: 10.1038/nn1276. PMID: 15220929.

WebMD. "Curcumin May Prevent Clogged Arteries." Heart Disease. Last modified
July 20, 2009. https://www.webmd.com/heart-disease/news/20090720/curcumin
-may-prevent-clogged-arteries.

Weiss, N. S., C. L. Ure, J. H. Ballard, A. R. Williams, and J. R. Daling. "Decreased
Risk of Fractures of the Hip and Lower Forearm with Postmenopausal Use of Estro-
gen." *New England Journal of Medicine* 303, no. 21 (1980): 1195–98. doi: 10.1056/
NEJM198011203032102. PMID: 7421945.

Wikipedia. "Bradford Hill Criteria." Last modified December 9, 2020. https://
en.wikipedia.org/wiki/Bradford_Hill_criteria.

Wiley, Christopher D., and Judith Campisi. "From Ancient Pathways to Aging Cells-
Connecting Metabolism and Cellular Senescence." *Cell Metabolism* 23, no. 6 (2016):
1013–21. https://doi.org/10.1016/j.cmet.2016.05.010.

Wilmoth, John. "In Search of Limits." In *Between Zeus and the Salmon,* edited by
Kenneth Wachter and Caleb Finch, 38–64. Washington, DC: National Academy
Press, 1997.

Witters, Lee A. "The Blooming of the French Lilac." *Journal of Clinical Investigation*
108, no. 8 (2001): 1105–7. https://doi.org/10.1172/JCI14178.

Wohlgemuth, Stephanie E., Arnold Y. Seo, Emmanuelle Marzetti, Hazel A. Lees, and
Christian Leeuwenburgh. "Skeletal Muscle Autophagy and Apoptosis during Aging:
Effects of Calorie Restriction and Life-Long Exercise." *Experimental Gerontology* 45,
no. 2 (2010): 138–48. doi: 10.1016/j.exger.2009.11.002. PMID: 19903516.

World Health Organization. "Ageing and Health." Fact Sheets. Last modified February 5, 2018. https://www.who.int/news-room/fact-sheets/detail/ageing-and-health.

———. "International Statistical Classification of Diseases and Related Health Problems (ICD)." Classification of Diseases. Last modified November 20, 2020. https://
www.who.int/classifications/icd/en/.

Writing Group for the PEPI. "Effects of Hormone Therapy on Bone Mineral Den-
sity: Results from the Postmenopausal Estrogen/Progestin Interventions (PEPI)
Trial." *Journal of the American Medical Association* 276, no. 17 (1996): 1389–96.
PMID: 8892713.

Yan, Riqiang, Qingyuan Fan, John Zhoum, and Robert Vassar. "Inhibiting BACE1 to
Reverse Synaptic Dysfunctions in Alzheimer's Disease." *Neuroscience and Biobehavioral Reviews* 65 (2016): 326–40. doi.org/10.1016/j.neubiorev.2016.03.025.

Yang, Ling, Danilo Licastro, Edda Cava, Nicola Veronese, Francesca Spelta, Wanda Rizza, Beatrice Bertozzi, Dennis T. Villareal, Gokhan S. Hotamisligil, and Luigi Fontana. "Long-Term Calorie Restriction Enhances Cellular Quality-Control Processes in Human Skeletal Muscle." *Cell Reports* 14, no. 3 (2016): 422–28. doi: 10.1016/j.celrep.2015.12.042. PMID: 26774472.

Yoshizawa, M., S. Maeda, A. Miyaki, M. Misono, Y. Saito, K. Tanabe, S. Kuno, and R. Ajisaka. "Effect of 12 Weeks of Moderate-Intensity Resistance Training on Arterial Stiffness: A Randomised Controlled Trial in Women Aged 32–59 Years." *British Journal of Sports Medicine* 43, no. 8 (2009): 615–18. doi: 10.1136/bjsm .2008.052126. PMID: 18927168.

Young, S. Stanley, and Alan Karr. "Deming, Data and Observational Studies. A Process Out of Control and Needing Fixing." *Significance* 8 (2011): 116–20.

Yousefzadeh, Matthew J., Marissa J. Schafer, Nicole Noren Hooten, Elizabeth J. Atkinson, Michelle K. Evans, Darren J. Baker, Ellen K. Quarles, et al. "Circulating Levels of Monocyte Chemoattractant Protein-1 as a Potential Measure of Biological Age in Mice and Frailty in Humans." *Aging Cell* 17, no. 2 (2018): e12706. doi: 10.1111/ acel.12706. PMID: 29290100.

Yu, Zhen, Rong Wang, Wilson C. Fok, Alexander Coles, Adam B. Salmon, Viviana I. Pérez. "Rapamycin and Dietary Restriction Induce Metabolically Distinctive Changes in Mouse Liver." *Journals of Gerontology. Series A, Biological Sciences and Medical Sciences* 70, no. 4 (2015): 410–20. doi: 10.1093/gerona/glu053. PMID: 24755936.

Zhang, Yuan, Yang Xie, Eric O. Berglund, Katie C. Coate, Tian T. He, Takeshi Katafuchi, Guanghua Xiao, et al. "The Starvation Hormone, Fibroblast Growth Factor-21, Extends Lifespan in Mice." *eLife* 1 (2012): e00065. https://doi.org/10.7554/ eLife.00065.

Zhao, Jia-Guo, Xien-Tie Zeng, Jia Wang, and Lin Liu. "Association between Calcium or Vitamin D Supplementation and Fracture Incidence in Community-Dwelling Older Adults: A Systematic Review and Meta-analysis." *Journal of the American Medical Association* 318, no. 24 (2017): 2466–82. doi: 10.1001/jama.2017.19344. PMID: 29279934.

Zheng, Shan-Qing, Xiao-Bing Huang, Ti-Kun Xing, Ai-Jun Ding, Gui-Sheng Wu, and Hui-Rong Luo. "Chlorogenic Acid Extends the Lifespan of *Caenorhabditis elegans* via Insulin/IGF-1 Signaling Pathway." *Journals of Gerontology. Series A, Biological Sciences and Medical Sciences* 72, no. 4 (2017): 464–72. doi: 10.1093/gerona/glw105. PMID: 27378235.

Zykovich, Aretem, Alan Hubbard, James M. Flynn, Mark Tarnopolsky, Mario F. Fraga, Chad Kerksick, Dan Ogborn, Lauren MacNeil, Sean D. Mooney, Simon Melov. "Genome-wide DNA Methylation Changes with Age in Disease-Free Human Skeletal Muscle." *Aging Cell* 13, no. 2 (2014): 360–66. doi: 10.1111/acel.12180. PMID: 24304487; PMCID.

Index

About the Author

Beth Bennett is a PhD geneticist with a background in evolutionary genetics and the science of aging. She has been published more than fifty times in peer-reviewed journals. She taught college biology for thirty years at the University of Colorado in Boulder, where she currently produces a radio show on science. She blogs on all things relating to aging.